STUDIES
IN
MEANING
4

Also available from Pace University Press

Studies in Meaning:
Exploring Constructivist Psychology
(2002)

Studies in Meaning 2:
Bridging the Personal and Social
in Constructivist Psychology
(2004)

Studies in Meaning 3:
Constructivist Psychotherapy in the Real World
(2008)

www.pace.edu/press

STUDIES IN MEANING 4: CONSTRUCTIVIST PERSPECTIVES ON THEORY, PRACTICE, AND SOCIAL JUSTICE

Edited by
Jonathan D. Raskin
State University of New York at New Paltz

Sara K. Bridges
The University of Memphis

and

Robert A. Neimeyer
The University of Memphis

Pace University Press
2010

Copyright © 2010 by
Pace University Press
41 Park Row, Room 1510
New York NY 10038

ISBN 0-944473-98-9

All rights reserved
Printed in the United States of America

Table of Contents

Contributors — viii
Preface — xi

PART I
THEORY

1. A Radical Constructivist View of Meaning and the Problem of Communication — 3
   Ernst von Glasersfeld

2. Meaning in Relationship — 9
   Kenneth J. Gergen

PART II
PRACTICE

3. Innovations in Psychotherapy: Tracking the Narrative Construction of Change — 29
   Miguel M. Gonçalves, Anita Santos, Marlene Matos, João Salgado, Inês Mendes, António Ribeiro, Carla Cunha, and Juliana Gonçalves

4. Reconstructing the Continuing Bond: A Constructivist Approach to Grief Therapy — 65
   Robert A. Neimeyer

5. The Dynamic Features of Love: Changes in Self and Motivation — 93
   Agnieszka Hermans-Konopka and Hubert J. M. Hermans

6. Asking and Answering Deconstruction Questions from within Counseling Dialogues — 125
   Tom Strong and Lara Schultz

PART III
SOCIAL JUSTICE

7. Doing Justice: A Witnessing Stance in Therapeutic Work alongside Survivors of Torture and Political Violence
   Vikki Reynolds — 157

8. Constructivist Mentoring as Social Justice
   Sara K. Bridges — 185

9. Gazing at Objectification Theory through a Social Constructionist Lens
   Melanie S. Hill — 205

10. The Integral Universe, Experiential Personal Construct Psychology, Transpersonal Reverence, and Transpersonal Responsibility
    Larry M. Leitner — 227

11. Constructing and Deconstructing Social Justice Counseling
    Jonathan D. Raskin — 247

PART IV
THEORY REVISITED

12. The Hierarchy of Epistemological Beliefs: All Ways of Knowing Are Not Created Equal
    Tabitha R. Holmes — 281

13. Psychotherapist-as-Philosopher-of-Science
    Dušan Stojnov — 317

14. The Status of the Individual in Pragmatism and Constructivism
    Trevor Butt — 361

About the Editors	381
Appendix: About the Constructivist Psychology Network	383
Index of Proper Names	385
Subject Index	395

Contributors

Sara K. Bridges, Department of Counseling, Educational Psychology and Research, The University of Memphis, Tennessee, USA

Trevor Butt, School of Human and Health Sciences, University of Huddersfield, United Kingdom

Carla Cunha, Department of Psychology, University of Minho, Braga, Portugal

Kenneth J. Gergen, Department of Psychology, Swarthmore College, Swarthmore, Pennsylvania, USA

Ernst von Glasersfeld, Scientific Reasoning Research Institute, University of Massachusetts Amherst, Amherst, Massachusetts, USA

Juliana Gonçalves, Department of Psychology, University of Minho, Braga, Portugal

Miguel M. Gonçalves, Department of Psychology, University of Minho, Braga, Portugal

Hubert J. M. Hermans, Department of Psychology, Radboud University, Nijmegen, Netherlands

Agnieszka Hermans-Konopka, International Institute for Dialogical Self, The Netherlands

Melanie S. Hill, Department of Psychology, State University of New York at New Paltz, New York, USA

Tabitha R. Holmes, Department of Psychology, State University of New York at New Paltz, New York, USA

Larry M. Leitner, Department of Psychology, Miami University, Oxford, OH, USA

Marlene Matos, Department of Psychology, University of Minho, Braga, Portugal

Inês Mendes, Department of Psychology, University of Minho, Braga, Portugal

Robert A. Neimeyer, Department of Psychology, The University of Memphis, Tennessee, USA

Jonathan D. Raskin, Department of Psychology, State University of New York at New Paltz, New York, USA

Vikki Reynolds, School of Psychology, City University, Vancouver, British Columbia, Canada

António Ribeiro, Department of Psychology, University of Minho, Braga, Portugal

João Salgado, Department of Clinical and Health Psychology, ISMAI, Maia, Portugal

Anita Santos, Department of Psychology, University of Minho, Braga, Portugal

Lara Schultz, Division of Applied Psychology, Faculty of Education, University of Calgary, Alberta, Canada

Dušan Stojnov, Department of Psychology, Faculty of Philosophy, University of Belgrade, Serbia

Tom Strong, Division of Applied Psychology, Faculty of Education, University of Calgary, Alberta, Canada

Preface

Our goal in this volume of *Studies in Meaning* is to share an array of provocative readings that highlight the diversity of viewpoints present within constructivist scholarship. Contributors were asked to write on one of three topics: theory, practice, or social justice. The rationale behind choosing three ostensibly discrete areas of focus was our belief—borne out in the completed volume—that new thinking in any one of these areas naturally and readily speaks to, amplifies, and informs developments in the others. Thus, the chapters stand as scholarly contributions in their own right even while readers are encouraged to identify areas of convergence and divergence amongst them.

Part I contains two brief but fascinating theoretical contributions from arguably the most influential figures in radical constructivism and social constructionism respectively, Ernst von Glasersfeld and Kenneth Gergen. Glasersfeld gets things started by exploring the problem of communication in radical constructivism; he addresses how communication is possible within a framework that sees human beings as closed systems only in touch with their own processes. Kenneth Gergen follows, offering a distinctly different take on the issue. Meaning, from his social constructionist viewpoint, is always relational rather than personal and private. The themes these two seminal thinkers introduce resonate, sometimes overtly and other times between the lines, throughout the rest of the volume.

Part II shifts attention toward clinical practice. Miguel Gonçalves and his colleagues set the stage by offering a systematic conceptualization of "innovative moments" (or i-moments) in psychotherapy, developing and applying a reliable coding system for tracking the instigation and consolidation of change in the discourse that arises between client and therapist. As they demonstrate, not only is it feasible to assess such i-moments at the levels of action, reflection, protest against an oppressive self-narrative, reconceptualization of the problem, and the projection of new experiences, but doing so also offers practical insights about processes that distinguish good and poor outcome cases. Next, Robert Neimeyer teases out the implications of constructivism for working with clients whose own lives are devastated by the loss of loved ones. Construing grieving as a process of reaffirming or rebuilding a world of meaning that has been challenged by the loss, he reviews the theoretical and empirical support for such a model, and then illustrates the use of several strategies for promoting sense-making through the use of narrative procedures, reconstructing the relationship with the deceased, and articulating tacit meanings that restore a sense of coherence and hope for the future. Counterbalancing Neimeyer's emphasis on grief, Agnieszka Hermans-Konopka and Hubert Hermans then explore a more positive but equally relational emotion, namely love, and offer practical insights deriving from research on its dynamic organization. Drawing on dialogical self theory, they find that love implies a greater change in the construction of self and motivation than a range of other positive and negative affective states, dispelling some of the traditional "mystery" that has surrounded this centrally important emotion. Finally, Tom Strong and Lara Shultz take the reader to the "shop floor" of psychotherapy, to reflect on the role counselor-client discourse plays in articulating both problems and solutions. Adopting a micro-analytic approach, they carefully "unpack" actual question-and-answer sequences from video recorded sessions that deconstruct the authority of problems and open up new horizons of possibility. Taken together, the research-informed contributions that comprise this section go some distance toward demonstrating the relevance of constructivism for the concerns that many clients bring to psychotherapy.

Part III turns to social justice. It opens with Vikki Reynolds' reflective essay on her therapeutic work alongside victims of politically sanctioned violence and torture. Positioning herself as an appreciative witness of their ethical resistance to such dehumanizing practices, she carefully spells out the assumptions that sustain her in this work, as well as the principles that help structure the sense of safety required for this form of social activism, that construct our collective accountability for the use of torture, that promote collaboration with the survivor, and that foster solidarity in opposing such practices on the political stage. Shifting directions, Sara Bridges describes the ways in which a constructivist approach to mentoring can be used to advance social justice for graduate students wading into the oftentimes murky political waters of academia. Using examples from her own experience as a mentor, she convincingly argues in favor of an egalitarian style of mentoring that seeks to help students chart their own developmental path. Subsequently, Melanie Hill employs concepts from social constructionism in examining the complex issue of sexual objectification. She seeks to position sexual objectification as a discourse, one with a multiplicity of social and personal implications. By becoming cognizant of the ways the discourse of sexual objectification operates, people can resist its more sinister implications. From there, Larry Leitner applies his experiential approach to personal construct theory in considering the idea of transpersonal reverence. He convincingly argues that damage results when people fail to reverently value their interconnectedness to one another and the wider social realm. Finally, Jonathan Raskin brings Part III to a close by examining social justice itself, specifically as it is embodied within counseling and psychotherapy. In a provocative essay, he argues that in order to guard against naïve realism and moral righteousness, social justice counselors must more fully articulate their theoretical approach and its implications for therapeutic practice. The papers in this section of the volume take divergent perspectives on social justice, but all demonstrate the powerful ways in which constructivist and social constructionist ideas can inform thinking in this area.

Finally, Part IV comes full circle, returning to the broader theoretical themes introduced at the beginning of the book. Tabitha Holmes provides a compelling examination of the often unstated hierarchy by which psychologists evaluate different styles of knowing. She endeavors to engender tolerance of the ways different epistemological beliefs serve different people under different circumstances, while also buttressing the case that the epistemological beliefs valued by psychology researchers are indeed preferable when operating within a research setting. Dušan Stojnov then explores Kelly's person-as-scientist metaphor and the elaborate personal science that researchers, clients and psychotherapists alike utilize to predict and make life meanings. Further he engages in an interesting and detailed appraisal of philosophy of science's connection to personal construct psychology and how logical mistakes could theoretically contribute to psychological distress. Trevor Butt brings the volume to a close by returning to the individual versus social debate reflected in Glasersfeld and Gergen's opening essays. Butt invokes philosophical pragmatism as a way to bridge the social-individual divide. His argument is that psychology can attend to the individual without resorting to mind/body dualism or the discourse of essential selfhood. Combining the philosophical pragmatism of Dewey, James, and Mead with the psychological pragmatism of George Kelly, Butt encourages us to move beyond the individual-social dilemma once and for all.

On a personal note, thank you to Mark Hussey, Steven Goldleaf, and Beth Scorzato at Pace University Press for all their help in the production of this volume. We also extend a hearty thank you to graduate student Alison Hickman for her assistance with indexing. Thank you also to our spouses and children, for supporting us and—you know—just being nice! Finally, to our readers: we sincerely hope you enjoy this fourth *Studies in Meaning* entry and find its chapters stimulate your thinking in new and innovative directions.

Jonathan D. Raskin
State University of New York at New Paltz

Sara K. Bridges
The University of Memphis

Robert A. Neimeyer
The University of Memphis

January 20, 2010

PART I

THEORY

☙ 1 ❧

A Radical Constructivist View of Meaning and the Problem of Communication

Ernst von Glasersfeld

When we ordinarily think of language and meaning, we tend to see words as the carriers of meaning and assume that both words and what they mean are shared by the speakers of our language. We take it for granted that they have an existence apart from ourselves. To some extent this is due to the fact that we acquired the use of language with the help of the adults among whom we grew up. We would not have any words or common language if we had grown up entirely by ourselves. Besides, when we acquired language we had not yet begun to reflect upon what we were doing and consequently we have no memory of what we did.

If we actually observe how children begin to use language, which usually happens just before their second year, we soon realize that it is a very intricate process. It is widely assumed that human children are genetically wired for the acquisition of language. Although I have difficulties with that assumption, I shall not argue against it here because, even if there is a genetic disposition, it is quite clear that genetic endowment can hardly include semantics. The words attached to specific meanings are different in every natural language. Children have to learn them individually and the way they accomplish this gives us a picture of what it is that constitutes meaning.

The first requirement on the way to language is that discrete items are isolated in the flow of experience. In many cases this happens when a displacement of the item is witnessed in the visual field. Dogs, cats, cockroaches, and, indeed, Mommy, become very special things, because they are observed to move by themselves.

The second requirement is that sound-images of words are isolated in the acoustic field of sensation. Only when individual sound-images have become recognizable as recurrent in the stream of sounds, can they be associated with other contiguous experiences.

The important thing to remember is that whatever an experiencer isolates in his or her sensory manifold is by definition part of experience and does not lead beyond the interface with an independently existing world. The traditional notion of reference, that is of words referring to things "in themselves," things that exist independently of the experiencer, is therefore turned into a myth. Wittgenstein expressed this in the clearest fashion when he likened language to a "Vorstellungsklavier," a piano the keys of which are ideas (1953, §6, p.4). The German word "Vorstellung" has always been translated with "representation." This is misleading because it inevitably suggests that there is an original of what is being presented. The German word has no such implication. It would be better translated as "imagination," "conception," or "idea."

Given that according to this view, words refer to what the individual language user has isolated in his or her experience, not to things that have an independent objective existence, there immediately arise three fundamental questions. One, where do these items of imagination come from? Two, if they are subjective constructs of individuals, how could we possibly communicate? Three, who are the "others" to whom we speak and from whom we have learned our language?

1. The Cybernetic Idea of Constraints Rather than Causes

The constructivist answer to the first question hinges on the cybernetic principle that the notion of constraints can replace the causal explanation of experience. The things, events, and relations that constitute the experiential world we live in are therefore not seen as representations of a "real" world but rather as constructs of our own that happen not to clash with the constraints of an inaccessible reality. We hold on to these constructs if we find them viable, that is, helpful in the pursuit of goals we have chosen. Our experience, therefore, is furnished not with conjectures about reality but with Vorstellungen (images, ideas, conceptions) that we keep or discard according to the way they serve us.

2. Social Adaptation, Language Games

When it first strikes a child that particular sounds may be linked with other parts of experience, these parts are usually fuzzy and either larger or smaller than they would be for an adult speaker of the language. They gradually become adapted in the course of interactions with others. That is how the impression is generated that meanings are the result of convention. After a while, when the child has begun to produce imitations of the sound-images of words in order to obtain things, they function so well that they create the belief that the association that links these sounds to specific experiences is shared by everyone. This kind of development is best explained by what Wittgenstein described as "language games" (1953, §§ 7-30, p.5-14).

3. The Construction of "Others"

It is important to realize that the others in our experience are no less our construction than everything else. In his *Critique of Pure Reason,* Kant formulated a fundamental principle: "It is obvious that, if I want to represent to myself a thinking being, I must put myself in his place, and thus substitute, as it were, my own subject for the object I am seeking to consider" (1780, A 354; Norman Smith Kemp translation).

You are led to this substitution when you realize that the items that are able to move by themselves are often predictable if you impute to them the ability to perceive, intentions, and methods for reaching goals that are like yours.[1]

Similar to your constructs of chairs, tables, and walls, "others" are useful in certain ways, but they also constitute constraints. Chairs, tables, and walls prevent you from walking through them. The others you construct not only prevent you from acting in certain ways, but also bring home the fact that the way you interpret what they do and say is frequently not viable. To a large extent such constraints are the effect of what Silvio Ceccato called "il consecutivo," that is, what follows from what you have already constructed (Ceccato, 1980, p. 55-56).

We learn to construct what others say according to the concepts and conceptual relations that have helped us to organize our own experience. But this interpretation of what they say does not always fit the patterns we expect. On the conceptual level this is analogous to hurting our shins on the edge of the coffee table. It shows that our construction of others is not ad lib. It is subject to constraints that may arise from the way we have initiated the specific construction: but they may also spring from the unknowable domain beyond our experience. Wherever they come from, these constraints force us to modify our interpretation of the other's use of language. We may do this by accommodating, by modifying what we consider the meaning of a word or by creating a new concept.

If linguistic communication is fraught with so much uncertainty, we cannot but wonder what it could be based on

---

[1] A more extensive analysis of how others may be constructed can be found in Chapter 6 of Glasersfeld (1995) and Chapter 3 of Larochelle (2008).

when we feel that we have understood an other's utterance. I would suggest that it is the result of fitting our interpretation of the utterance without difficulty into our conceptual world; and this fit may subsequently be confirmed by the fact that the other says or does nothing that contradicts our expectations.

Claude Shannon, who published the first formal theory of communication (Shannon, 1948), made it very clear that signals sent from a source to a receiver do not convey meaning in the linguistic sense. The only information they carry is an indication where, in an agreed pre-established code, their convened interpretation can be found. Without such a code, signals are meaningless—just as words of a language that is foreign to you have no meaning for you. Even if you have perceived their sound-images correctly, you do not possess the semantic "code" in which they might be linked to items of your experience. The semantic code of a language is initially built up by incipient individual speakers and consists of associations in the way I described above. Once a basic vocabulary has been created, new meanings can often be generated with their help. Even then, in spite of all social interaction, meaning remains subjective, not only as regards the basic experiential elements but also in the way the learner has combined them to form complex ideas by means of conceptual relations.

Shannon's theory is frequently and erroneously referred to as "information theory" and this opens the way to notions of "information transfer" that are incompatible with the original theory. What is transferred by the signals in communication systems, including natural languages, are selection instructions relative to a code that must be available to both sender and receiver; the meanings linked to signals in the code are not transmitted. With a message sent in Morse code, this is perfectly obvious: if you do not know how dots and dashes are linked to letters of the alphabet, you cannot read the message. In human communication this is not so obvious. Imagine that you go to the "Information" counter in an airport and ask "When is the plane from Boston supposed to arrive?" You may get the answer "6:30" and you are likely to think that this is the answer to your question. You are unaware of the fact that it is no more than the instruction to select a particular spot in a temporal scheme of hours and minutes that you have learnt long ago. Without that scheme, "6:30" would have no meaning.

Linguistic communication is made uncertain by the fact that the meanings of words are acquired, but not from a pre-established code that could be handed to beginners. Rather, the meanings of words have to be abstracted by each individual child from his or her own experience. In spite of dictionaries and encyclopedias, meanings remain subjective because—no matter how detailed these reference books may be—they are composed of words that, ultimately, can be interpreted only on the level of experience.[2]

REFERENCES

Ceccato, S (1980). *Il punto* (Vol.1). Milan: Ipsoa informatica.
Glasersfeld E. von (1995). *Radical constructivism: A way of knowing and learning.* London: Routledge/Falmer Press.
Kant, I, (1780). *Critique of pure reason* (N. Smith Kemp, trans.). London: Palgrave Macmillan.
Larochelle, M. (Ed.). (2008). *Key works in radical constructivism.* Rotterdam: Sense Publishers.
Shannon, C. E. (1948). The mathematical theory of communication. *Bell Systems Technical Journal, 27,* 379-423 & 623-656.
Wittgenstein, L. (1953). *Philosophical investigations.* Oxford: Basil Blackwell.

---

[2] This connection to experience unsettles the notion of translation implied by bilingual dictionaries: they seem to take for granted that the words they suggest for foreign words are linked to identical experiences. It does not take much familiarity with a foreign culture to know that frequently this is not the case.

❧ 2 ☙

Meaning in Relationship
Kenneth J. Gergen

A mist of ambiguity has always hovered about the concept of meaning. Differing schools of philosophy, theology, psychology, literary theory, communication, and linguistics have variously attempted to control the cacophony. Even the classic work of Ogden and Richards (1979), *The Meaning of Meaning*, did not serve to silence the competing dialogues. However, somewhere toward the center of the controversy is the a shared assumption that the essence of meaning is to be found within the individual person. Whether viewed as symbolic process, subjectivity, intentionality, mental representation, interpretation, or cognitive schema, meaning is held to be a private matter. Words and actions do not contain meaning in themselves. Rather, the meaning lies somewhere behind—in the mind of the speaker or actor, at the outset, and then with discernment, in the mind of the interpreting agent. In the present chapter I wish to challenge the traditional view of meaning. More importantly, I wish to outline an alternative view of rich potential. This relational view of meaning moves the focus of concern away from the minds of single individuals to the processes of relationship in which individuals are embedded.

The development of this view emerges from a long-standing engagement in dialogues on the social construction of knowledge (see summaries in Gergen, 1994, 2009). As these dialogues suggest, what we accept or embrace as objective knowledge is not the product of individual observation and reason, but issues from communicative interchange. Until there is negotiated agreement on "what there is," research into the nature of the world is precluded. Or to put it in terms of Thomas Kuhn's (1970) classic work, it is only within a communally shared paradigm that scientific facts can be produced. Yet while there is widespread agreement in the view that knowledge issues from communal relationships, it is traditionally presumed that relationships are constituted by individual, or psychological, subjects. In effect, the presumption of meaning as internal to the individual remains pervasive and unaddressed. It is to a relational alternative that the present paper is devoted.

Preparing the Way: Impasse and Ideology

There are many reasons for abandoning the presumption of meaning as an internal or psychological phenomenon. Among the most significant are shortcomings both conceptual and ideological. In the case of conceptual problems, philosophers have labored for centuries with the enigmas created by distinguishing between an inner or subjective world as against an external world of facts. As perennially asked, how do events in the objective realm make their way into the psychological world; and conversely, how do psychological events cause the physical activity of the body? These are essentially the problems of epistemology, in the first instance, and the mind-body problem in the latter. Despite centuries of philosophic deliberation on these problems, no viable answers have been forthcoming. As twentieth century philosophers such as Wittgenstein, Austen, and Ryle began to demonstrate, the very presumption of a mind within a body—"the ghost in the machine"—leads to a philosophical impasse. In what may be viewed as a summary conclusion, Richard Rorty (1979) proposed these insoluble enigmas are essentially a byproduct of a Western language game.

These philosophic problems are accompanied by a further dilemma: how to account for human understanding. We traditionally view words, in particular, as outward expressions of internal or psychological states. However, we now confront the difficult challenge of determining how it is that we understand each other. How do we penetrate the meaning underlying the words? Obviously no one has direct knowledge of another's mind. One can never peer behind the veil of the eyes. So, how is one to draw conclusions about another's inner world, what the other actually feels, or is trying to say? Hermeneutic theorists, concerned with how it is we can accurately understand the intentions behind the words of the Bible or holy writs, have worried about the problem of "inner access" for over three centuries now. A satisfactory answer to this question has never been forthcoming. In Hans Georg Gadamer's (1975) pivotal work, the major emphasis shifts to the "horizon of understanding" which the reader inevitably brings to the text. As Gadamer reasoned, all readings must necessarily draw from this forestructure of understanding—what it is the reader presumes about the world, the writing, the author, and so on. And reading must inevitably take place from this horizon. Much the same conclusion is reached by a host of "reader response" theorists in literary studies. As Stanley Fish (1980) has put the case, every reader is a member of some interpretive community, a network of people who understand the world in certain ways. And whatever interpretation of the text is made will inevitably rely on these understandings. In effect, the reader never makes authentic connection with the subjectivity of the writer; there is no escape from the standpoint one brings to the interpretation. The dismal conclusion of this line of criticism is that we never gain access to the other's subjectivity; we never understand each other! We shall revisit the problem of understanding shortly.

In addition to these insoluble problems, there is a second

line of criticism that is more ideological in nature. Here it is variously proposed that by placing such importance on individual subjectivity we give further support to an individualist ideology, an ideology detrimental to our cultural future. To reiterate some of these critiques, when we hold individual subjectivity as the essential ingredient of humanity, we simultaneously construct a world of fundamentally isolated individuals, each locked within their own private world. All we have to count on, ultimately, is ourselves. Others are by nature alien, and because self-seeking is the obvious choice under such conditions, others may indeed be seen as potential enemies. When the quality of individual subjectivity is paramount, all forms of relationship—marriage, friendship, family, community—are necessarily artificial and secondary. If this form of ideology retains its pervasive grip on cultural life, the future seems grim. In effect, by placing the origin of meaning within the individual, there are injurious effects on society. For a more extensive account of these problems with the traditional view, and the alternative that follows, the reader may consult my recent book, *Relational Being: Beyond the Individual and Community* (Gergen, 2009).

MEANING AS COORDINATED ACTION

How are we to make sense of the proposal that meaning is a byproduct of relationship? Can such a conception avoid repeating the problems inherent in the earlier traditions? My belief is that a new view of human communication can indeed be drawn from the constructionist dialogues, not only as they are taking place within therapeutic circles but as they have developed in the neighboring domains of ethnomethodology, the history of science, the sociology of knowledge, discursive psychology, literary theory, and communication theory.[1] In each of these cases there is a strong tendency to place the locus of

---

[1] See, for example, Garfinkel, 1967; Kuhn, 1970; Latour & Woolgar, 1986; Edwards & Potter, 1994; Fish, 1980; and Shotter, 1993.

meaning within the process of interaction itself. That is, the individual agent is de-emphasized as the source of meaning; attention moves from the *within* to the *between*.

Although recognition of the jointly constructed character of meaning has become increasingly widespread, there is as yet no comprehensive account of how such a process occurs. If we accept such an orientation, what are the action implications? What new conceptual resources can be mobilized? What new questions are raised? For purposes of furthering the dialogue, in what follows I shall make a preliminary incursion into these domains. I offer here a series of rudimentary propositions that place meaning squarely within the relational matrix.

An Individual's Utterances in Themselves Possess No Meaning

We pass each other on the street. I smile and say, "Hello Anna." You walk past without hearing. Under such conditions, what have I said? To be sure, I have uttered two words. However for all the difference it makes I might have chosen two nonsense syllables. You pass and I say "Umlot nigen." You hear nothing. When you fail to acknowledge me in any way, all words become equivalent. In an important sense, nothing has been said at all. I cannot possess meaning alone.[2]

The Potential for Meaning is Realized through Supplementary Action

Lone utterances begin to acquire meaning when another (or others) coordinate themselves to the utterance, that is, when they add some form of supplementary action (whether linguistic or otherwise). Effectively, I have greeted Anna only by virtue of her response. "Oh, hi, good morning" brings me to life as one who has greeted. Supplements may be very simple, as simple

---

[2] You may object: "Well, even if not acknowledged, what I say might mean something to me personally," and that may be. But the question then becomes, how did your utterances come to have personal meaning? We take up this issue shortly.

as a nod of affirmation that indeed you have said something meaningful. It may take the form of an action, such as shifting the line of gaze upon hearing the word "look!" Or it may extend the utterance in some way, as in "Yes, but I also think that . . . ." We thus find that to communicate at all is to be granted by others a privilege of meaning. If others do not treat one's utterances as communication, if they fail to coordinate themselves around the offering, one is reduced to nonsense.

To combine these first two proposals, we see that meaning resides within neither individual, but only in relationship. Both act and supplement must be coordinated in order for meaning to occur. Like a handshake, a kiss, or a tango, the individual's actions alone are empty. Communication is inherently collaborative. In this way we see that none of the words that comprise our vocabulary have meaning in themselves. They are granted the capacity to mean by virtue of the way they are coordinated with other words and actions. Indeed, our entire vocabulary of the individual—who thinks, feels, wants, hopes, and so on—is granted meaning only by virtue of coordinated activities among people. Their birth of "myself" lies within relationship.

Supplementary Action is Itself a Candidate for Meaning

Any supplement functions twice, first in granting significance to what has preceded, and second as an action that also requires supplementation. In effect, the meaning it grants remains suspended until it too is supplemented. Consider a client in therapy who speaks of her deep depression; she finds herself unable to cope with an aggressive husband and an intolerable job situation. The therapist can grant this report meaning as an expression of depression, by responding, "Yes, I can see why you might feel this way; tell me a little more about your relationship with your husband." However, this supplement too stands idle of meaning until the client provides the supplement. If the client ignored the statement (for example, going on to talk about her success as a mother), the therapist's words would be denied significance. More broadly, we may say that in daily life there are no *acts in themselves,* that is, actions that are not simultaneously supplements to what has preceded. Whatever we do or say takes place within a temporal context that gives meaning to what has preceded, while simultaneously forming an invitation to further supplementation.

Acts Create the Possibility for Meaning but Simultaneously Constrain its Potential

If I give a lecture on psychoanalytic theory, this lecture is meaningless without an audience that listens, deliberates, affirms, or questions what I have said. In this sense, every speaker owes to his or her audience a debt of gratitude; without their engagement the speaker ceases to exist. At the same time, my lecture creates the very possibility for the audience to grant meaning. While the audience creates me as a meaningful agent, I simultaneously grant to them the capacity to create. They are without existence until there is an action that invites them into being.

Yet it is also important to realize that, in practice, actions also set constraints upon supplementation. If I speak on Freud, as an audience member you are not able to supplement in any way you wish. You may ask me a question about object relations theory, but not astrophysics; comment on the concept of repression, but not on taste of radishes. Such constraints exist because my lecture is already embedded within a *tradition of act and supplement.* It has been granted meaning as a "lecture on Freud," by virtue of previous generations of meaning givers. In this sense, actions embedded within relationships have *prefigurative* potential. The history of usage enables them to invite or suggest certain supplements as opposed to others—because only these supplements are considered sensible or meaningful within a tradition. Thus, as we speak with each other, we also begin to set limits on each other's being; to remain in the conversation is not only to respect a tradition, but to accede to being one kind of person as opposed to another. If you tell me that I have not been a good friend, I will scarcely be recognizable unless I ask you to tell me why you feel this way, and what have I done. Your very comment constrains my potentials.

Supplements Function Both to Create and Constrain Meaning

As we have seen, supplements "act backward" in a way that creates meaning of what has preceded. In this sense, the speaker's meaning—his or her identity, character, intention, and the like—are not free to "be what they are," but are constrained by the act of supplementation. Supplementation thus operates *postfiguratively* to create the speaker as meaning this as opposed to that. From the enormous array of possibilities, the supplement gives direction and temporarily narrows the possibilities of being. Thus, for example, for a therapist to inquire into a client's depression is to establish a form of constraint. If the client is to remain sensible, he or she may readily accede to being depressed. A therapeutic question can harbor implications for an entire life trajectory.

While Acts/Supplements are Constraining, They Do Not Determine

As proposed, our words and actions function so as to constrain the words and actions of others, and vice versa. If we are to remain intelligible within our culture, we must necessarily act within these constraints. Such constraints have their origins in a history of preceding coordinations. As people coordinate actions and supplements, and come to rely on them in everyday life, they are essentially generating a way of life. If enough people join in these coordinated activities over a long period, we may speak of a cultural tradition. Yet it is important to underscore that our words and actions function only as *constraints* and *not as determinants*. This is so for two important reasons: First, the conditions under which we attempt to coordinate our actions are seldom constant. We are constantly faced with the challenge of importing old words and actions into new situations. As we do so, such words and actions acquire new possibilities for meaning. For example, you are visiting a farm and you point out to your child, "Look. That is a chicken." The word "chicken" thus gains its meaning from the way it is embedded in this configuration of events. Later that day, the farmer's wife comes to the dinner table bearing a large platter, and announces, "We are having chicken for dinner tonight." Now the word used in referring to the live and clucking animal refers to the individual pieces of cooked meat. As new situations develop, so will the same word acquire other potentials for meaning. More formally, we say that all words are *polysemic*; they may be used in many different ways.

A second important reason for our relative freedom of action lies in the fact that meaning making is always local. That is, coordination is always located in the here and now, in momentary and fleeting conditions—in the kitchen, the boardroom, the mine, the prison, and so on. These local efforts to coordinate give rise to local patterns of speaking and action—street slang, academic jargon, baby talk, jive talk, signing, and so on. And because those who enter into such coordinations may issue from different cultural traditions, new combinations are always under production. In effect, we inherit an enormous potpourri of potentially intelligible actions, each arising from a different form of life—and the repository is under continuous motion. Our actions may be invited by history, but they are not required. In this sense, we can indeed "step over our shadows," and in order to function adequately in continuously changing circumstances, creative combinations will always be necessary. As we speak together now we have the capacity to create new futures.

Traditions of Coordination Furnish the Major Potentials for Meaning, but Do Not Circumscribe

To amplify a preceding line of reasoning, it is important to recognize that the words and actions upon which we rely to generate meaning together are largely byproducts of the past. If I approached you and began to utter a string of vowels, "ahhh, ehhhh, ooooo, uuuu," you would surely be puzzled; perhaps you would make for an exit, as I might well be dangerous. This is so because this utterance is nonsense, or to put it another way, not recognizable as a candidate for meaning within Western traditions of coordination. Similarly, if we began to dance and you suddenly crouched and gazed at the floor, I would scarcely continue dancing. Your actions are not part of any coordinated sequences with which I am familiar. Our capacity to make meaning together today thus relies on a history, often a history of centuries' duration. We owe to traditions of coordination our capacities for being in love, demonstrating for a just cause, or taking pleasure in our children's development.

This is not to say that there is no room for novel words and actions. Indeed, in the past century we have witnessed an explosion in new vocabulary terms, sporting activities, dance steps, and so on. Because we are not determined by the past, we are free to play, to violate expectations, to explore the outrageous. And when we confront the novel word or act, we can with effort bring it into meaning. To return to our dance, I might well have stopped dancing when you crouched on the floor. However, if I understood you to be playing, inviting, challenging, I would do my best to find a means of coordinating with you. Perhaps I would also crouch, and begin to sway forward in your direction. Thus, an adolescent who wears something "weird" to school may give rise to a fad. And therapists who believe the schizophrenic's "word salad' is meaningful will find ways to render such utterances meaningful.

Thought and Feeling Consist of Public Meaning-Making Conducted Privately

As offered earlier, we do seem to experience what might be called "private meaning." If an intimate friend expresses anger toward us, we may lapse into silence, unable to respond. However, this does not mean that the word has no meaning to us. A dozen replies may buzz through our head; we ride an emotional roller-coaster. Let us not deny the significance of such an event. However, the existence of unspoken replies does not simultaneously mean a reinstatement of the subjectivity assumption, the view that meaning originates in private minds and is expressed outwardly in words. We must avoid the problems inherent in the view that there is an internal agent inside who can rise above cultural meaning, who possesses the capacity to generate meaning prior to any immersion in a relational world. Let us, rather, reconstruct the meaning of subjectivity—the "inner world." Consider: you have agreed to take part in a play, and you must master your lines before tonight's rehearsal. With the script before you, you speak the lines; when they are familiar you put the book down and perform them more fully, perhaps with a laugh or a shout. You decide to take a shower, and while you are showering you try to recall the lines silently. During the silent rehearsal you move through a clever line and a smile crosses your face. You "feel" the mirth. Here we see that the distinction between the internal and external world breaks down. What takes place internally is essentially an action in the external world, only conducted without full expression. The internal activity is effectively a reduced form of making sense in our common relationships. As some scholars put it, thought is a form of internal speech—a public act simply carried out in private.

In much the same way, we may usefully reconfigure the concept of intention. We commonly speak about our intentions as causing our actions. For example, we say to ourselves, "I must apologize," and then we proceed to do so. To be sure, the apology may not be defined that way by others; in this sense I need them to make it an apology. However, I did know what I was doing at the time, from my perspective, and this knowing *preceded* the supplementation. Such common events are often used to support the assumption of conscious agency: I chose my actions; I intended certain meanings and not others. This concept of a free, internal agent that directs the traffic of one's words and deeds has a long tradition, and much contemporary support from humanistic scholars. Yet in spite of its attraction ("I am the god of my action"), the concept has faired poorly both philosophically and ideologically. The notorious problem of free will on the one hand, and the politics of narcissism on the other, are only two of the knotty issues. How can we sustain the conception of conscious intention without falling into these traditional traps?

We find a promising answer by extending the view of thought and feeling as the private recirculation of public life. If I am an actor who does what we call "playing the part of Hamlet," I can readily tell someone that "I am playing Hamlet tonight." Public life provides me then with a pattern of action and an acceptable construction of that action. It allows me to tell others that "this is what I will do." Of course, I may silently say this to myself as well, as in: "Hmmm, I really shouldn't take this drink because I will be playing Hamlet tonight." These private constructions, resulting from my participation in public life, are what we may call intentions. They do not direct the action so much as comment upon its occurrence. In this way I can say "I intended that remark as an apology." I can say this with full assurance because my immersion in public life gives me grounds for knowing that the words I have uttered are commonly defined as an apology. By the same token, we can say "he intended to commit the murder," not because we have insight into his conscious state, but because his experience in cultural life furnished him with just this construction of the act in question.

Meanings are Subject to Continuous Reconstitution Via the Expanding Sea of Supplementation

In light of the above, we find that what an utterance means is inherently undecidable. No amount of discussion, discourse analysis, conversation analysis, or other attempt to determine what has been said, can be determinative. The meaning of any utterance is a temporary achievement, born of the collaborative moment. Further, as relations continue over time, what is meant stands subject to continuous alteration through an expanding arena of action/supplements.

Sarah and Robert may find themselves frequently laughing together—affirming each other as humorous persons—until Robert announces that Sarah's laughter is "unnatural and forced," just her attempt to present herself as an "easy going person" (in which case the definition of the previous actions would be altered). Or Sarah could announce, "This is all very pleasant, Robert, but really you're a superficial guy; we really don't communicate at all" (thus reducing Robert's humor to banality). At the same time, these latter moves within the ongoing sequence are subject to further reconstitution. (In reply to Robert's accusation of being unnatural, Sarah replies, "Robert, are you worried about your job again? What's bothering you?") Or Robert replies to Sarah's ascription of superficiality with "Now I see. You are only saying that, Sarah, because you find Bill so attractive.") Such instances of alteration may also be far removed from the interchange itself (e.g., consider a divorcing pair who retrospectively redefine their entire marital trajectory), and are subject to continuous change through interaction with and among others (e.g., friends, relatives, therapists, the media etc.).

In summary, we find the exclusive focus on the face-to-face relationship is far too narrow. For whether "my words are meaningful" is not under my control; nor is it determined by you, or the dyadic process in which meaning struggles toward realization. At the outset, we largely derive our potential for coordination from our previous immersion in a range of other relationships. We arrive in the relationship as extensions of the past. And as the current relationship unfolds, it serves to reform the potentials of the past. These interchanges may be supplemented and transformed by still others in the future. In effect, meaningful communication in any given relationship ultimately depends on an extended array of relationships, not only "right here, right now," but how it is that you and I are related to a variety of other persons, and those persons to others still—and ultimately, one may say, to the relational conditions of society as a whole. We are all in this way interdependently interlinked—without the capacity to mean anything, to possess an "I"—except for the existence of an extended world of relationship.

THE QUESTION OF UNDERSTANDING MINDS

Although briefly outlined, the present account of meaning avoids the perennial problems inherent in the dualistic and individualist vision of the person. However, this account also raises a variety of challenging questions. In addressing two of these questions, I will complete the present analysis. At the outset there is the question of understanding. Recall the preceding discussion of the problems inherent in trying to penetrate "what's on someone's mind." As we found, there is no means of gaining access to others' psychological states. One could do no more than guess. Any accumulation of evidence would constitute no more than a multiplication of further guesses. Thus, if understanding were a process of inter-subjective connection, understanding would scarcely occur. However, this critique left us with an impasse. What account can now be given about the way in which we understand (or misunderstand) each other?

To explore the presumption of understanding as a relational phenomenon, the metaphor of the dance is useful. Consider, for example, the movements of skilled tango dancers. Each movement of the one is coordinated with the other; their actions are wholly synchronized. I propose that such synchronic coordination is the essence of mutual understanding. If one of the partners moved in such a way that the other fell to the floor, he or she would be discredited. Now, consider: If you tell me tearfully of the untimely death of a family member, how shall I respond? Let's say I reply with a hearty "Well, that's that. No sense in crying over spilled milk. Let's get a beer." Chances are you will be startled. How could I respond in this way? You are supposed to be my friend, but seem to have no comprehension of the importance of this loss to me. Now, contrast this with my responding with silence and then uttering quiet words of consolation. Here you may well credit me with understanding. In effect, to understand each other is to coordinate our actions within the common scenarios of our culture.[3] A failure to understand is not a failure to grasp the essence of the other's psyche, but an inability to participate in the kind of scenario the other is inviting.

There is a final and related issue that demands attention. Specifically, how can we account for the claim that we know that we do not understand something, and this knowledge is a feeling that registers within? For example, at some time in our lives, most of us have experienced failure in understanding the words of a teacher or professor. And we do not seem to require the supplement of another's telling us that we fail to understand. We seem to know it directly. To account or this "feeling of misunderstanding" as a relational phenomenon, we must first eliminate the binary upon which this question rests, the distinction between an "in here" and an "out there." Rather, let us view the judgment of understanding (or misunderstanding) as an action within a relationship. To appreciate this possibility,

---

[3] See also J.L. Austin's discussion of the "felicity conditions" for meaningful communication. Austin, J.L. (1962) *How to do things with words.* Oxford: Clarendon.

return to the case of the student attempting to understand the teacher. If understanding is coordinated action, as just proposed, then understanding a teacher is the ability to respond to a lecture in a way that the teacher would approve. Or, roughly put, when students can respond to their teachers' questions about their lecture by repeating or extending its content, they may be credited with understanding. If they are unable to perform according to the teachers' criteria, they have not understood. The feeling, then, that one does not understand is the recognition that one cannot adequately respond to what has been said. It is a social action carried out silently. Michael Billig (1996) points in this direction when he asks us to consider thinking as a "silent argument." In effect, it is a social performance on a minimal scale. Instead of uttering the words out loud to another, one utters them to an implied audience and without sound. In the same way an actor may rehearse his lines silently, or one may hum to herself. What we do privately is not taking place in an "inner world" called mind, but is to participate in social life without the audience physically present.

REFERENCES

Austin, J. L. (1962) *How to do things with words.* Oxford: Clarendon.
Billig, M. (1996). *Arguing and thinking: A rhetorical approach to social psychology.* Cambridge, UK: Cambridge University Press.
Edwards, D., & Potter, J. (1992). *Discursive psychology.* London: Sage.
Fish, S. (1980). *Is there a text in this class? The authority of interpretive communities.* Cambridge, MA: Harvard University Press.
Gadamer, H. (1975). *Truth and method* (G. Barden & J. Gumming, Trans.). New York: Seabury.
Garfinkel, H. (1967). *Studies in ethnomethodology.* Englewood Cliffs, NJ: Prentice-Hall.
Gergen, K. J. (1994). *Realities and relationships: Soundings in social construction.* Cambridge, MA: Harvard University Press.
Gergen, K. J. (2009). *Relational being: Beyond the individual and community.* New York: Oxford University Press.
Kuhn, T. (1970). *The structure of scientific revolutions.* Chicago: The University of Chicago Press.

Latour, B., & Woolgar, S. (1986). *Laboratory life: The construction of scientific facts*. Princeton, NJ: Princeton University Press.

Ogden, C. K., & Richards, I. A. (1979). *The meaning of meaning: A study of the influence of language upon thought and of the science of symbolism*. Orlando: Harcourt.

Rorty, R. (1979). *Philosophy and the mirror of nature*. Princeton, NJ: Princeton University Press.

Shotter, J. (1993). *Cultural politics of everyday life: Social constructionism, rhetoric, and knowing of the third kind*. Milton Keynes: Open University Press.

PART II

PRACTICE

3

Innovations in Psychotherapy: Tracking the Narrative Construction of Change[1]

Miguel M. Gonçalves, Anita Santos, Marlene Matos, João Salgado, Inês Mendes, António P. Ribeiro, Carla Cunha, and Juliana Gonçalves

This chapter presents a research program on narrative change processes that is under development at our research center. It developed from the study of narrative therapy, following White and Epston's (1990) model of re-authoring narratives, in which the notion of "unique outcome" is central. Unique outcomes are defined as all the details that fall outside the domain of the dominant narrative, namely episodes in which the person did, thought, imagined or felt something different, or related to others in a new way, from what the problematic narrative "prescribes" for his or her life (see also White, 2007).

We started studying how "unique outcomes" developed throughout the process of narrative therapy, and then wondered if developing these narrative details outside the main problematic story could be, in a sense, a common factor of all different kinds of psychotherapies, even if this is something that therapists outside the narrative tradition do not emphasize explicitly. If one assumes that all therapists wish to produce novelties in different forms (cognitive, affective, behavioral) it is not hard to

---

[1] This chapter was supported by the Portuguese Foundation for Science and Technology (FCT), by the Grant PTDC/PSI/72846/2006 (Narrative Processes in Psychotherapy). We are grateful to Gena Rodrigues for the revision of the English and to Carla Machado for the suggestions done on the first draft of this chapter.

imagine that "unique outcomes" must emerge in every form of successful psychotherapy, independently of the means that are used to achieve them.

The target of this chapter is to provide an overall view of the studies on the role of these unique outcomes in psychotherapy change. We organized this chapter in four parts. We start by discussing the theoretical and methodological foundations of our research, highlighting its narrative frame. After presenting our current main findings, a heuristic model of change is presented. Working from this model, we reflect upon how change is prevented from occurring in poor-outcome cases. We then discuss the new paths of research that we are developing: namely intensive case-study research of these models of change and stability. This chapter ends with some provisional reflections about how this research can inform therapists, contributing in this way to the development of psychotherapy as a practice.

THEORETICAL ASSUMPTIONS

Bateson (1979) once suggested that if we were able to ask a computer if it would one day be able to think as a human being (and if the computer could in fact model the way humans think), the output would begin, after some difficult processing, "That reminds me a story" (p. 22). Congruent with this idea from Bateson, our first assumption is that human beings organize reality in a narratively structured way (Bruner, 1986; McAdams, 1993; Polkinghorne, 1988; Sarbin, 1986). Emotions, feelings, relations and behaviors acquire meaning through their integration in stories that are narrated to the self and/or to others. In the uninterrupted flow of our life we create meaning out of events by "cutting" the flow of timely experience into discrete pieces and by constructing meaning by elaborating narrative themes (Kelly, 1955). We have here two interrelated processes: the event, that is something that happened, and the action of narrating it to a meaningful audience (the self, the therapist, meaningful others). This means, as Hermans (1996) said, that the self is simultaneously the content of the story and the act of telling it. Or, as suggested by Wortham (2001), the articulation between the narrative content and the act of telling is a powerful tool for self-construction. Moreover, narrative always has a dimension of enactment, since it is quite related with our action, as human agents, in the physical and social world. Narratives, in a way, are performative acts—not simply self-contained performances—and, as such, they produce relational results to which, in return, we adapt to. Through the use of these symbolic means we are thrown into a constant dynamic of narrative positioning and repositioning (Hermans & Dimaggio, 2004; Valsiner, 2002; Salgado & Gonçalves, 2007).

Congruently, therapists have been developing a diversity of techniques to allow the transformation of life-narratives, but it is our suggestion, inspired by the re-authoring therapy of White and Epston (1990), that at least part of this transformation occurs through the expansion of unique outcomes. New self-stories are constructed from the narration of novelties, since these innovative stories create new paths of further development and free the person to engage in new forms of authorship. To tell new viable stories means to live new narratives. Indeed, as we argued previously, new forms of narrative are intermingled with new forms of relating with (and within) our world.

However, as our research has developed, so too has our terminology. Instead of "unique outcomes," we prefer to use the term "innovative moments" (or *i-moments*), for two main reasons. First, as we shall see, unique outcomes are not unique events; they occur frequently in psychotherapy, even in poor outcome cases. Of course, the idea of "unique" in White and Epston's (1990) work does not refer literally to the frequency of the events, but to their exceptionality in relation to the problematic narrative. However, for the unfamiliar reader the idea of uniqueness may be misleading. Another problem has to do with the term "outcomes." "Unique outcomes" are more than a result or an output, and as we will illustrate, they reflect a developmental process. Hence, in this research we are truly concerned with the processes involved in narrative transformations and that is why we prefer the idea of innovative moments (or i-moments) over unique outcomes.

Before moving to a consideration of psychotherapy let us illustrate the concept of i-moment at a more elementary level, using for that purpose the developmental research of Fogel, Garvey, Hsu and West-Stroming (2006) on the relationship of mothers and babies in infancy. Fogel et al. study how a relationship develops by using the concept of *frames*, understood as "segments of co-action that have a coherent theme, that take place within a particular location (in space or in time), and that involve particular forms of mutual co-orientation between participants" (p. 3). These frames evolve in time, in particular forms of sequence of mutual action and response, creating a kind of lived narrative. By their turn, in our view, narratives themselves operate as basic guidelines of social coordination—in a sense, as frames. These frames can also be studied in their developmental dynamics, as it happens with narratives.

One typical frame in the first 6 months of life is the *guided object frame*, in which the caregiver and child play with objects. Let us imagine that in one situation the mother shows different objects to the child while the infant observes, but in another the mother attempts to put the toy in the infant's hands or the infant tries to reach for the object. These last occurrences open the possibility for development to occur, given that they bring an innovation to the system. From here the child may start grabbing objects and playing with them, without the help of the mother, giving rise to a new frame, which Fogel et al. (2006) term *non-guided object frame*.

We have in this simple example three types of change that are characterized by Fogel et al. (2006), namely:

- Level 1 change, which occurs when there is variability inside the same frame (e.g., mother shows different objects);

- Level 2 takes place when an innovation occurs (in our terminology, an i-moment), for instance when the infant for the first time reaches for the toy;
- Level 3, the final level, in which there is a clearly developmental change; for instance when the non-guided frame emerges and stabilizes out of level 2 (we equate this in psychotherapy with the expansion of i-moments into a new narrative).

To Fogel et al. (2006) although level 1 change is always present given the dynamic nature of open systems, level 2 innovations can lead to more enduring changes, through developmental change (i.e. level 3):

> The successful innovations, the ones that get noticed, remain in the system, and ultimately provoke a level 3 change, must somehow be perceived as "interesting", or "better", or "exciting", or "worthwhile". This implies that there is an inherent valuation of changes that is, an emotional aspect to the information of what makes a difference. (p. 238)

The reality of therapy is far more complex than that of the early interaction between caregivers and infant, however it is our suggestion that the same kinds of changes are also present in therapy. Whenever the client tells a redundant story—let us take as an example a story of pain for not being valued and loved as a child—we notice the same themes present over and over[2]. White and Epston (1990) call this redundancy a problem-saturated story and Neimeyer (2000), in his conceptualization of narrative disruption, equated this with narrative dominance. Whatever the term used to describe this, the process present in this kind of narrative organization is the repetition of the same theme, over and over again. With this client, independently of what we ask, we will hear stories of pain, shame, low self-esteem, loneliness and rejection and so on. In other words, we

---

[2] This example is inspired by a psychotherapy conducted by the first author with a woman in her mid-thirties.

will hear variations under the same general theme or narrative pattern. This is akin to level 1 change. It is variability without any meaningful psychological change. From this variability is very difficult to construct a new self-narrative. In fact, clients and therapists hardly perceived this variability as "change."

Sometimes in good outcome therapy, instead of this variability something different emerges. Let us say that the therapist invites the client to write an "unsent letter" to her parents telling what she feels about them. When reading the letter in the session a new idea and a strong feeling emerges: she was unable to figure out why her parents' behavior was so rejecting. After all she is a mother herself and she feels oppressed by her inability to understand the rejection that she was a victim of. Until now she was unaware of this urge to understand, because she felt that she was the guilty one. Somehow she was not good enough to be loved. This was a very important innovation in the therapeutic process—a level 2 change in Fogel et al. (2006) model.

Taking level 2 changes as a starting point, therapist and client can work towards the construction of level 3 changes. A sign of this level of change is, for instance, the fact that the client started seeing her relation with her family in a different light. Instead of continuing fighting for her family's attention, being nice and a "good girl", she decided that she needed to let the past stay in the past and mourn for the lost family. She now faces a very difficult feeling: in fact she never had a family in the true sense of the word; she never had someone who really cared. As an adult, she also wouldn't have the love of the family as she wished, but she started feeling the need to move forward with her life, and, perhaps more important, her present difficulties (e.g., raising a child alone) were not a sign of her inability in living. This feeling was liberating and initiated a cascade of other innovations (e.g., in her relationship with her own son, in her relationship with the rest of the family, and so on). As in the previous example with mother-infant interaction, from the expansion of level 2 changes the developmental change emerges. Thus, i-moments are all the moments in which level 2 change emerges. We will discuss below how level 3 change can be constructed from these kinds of innovations or how they can be minimized or trivialized, maintaining in this way the problematic narrative. However, it is our hypothesis that level 3 change is constructed by the accumulation of level 2 change, creating a new gestalt, able to compete with the previous problematic narrative (see Gonçalves, Matos, & Santos, 2009).

The narrative background that supports our research inspired us to look at i-moments as processes in which level 2 change emerges and also allowed us to identify an empirical way of doing so. Given its complexity, it is harder to identify level 2 changes in psychotherapy (as was illustrated by the example above) than in more elementary interactions, such as those between a caregiver and an infant in which there is a restricted behavioral repertoire, without the intricacies of discursive interactions. Thus, we track i-moments by identifying the problematic narrative that shapes the life of the person and define i-moments as all those occurrences in which this narrative is implicitly or explicitly defied or rejected. While the problematic narrative is the "rule," the i-moment is the "exception to the rule."

In our research we began by studying a sample of narrative therapy and discovered five different types of i-moments (Matos & Gonçalves, 2004; Matos, Santos, Gonçalves, & Martins, 2009). From this first research we developed a coding system (Gonçalves, Matos, & Santos, 2009; Gonçalves, Ribeiro, Matos, Santos, & Mendes, in press) and checked if this system was applicable to different types of psychotherapy (e.g., experiential, client-centered, cognitive-behavioral). In individual therapy, this coding system seems applicable and reliable as we will discuss below. To this point the only difficulty we have encountered is related to its application to marital and family therapy given the multiplicity of authors involved (Batista, 2008).

The five different types of i-moments that emerge in psychotherapy are action, reflection, protest, re-conceptualization and performing change (see Table 1). We will therefore present these five types as well as a clinical vignette illustrating each of them (Gonçalves et al., 2009; Gonçalves et al., in press).

Action i-moments refer to specific actions or behaviors that challenge the dominance of the problematic narrative.

> *Clinical vignette (Problematic narrative: agoraphobia)*
>
> *Therapist*: Was it difficult for you to take this step (not accepting the rules of "fear" and going out)?
> *Client*: Yes, it was a huge step. For the last several months I barely went out. Even coming to therapy was a major challenge. I felt really powerless going out. I have to prepare myself really well to be able to do this.

Reflection i-moments involve the emergence of new understandings or thoughts that are not congruent with the dominant plot. The cognitive challenge to the problem, envisioning new perspectives on the problem and defying cultural prescriptions that facilitate the development of the problematic narrative are examples of these i-moments. They involve cognitive outcomes that create a different landscape of consciousness, to paraphrase Bruner (1986), from the usual one associated with the problematic narrative.

> *Clinical vignette (Problematic narrative: depression)*
>
> *Client*: I'm starting to wonder about what my life will be like if I keep feeding my depression.
> *Therapist*: It's becoming clear that depression has a hidden agenda for your life?
> *Client*: Yes, sure.
> *Therapist*: What is it that depression wants from you?
> *Client*: It wants to rule my whole life and in the end it wants to steal my life from me.

Protest i-moments are present when there is some sort of protest against the problem, against its specifications and also against the persons who are somehow the problem's supporters. It can take the form of an action or a reflection, but it necessarily involves an active form of resistance, repositioning the self towards the problematic narrative and through this, a more proactive process emerges (e.g., deciding something relevant about the problem that reduces its power over the client's life). In these i-moments we can discern, implicitly or explicitly, two positions: one that supports the problematic narrative and another one that defies it. In a protest i-moment the latter position gains more power than the former.

> *Clinical vignette (Problematic narrative: feeling rejected and judged by her parents)*
>
> *Client*: I talked about it just to demonstrate what I've been doing until now, fighting for it...
> *Therapist*: Fighting against the idea that you should do what your parents thought was good for you?
> *Client*: I was trying to change myself all the time, to please them. But now I'm getting tired, I am realizing that it doesn't make any sense to make this effort.
> *Therapist*: That effort keeps you in a position of changing yourself all the time, the way you feel and think...
> *Client*: Yes, sure. And I'm really tired of that, I can't stand it anymore. After all, parents are supposed to love their children and not judge them all the time.

Re-conceptualization i-moments involve a meta-reflective level, meaning that the person not only understands what is internally different in her or him (which would be coded as reflection or protest), but also is able to describe the processes involved in that transformation. These i-moments involve three components: the self in the past (problematic narrative), the self in the present and the description of the processes that allowed the transformation from the past to the present. The client not only understands something new but can also establish a distinction from a previous condition and has access to the processes by which the transformation took place.

> *Clinical vignette (Problematic narrative: partner's abuse and its effects)*
>
> *Client*: I think I started enjoying myself again. I had a time... I think I've stopped in time. I've always been a person that liked myself. There was a time... maybe because of my attitude, because of all that was happening, I think there was a time that I was not respecting myself... despite the effort to show that I wasn't feeling... so well with myself... I couldn't feel that joy of living, that I recovered now... and now I keep thinking "you have to move on and get your life back."
> *Therapist*: This position of "you have to move on" has been decisive?
> *Client*: That was important. I felt so weak at the beginning! I hated feeling like that.... Today I think "I'm not weak." In fact, maybe I am very strong, because of all that happened to me, I can still see the good side of people and I don't think I'm being naïve... Now, when I look at myself, I think, "No, you can really make a difference, and you have value as a person." For a while I couldn't have this dialogue with myself, I couldn't say, "You can do it" nor even think, "I am good at this or that"...

Performing Change i-moments refers to the anticipation or planning of new experiences, projects or activities. In these i-moments the client may apply newly learned skills to daily life, performing new ways of acting, getting back to former and abandoned projects and activities, or think about what he or she has learned with the problematic story that could make the next change in his or her life meaningful.

> *Clinical vignette (Problematic narrative: partner's abuse and its effects)*
>
> *Therapist*: You seem to have so many projects for the future now!
> *Client*: Yes, you're right. I want to do all the things that were impossible for me to do while I was dominated by fear. I want to work again and to have the time to enjoy my life with my children. I want to have friends again. The loss of all the friendships of the past is something that still hurts me really deeply. I want to have friends again, to have people to talk to, to share experiences and to feel the complicity of others in my life again.

Bruner (1986) suggested that narratives are constructed in two landscapes, one of action and another one of consciousness. Landscape of action refers to the development of the plot, the actions taking place, the actors involved and the setting where action occurred. Landscape of consciousness refers to what actors know, feel and think, or what are their projects, values or intentions. Although one landscape can transform the other, "they are essential and distinct: it is the difference between Oedipus sharing Jocasta's bed before and after he learns from the messenger that she is his mother" (p. 14).

Action and reflection i-moments are "pure" representatives of action and consciousness landscapes. As we said before, protest can occur in one landscape or in the other, or can even have elements of both. Likewise, performing change can be situated in both landscapes, being a new way of feeling or thinking, or a new action. Re-conceptualization as a meta-level typically has elements of both landscapes, integrating them.

The coding system we constructed (Gonçalves et al., 2009; Gonçalves et al., in press) from this variety of i-moments allows the study of a diversity of psychotherapy cases, from small samples to single-cases. Our findings and the heuristic model of change that we have constructed from our data will be described below. Before we proceed, we need to clarify some methodological details. Readers who wish to learn more about this coding system may order it directly from the authors (free of charge).

METHODOLOGICAL PROCEDURES

In order to systematize the procedures of i-moment coding we developed the *Innovative Moments Coding System* (IMCS, Gonçalves et al., 2009; Gonçalves et al., in press). The IMCS is a qualitative method of data analysis applicable to studies where the aim is to understand change processes beneath different life situations; for instance, therapeutic and non-therapeutic change, specific life transitions and adaptations to new health situations. In this sense, it is applied to qualitative data, namely discourse or conversation, such as therapeutic sessions, qualitative in-depth interviews or biographies, predominantly through video/audio systems or transcript support. We will further describe the procedures that are applied in such analyses.

After establishing the IMCS, we developed a training program for reliable coding of i-moments. Within this training, coders are first familiarized with the data collection and participants, but are not aware of the hypothesis being studied or the group (good or poor outcome) to which a particular case belongs. After this training, coders can engage in coding research material.

The codification procedure requires analysis by two coders. The first contact with materials (e.g., sessions, interviews transcripts) is reading/visualizing/listening to the data (e.g., one entire therapeutic case) to get familiar with the material under analysis. After this initial procedure, coders must gather and discuss their views on participants' problematic narrative, and the different facets of it (e.g., intrapersonal, interpersonal problems, work, family). After this discussion, the problems should be identified consensually and their definition must be as close as possible to the client's/ interviewee's narrative. This procedure sets the stage for i-moment identification, as they involve every moment when the participant engages in novel or different actions, thoughts or emotions, from the identified problem(s). For instance, the act of *"walking away from the problematic situation"* can be coded as an action i-moment if the problem is intimate abuse, even though an equivalent act can be part of the problem if it is viewed as avoidance behavior involved in an anxiety disorder. Then, 100% of the material is independently coded by the pair of judges, allowing for reliability calculation (percentage of agreement and Cohen's Kappa).

The coding procedure is conducted by reviewing the material in a sequential fashion (session one, two, three and so forth). Each session is analyzed and coders have to identify each i-moment excerpt, categorize it and record its duration (the beginning and the end of each i-moment, to the nearest second).

In sum, i-moments coding involves the analysis of three main indexes:
- *The type of i-moment:* Action, Reflection, Protest, Re-conceptualization and Performing change.
- *The temporal salience of i-moments,* representing the percentage of time occupied by each i-moment in the session. It is computed from the duration of telling the specific i-moment, related to the total duration time of the session. Alternatively, to code transcripts, the temporal salience could be measured by the quantity of text occupied by each i-moment, in reference to the full text (measured in the number of words). In each session an index of

temporal salience is computed for each of the five i-moments, as the percentage of time in which a specific i-moment was narrated in the session. We also computed an index of overall temporal salience of i-moments as the sum of the saliencies' of the five i-moments for each session. The index of each case temporal salience is obtained through a mean score of temporal saliencies of all sessions.

- *Emergence of i-moments*, indicating if an i-moment is brought to the conversation by the therapist/interviewer or the client/interviewed. Basically, there are three possibilities: (1) the i-moment is produced by the therapist (e.g., through a question or commentary), but is accepted and elaborated by the client; (2) the i-moment results from a therapist's question which does not refer clearly the i-moment, facilitating its emergence (e.g., T: What can you learn from this experience?; C: I learned that...[a specific i-moment]); or (3) the i-moment is spontaneously produced by the client, not being triggered by any specific question made by the therapist. This topic should be addressed after the codification of the i-moments.

Thus, the coding process involves four steps: (1) identifying one i-moment, (2) deciding what type it is, (3) marking the beginning and the end of it, and (4) identifying if it was asked directly or indirectly by the therapist, or if it was spontaneously produced by the client.

For reliability purposes the coding requires, as we mentioned before, two trained coders. Interjudge percentage of agreement on overall temporal salience is calculated as the temporal salience of i-moments identified by both judges (agreement) divided by the time identified by either judge (or, equivalently, twice the time spent on agreed i-moments divided by the sum of i-moments times independently identified by the two judges).

After identifying the passages (through temporal salience agreement) where both coders agreed that it corresponded to an i-moment, the reliability for distinguishing i-moment categories is calculated by Cohen's kappa.

Major Findings

Given the fact that the coding of all sessions of a case, second by second, is so arduous we have been working with relatively small samples (e.g., $N = 10$ comparing good and poor outcome cases) or intensively analyzing case studies. To this point we have results from one sample of narrative therapy with victims of partner's abuse (Matos et al., 2009) and another one of major depression treated with emotion-focused therapy (Mendes, Gonçalves, Ribeiro, Angus, & Greenberg, 2008) from the York I Depression Study (Greenberg & Watson, 1998)[3]. Besides these two main samples we have been conducting several intensive case-studies, which allow us to investigate change processes at a more microanalytic level. Summarizing the most important data from these two samples, several findings are particularly interesting and will be targeted in the models presented below.

Good outcome cases are clearly different from poor outcome cases, as can be seen in Figures 1, 2 and 3. All these figures show the average of i-moments in each case, the first two from the sample of narrative therapy and the third one from the emotion-focused therapy sample. These findings are also congruent with the case-studies we have done to this point.

---

[3] We are grateful to Lynne Angus and Leslie Greenberg for allowing us to work with their sample from EFT.

FIGURE 1. GOOD OUTCOME CASES IN NARRATIVE THERAPY

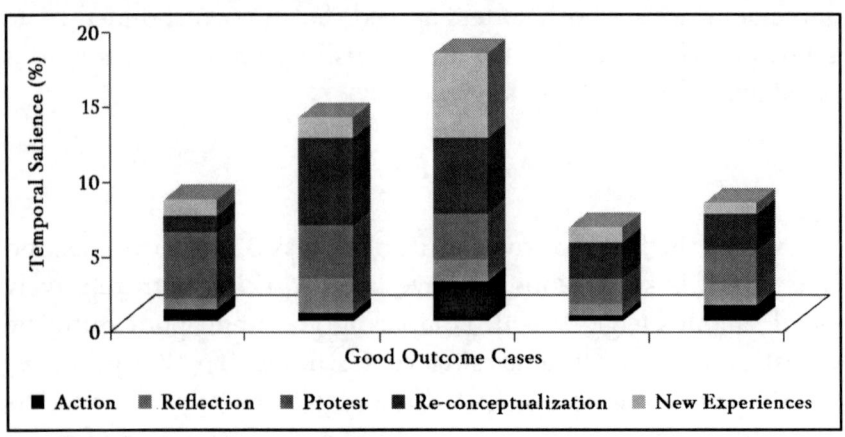

FIGURE 2. POOR OUTCOME CASES IN NARRATIVE THERAPY

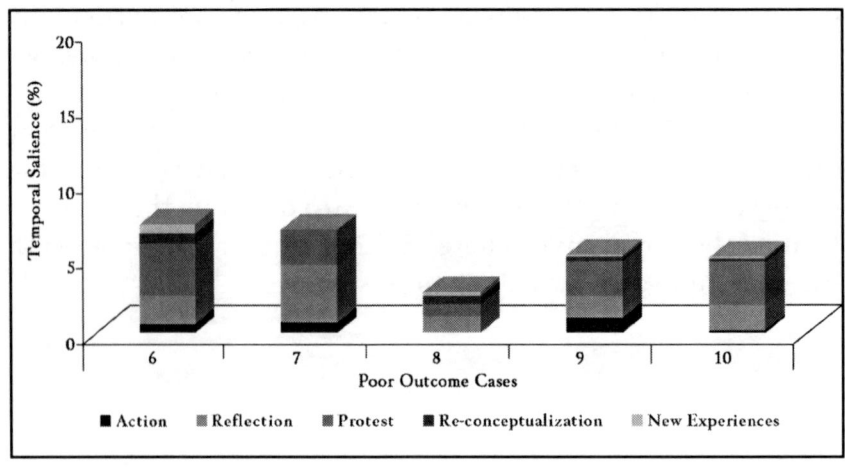

Figure 3. Good and poor outcome cases in EFT

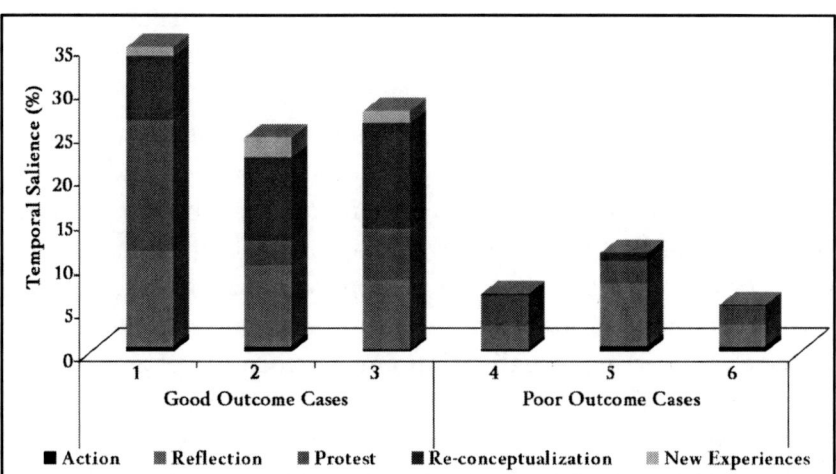

An initial examination of these figures shows that the temporal salience of i-moments is significantly higher in good outcome cases, but curiously i-moments occurred also in poor outcome cases. This means that level 2 changes occur in psychotherapy even when the outcome is poor. We will discuss below what processes may be involved in preventing the development of a level 3 change.

A closer look makes it clear that in narrative therapy re-conceptualization and performing change are almost absent in the poor outcome sample. Something similar, although not so clear in the case of performing change, also occurs in the emotion-focused sample. Clearly, re-conceptualization is very infrequent in or absent from the poor outcome sample in both therapeutic models.

In order to have a more process-oriented view of the development of i-moments throughout therapy, Figures 4 and 5 show the evolution session by session of one good and one poor outcome case from the first sample.

There is a tendency of i-moments to increase throughout the psychotherapy process in good outcome cases, appearing as a high diversity of types of i-moments almost from the beginning.

For instance in session 2 there is already action, reflection and protest i-moments; and after session 4 all i-moments are present, continuing to occur until the end of therapy (Santos, Gonçalves, Matos, & Salvatore, 2009).

In poor outcome cases the diversity of i-moments is usually much reduced. Along the therapy one can see action and protest, or protest and reflection; but there are hardly any sessions in which the five types occur. Thus, most of the times two or three types of i-moments appear in poor outcome cases (with a clear prominence for action, reflection and protest). Also, as we said before re-conceptualization and performing change have a reduced presence, if they are not absent entirely (Matos et al., 2009). Re-conceptualization i-moments usually emerge in the middle of the psychotherapy process and increase until the end. The majority of performing change i-moments occur after the development of re-conceptualization.

FIGURE 4. A GOOD OUTCOME CASE IN NARRATIVE THERAPY (11 SESSIONS PLUS FOLLOW-UP)

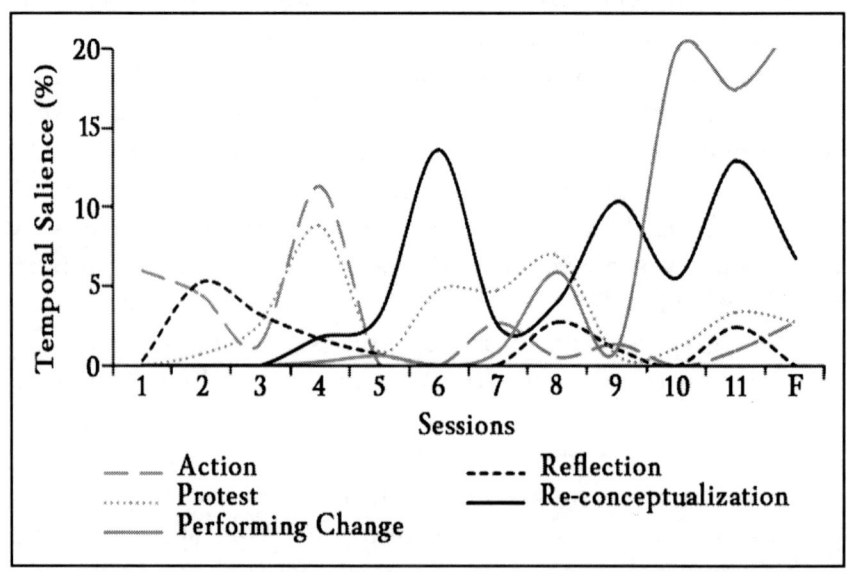

FIGURE 5. A POOR OUTCOME CASE IN NARRATIVE THERAPY
(15 SESSIONS PLUS FOLLOW-UP)

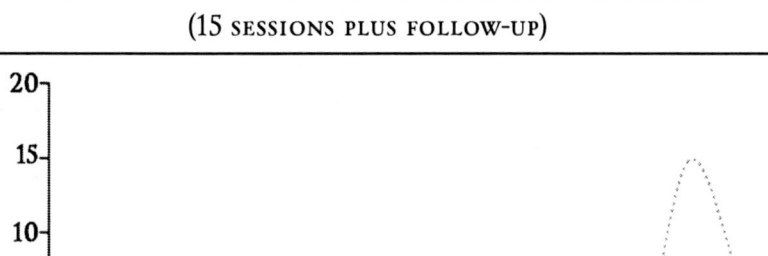

So, let us briefly summarize what we have found in the two samples presented here, which are also congruent with several intensive case studies (e.g., Gonçalves, Mendes, Ribeiro, Angus, & Greenberg, 2008; Ribeiro, Gonçalves, & Ribeiro, 2008).

The global picture of good-outcome cases is characterized by a progressive tendency toward the generation of i-moments from the beginning to the end of therapy; action, reflection and protest being more salient at the beginning than at the end. Re-conceptualization emerges in the middle phase of therapy and increases until the end, seeming to be an important marker of successful psychotherapy. Performing change tend to appear after re-conceptualization, representing a performance of the change process.

The global picture of poor-outcome cases is characterized by a lower temporal salience of i-moments, taking the form of action, protest and reflection without a clear increasing tendency. Re-conceptualization and performing change are absent or have a very low temporal salience.

An interesting communality between good and poor outcome cases, despite all the differences found, is the presence of i-moments from session 1 onward. This reinforces the idea that level 2 changes take place even when people are dominated by problematic narratives, and that potential openings to new narratives are present, even if they are later on dismissed, ignored or trivialized.

Curiously we have also results from a project that studied "spontaneous" change that reproduces these results. In an exploratory study (Cruz & Gonçalves, 2008) we asked the participants ($N = 27$) to identify three types of difficulties in their lives: past (and solved), present (at the moment of the interview) and persistent (present for more than 6 months). The interviews were coded for the presence of i-moments with the IMCS (Gonçalves et al., 2009; Gonçalves, et al., in press) and significant differences were found between solved and non-solved difficulties in re-conceptualization i-moments. This kind of i-moment was the only one that significantly differentiated solved from present difficulties. A similar study, but with a longitudinal design, replicated these findings concerning re-conceptualization (Meira, Gonçalves, Salgado, & Cunha, 2008).

The results presented here suggest that re-conceptualization seems to be a critical ingredient in the process of sustaining change. In the next section we will discuss not only a model of change based on these results, but also a model that explains the persistence of problematic narratives.

A Heuristic Model of Therapeutic Change

From the results briefly presented we have suggested a general model of narrative change (Gonçalves et al., 2008; Gonçalves et al., 2009; Matos et al., 2009), in which i-moments have a pivotal role.

Of course we know that there are several ways to abort this emergence of novelty. The person can implicitly or explicitly refuse the meaningful nature of these events, as it happens frequently in clinical practice. The novelty can be turned into something similar to the old narrative. Cognitive therapists have described this process as a cognitive distortion (e.g., Beck, Rush, Shaw, & Emery, 1979) and constructivist theorists (e.g., Mahoney, 1991) have referred to this process as a form of protecting and maintaining the core-ordering processes within the person. We argue that this process is fed by several forms of narrative invalidation, in which the power of the problematic narrative is so strong that even what appears as novelties and exceptions to the rule are transformed accordingly to the problematic narrative. We will return to these forms of invalidation later in this chapter. Sometimes, even if the person is validating to him or herself the change that is taking place, significant others can have a powerful impact in deflecting the novelties, making them non-meaningful (e.g., "you're better because of your medication"), false (e.g., "in reality you're doing/thinking X (a novelty), but what you mean is Y (problematic narrative)"), or trivial (e.g., "you're doing/thinking differently, but later you'll do/think as usual"). Our life-narratives, as White (2007) recently emphasized, and as a long tradition of systemic thinking reinforces (e.g., Minuchin, 1974/1999; Watzlawick, Bavelas, & Jackson, 1967), have to be validated by significant others. Sometimes the others in our lives don't really believe that we can change and this can be a very strong obstacle to attain that goal, becoming in this way a self-fulfilling prophecy (Watzlawick, Bavelas, & Jackson, 1967). Thus, our claim is that these novelties, to be sustained, need to be intrapersonally and interpersonally validated, meaning that self and significant others need to conceptualize somehow these novelties as personal changes, and not as the same story.

From our view action and reflection i-moments are the more elementary forms of innovation. As people start to act differently and think differently about the problematic narrative these i-moments can be signs to the self and others that something different from the "old story" is taking place. Cycles of action and reflection (or the other way around from reflection to action) may be needed to assure the person and to others that something really different from the problematic narrative is occurring.

Curiously, in the cases studied so far, most of the times reflection has a stronger temporal salience than action. We do not know at this stage if the opposite scenario (action higher than reflection) is common. In any case, it seems that even if the beginning of the change process occurs with action i-moments, the reflection of the client about them, spontaneously produced or triggered by therapist questions, allows the elaboration of these action i-moments in the landscape of consciousness (triggering more reflection i-moments). The future study of cases with a theoretical orientation that favors action rather than meaning (e.g., early stages of cognitive-behavioral therapies) could be an interesting way to empirically address this issue.

In some cases several cycles of action-reflection i-moments occur before protest i-moments surface, whereas at other times protest appears from the beginning of therapy (see Gonçalves et al., 2008). We consider that protest i-moments are very important since they represent a strong attitudinal movement against the problematic narrative. They can occur as forms of action or as reflection, but they are more proactive, given the meaning implied in them, as the person strongly refuses the problematic narrative.

We have identified two different types of protest i-moments with two apparently different functions in the change process. Protest can address the problematic narrative and the people who support them (e.g., "my husband is responsible for his actions, he should not blame me all the time") or protest can be directed to changes in the self (e.g., "I want to be loved, I need that"). It is our hypothesis that the first form of protest may be needed at the beginning, but if the person is not able to center in the self later on, protest becomes a mere opposition to the problematic narrative. The transition to protest centered on the self is a way to assert the needs that the person is feeling, and from here a new position can emerge, different from the mere opposition towards the problem. We found that this second kind of protest (centered on the self) is sometimes deeply associated with the emergence of re-conceptualization (Gonçalves et al., 2008; Santos et al., 2009).

In fact, we suspect that a new narrative of the self may be not sustained only by these three kinds of i-moments (action, reflection and protest) and perhaps one of the reasons is that they can be a mere opposition to the problem, which means that they can operate inside the same constructs that are responsible for the problematic narrative (more about this latter). That way the problem is present even in its absence, given that the client operates inside a dichotomy between the problem and its negation (e.g., "I'm depressed ... I want to be happy"). Perhaps this is an important reason that makes re-conceptualization vital in the process of change: its ability to integrate old and new, the former problematic narrative and the emergent one. In fact, when coding re-conceptualization one needs to have some description of the process of change, and also the contrast between past and present self. Thus, re-conceptualization must be more than some form of negation of the problem, as it has to have new dimensions outside the dichotomy of "problem / negation of the problem." We will return to this topic later when discussing the stability of the problematic narrative.

Another important reason for the inability of action, reflection and protest to produce stable narrative change is that they are most of the times episodic and unstructured, and hence, unable to create a structure that can organize the diversity of innovations. Re-conceptualization, emerging in the middle stage of successful psychotherapy, is in our view responsible precisely for this organization. Given its narrative structure it can give coherence to what otherwise would be disperse occurrences of novelties. That way, re-conceptualization acts like a gravitational narrative field, attracting and giving purpose and meaning to other i-moments.

Finally, with re-conceptualization i-moments the client posits herself or himself as the author of the change process. The client is not only an actor, but given his/her access to the way the plot is changing he or she is authoring it (to use a distinction from Sarbin, 1986).

After some elaboration of re-conceptualization i-moments, new cycles of novelty exploration occur again in the form of action, reflection and protest; this time, consolidating and being consolidated by re-conceptualization i-moments. Several cycles may be needed to sustain change. Finally, performing change i-moments expand the change process into the future since, as several authors suggested (Crites, 1986; Omer & Alon, 1997; Slusky, 1998), good new stories have to have a future.

Figure 6 shows the process of change that we have just described.

FIGURE 6. MODEL OF I-MOMENT CHANGE IN PSYCHOTHERAPY

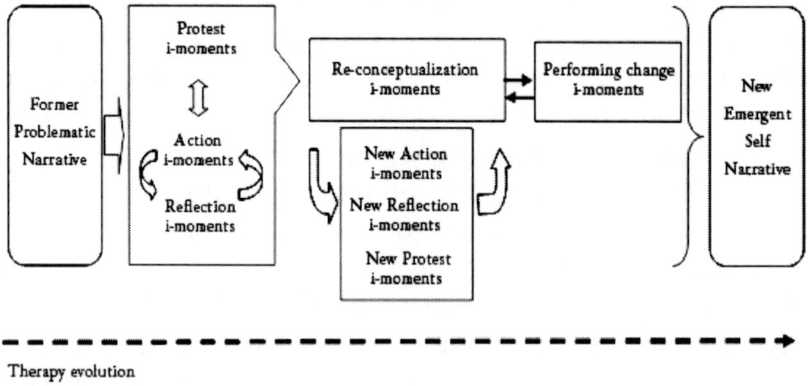

Therapy evolution

We have previously suggested (Gonçalves et al., 2008; Gonçalves et al., 2009; Santos et al., 2009) that several other models of change can help us make sense of the role that re-conceptualization plays in the change process. For instance, re-conceptualization has some overlap with the concept of insight (Castonguay & Hill, 2007), which has a central role in change according to a diversity of therapeutic models. However, we argue that insight is related not only to re-conceptualization, but also to reflection and protest as these are defined in our model. Thus, it is interesting that reflection and protest as possible forms of insight do not discriminate good from poor outcome cases, while re-conceptualization does so.

The model of assimilation of voices proposed by Stiles can also highlight the role of re-conceptualization in therapeutic change. For Stiles and colleagues (Honos-Webb & Stiles, 1998; Stiles, 1999; Stiles et al., 1990; Stiles, Meshot, Anderson, & Sloan, 1992) the self can be conceptualized as a community of voices that represent former experiences of the person. Each experience leaves an active trait in the form of a voice. Most of the times these voices are resources for dealing with new experiences, but other times painful experiences make some voices difficult to accept by the community (that is, the self). Stiles and his team have been studying the assimilation of problematic experiences with this model and have developed a coding process to identify the status of the problematic voices in reference to the other voices of the self—the assimilation of problematic experiences scale (APES). The APES (see Honos-Webb & Stiles, 1998; Osatuke & Stiles, 2006) identifies voices from the level 0 (warded off dissociated), in which the person is unaware of the problem and the problematic voice is dissociated; to level 7 (integration–mastery), in which the client generalizes solutions to new problems and the previous poorly integrated experience so that the voice is now part of the community of voices. The intermediate level (4) seems very important and marks the level that is not attained in poor outcome cases (Detert et al., 2006). This level is precisely the one in which understanding and insight is possible. Although we have no empirical data confirming this, we can speculate that re-conceptualization operates at level 4 or higher in the APES scale. Empirical studies that use both the APES and the IMCS with the same cases can clarify this issue in the future.

From a different perspective, the therapeutic cycles mode from Mergenthaler (see Lepper & Mergenthaler, 2007;

Mergenthaler, 1996) proposes that change takes place in cycles of reflection (abstraction) and emotional processing (emotional tone). According to this model of change, the following pattern of four stages can be identified: *relaxing* (low abstraction and low emotional tone), *experiencing* (high emotional tone and low abstraction), *connecting* (high abstraction, high emotional tone), *reflecting* (high abstraction, low emotional tone). Each four stage cycle gives place to another cycle, starting again with relaxing, and so on. In the i-moments system, we do not explicitly track emotional experience, although it is likely that what we call re-conceptualization may fall under connecting and reflecting modes. So what we suggested about the cross-fertilization between the IMCS and the APES may be applicable to the study of the IMCS with the therapeutic cycles model.

Finally, the narrative research from Angus and her team (Angus, Lewin, Bouffard, & Rotondi-Trevisan, 2004) also has some important connections with our program. Angus and colleagues have identified three different narrative modes: external, internal and reflexive. This model conceptualizes change "as entailing a process of dialectical shifts between narrative story-telling (external narrative mode), emotional differentiation (internal narrative mode), and reflexive meaning-making modes of inquiry" (Angus et al., 2004, p. 88). However, the narrative process model is very different from our IMCS, as the latter is a system of tracking novelties in the process of change. So, while the model proposed by Angus and colleagues addresses the way narratives are elaborated and assimilated in psychotherapy by integrating external, internal and reflective dimensions, the IMCS focuses on the way novelties emerge and are elaborated in psychotherapy.

From our perspective, and assuming as a solid result that re-conceptualization clearly discriminates good from poor outcome cases, an interesting question arises: what blocks the development of re-conceptualization in poor outcome cases? Or in other words, what prevents level 3 change after some level 2 changes have occurred? We will address this topic in the next section.

A Heuristic Model for Therapeutic Stability

We suggest that one important way of impeding re-conceptualization is the process of mutual in-feeding (Valsiner, 2002). Valsiner described this as an ambivalent process in which two opposite voices (e.g., "life is good", "life is bad") feed each other, thus stabilizing the dialogical self from further change. Take the following hypothetical example, in which voice A is "I'm sad" and voice B is "I want to be happy." According to IMCS voice A could be the problematic voice and voice B would be an i-moment (in this case a reflective one). Imagine that we have the sequence of voices depicted in Figure 7.

In this example, we have two opposite voices that feed each other virtually *ad eternum.* Actually, this is an extreme example of mutual in-feeding, because the two voices, as time goes by, are becoming more polarized, a process that Valsiner (2002) terms escalating of voices. The most interesting thing in this example is that what maintains stability is a dynamic process in the relationship between the initial voices.

FIGURE 7. DYNAMIC STABILITY BETWEEN TWO OPPOSITE VOICES THROUGH MUTUAL IN-FEEDING

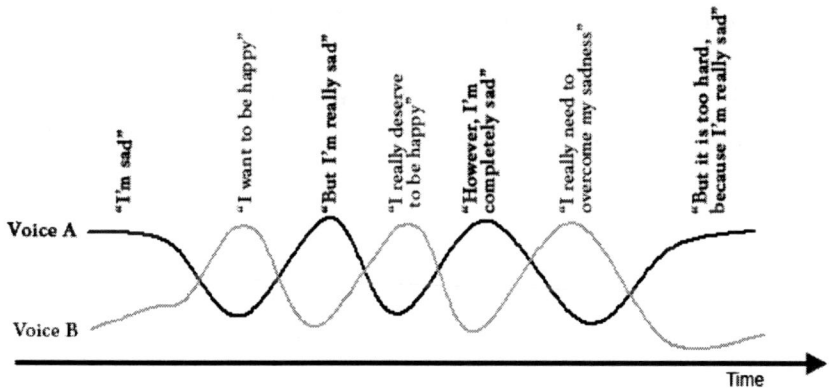

From the perspective of IMCS the problematic narrative and the emergence of action, reflection and protest i-moments can be related in a way that they feed into each other, resulting in a stable feedback loop, similar to the one depicted in Figure 8. We suggested that this can only happen in these i-moments and not in re-conceptualization i-moments, because in this last one the contradiction between the problem and innovation is already dialectically integrated inside the i-moment (past and present self). The other i-moments can be a mere opposition of the problem, facilitating in this way the return to it.

New experiences, by their nature (generalization of the change process into several life domains) can hardly be involved in mutual in-feeding. Also, they tend to occur later in the process of change and, in principle, mutual in-feeding in good outcome cases should occur more at early stages of therapy.

When mutual in-feeding occurs in action, reflection and protest i-moments they temporally free the person from the problem, but facilitate the return to it, given that the negation of the problem makes it present even when it is absent. If I want to be happy, and this is the contrary of feeling depressed, then if I can't be happy as I dreamt, this means that I'm really miserable! Clinically this process is also clear in the counter-phobic reactions of fearful clients: dreaming about freeing themselves from fear makes them be "courageous" to a point that they get paralyzed by fear again. Thus, novelties are created but soon are bypassed given the return to the problematic narrative.

The process of mutual in-feeding can be conceptualized from other theoretical perspectives. For instance, from a personal construct perspective the same process can be described as the dance between two poles of the same construct, which Kelly (1955) called "slot rattling." In strategic therapy this is akin to what was termed an "ironic process" (Shoham & Rohrbaugh, 2002), in which the more the person tries to get free from the problem the more the problem stays strong (Watzlawick, Weakland, & Fisch, 1974). Or in Stiles' model of assimilation (Brinegar, Salvi,

Stiles, & Greenberg, 2006) these exchanges between voices can be theorized as a process of "rapid crossfire," in which the person oscillates between two contradictory voices. Gustafson (1992; see also Omer, 1994) refers to a similar process: "these [dominant] stories seem inescapable because what is viewed as the only alternative (the *shadow* story) turns out to be a loop that reintroduces the main line" (Omer, 1994, p. 47).

Whatever the theoretical perspective from which one conceptualizes this phenomenon, from a dialogical framework this is a dynamic process responsible for a monological, closed outcome (see Gonçalves & Guilfoyle, 2006). Figure 8 illustrates this process of mutual in-feeding. Thus, it is our hypothesis that re-conceptualization leads to the overcoming of the mutual in-feeding process, by integrating the two conflicting positions.

FIGURE 8. MUTUAL IN-FEEDING IN PSYCHOTHERAPY

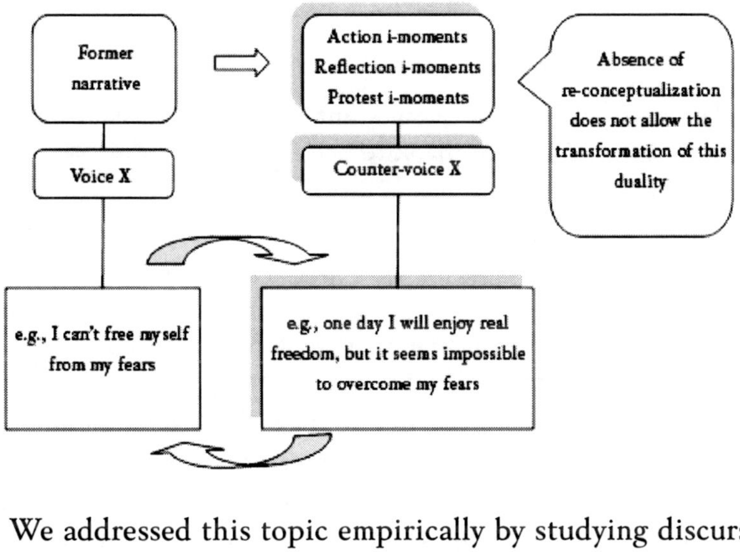

We addressed this topic empirically by studying discursive markers of return to the problem, after the emergence of an i-moment. The results that we present below were obtained in the sample previously described of narrative therapy with women victims of partner abuse. However we currently have only preliminary results from 6 cases: 3 good outcome and 3 poor outcome cases. The way we operationally defined the theoretical concept of mutual in-feeding was by identifying all the times an i-moment emerged and was immediately followed by a return to the problem. Let us illustrate this with two examples from our sample (poor outcome cases):

> *First Session*
>
> *Therapist*: You said that "in part" you have a voice that says you don't have to make any effort because you would never get anywhere. But is there another voice?
> *Client*: Yes, there's other part that seems that I can do everything! *(Reflection i-moment)* But suddenly, it falls down! Like a house of cards that we build and then suddenly falls! *(Return to the problematic narrative)*

> *Fourth Session*
>
> *Therapist*: What do you want to do to this "wave" *(Externalized label for depressive symptoms)*? Today you've defied it ...
> *Client*: End with it completely, *(Protest i-moment)* but it seems very difficult to me... *(Return to the problematic narrative)*
> *Therapist*: End with it...! You´re ambitious!

In these examples the client describes the i-moment but immediately returns to the problematic narrative. Thus, these markers appear immediately after the i-moment or during its description. It is clear that the use of linguistic connectors (e.g., but, however, but still, it's just that) represents opposition or denial of what has just been asserted.

In terms of procedures the coding of the return to the problem markers was made by two independent judges, unaware of the status of the case (poor or good outcome). For each session the judges coded the presence or absence of the return to the problem for each i-moment previously identified in the former research (Cohen's Kappa was .85). Over 20% of i-moments in poor outcome cases had markers of returning to the problem, whereas these markers occurred in only about 2% of good outcome cases.

If we now take a closer look at what type of i-moments had returned to the problem markers, it is clear that this only occurred in action, reflection and protest—as we have predicted. Another question is, of course, what is the possible causality between return to the problem markers and re-conceptualization i-moments. If the data obtained with this sample is replicated, it seems that the return to the problem (or mutual in-feeding) impedes the emergence of re-conceptualization, given the low occurrence of this dance between the problem and the innovations in good outcome cases[4]. However, if we take into account intensive case-studies perhaps one could hypothesize that re-conceptualization may also prevent the return to the problem. Figure 9 below shows an evolution along twelve sessions of a constructivist therapy process. In the figure we have represented the evolution of i-moments with and without return to the problem markers. In this case, curiously, the amount of presence and absence of these markers is almost the same until session five, after which the tendency is clearly different: the presence of the problem marker clearly diminishes, while i-moments without the markers clearly increase. Interestingly, it was precisely at session six that re-conceptualization emerges, which suggests some relationship in this case between these two processes.

---

[4] Of course, we don't know at this moment if other processes prevent both the resolution of mutual in-feeding and the emergence of re-conceptualization.

Figure 9. Return to problem markers in one good-outcome case of constructivist therapy

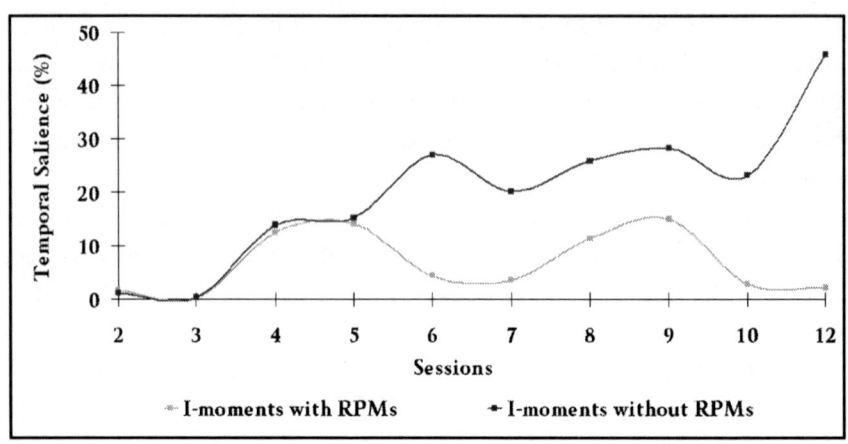

Of course, it is not possible at this time to infer any causal relationships between mutual in-feeding and re-conceptualization, but from these data it is clear that the return to the problem plays an important role in poor-outcome psychotherapy. Also, the absence of these indicators in re-conceptualization reinforces the idea that these i-moments may be pivotal in the process of change.

Some Implications for Practice

In our view it is too early to infer from our research program clear implications for psychotherapeutic practice. We need to study these processes in other samples and expand the research with more intensive cases studies. However, the results found until now suggest that i-moments can be a relevant strategy to track and analyze the therapeutic change.

Also, it is clear through the heterogeneous nature of i-moments that some can be more "potent" than others in the promotion of level 3 change. Therapists can dedicate some effort in the middle of therapeutic process to the elaboration and expansion of i-moments, mainly in the form of re-conceptualization. Of course, the other types, according to our model, may be needed to achieve re-conceptualization.

It also may be important in therapy to elaborate novelties outside the dichotomy problem–opposition to the problem. In this context the attention of therapists can be focused in the processes of mutual in-feeding and conversational strategies to bypass it. Of course, we need to contrast poor and good outcome cases in what concerns mutual in-feeding to learn what conversational strategies prevent or facilitate getting out of this process. In this sense, we are starting to explore if there is a link between specific therapist response modes and client response modes preceding or associated with the appearance of i-moments in different kinds of therapeutic modalities. This might indicate some "preferred" client-therapist conversational interactions that are more associated with the amplification of i-moments into a new self-narrative.

REFERENCES

Angus, L. E., Lewin, J., Bouffard, B., & Rotondi-Trevisan, D. (2004). "What's the story?" Working with narratives in experiential psychotherapy. In L. E. Angus & J. McLeod (Eds.), *The handbook of narrative psychotherapy: Practice, theory and research* (pp. 87-102). London: Sage

Bateson, G. (1979). *Natureza e espírito.* [*Mind and nature: A necessary unity*]. Lisboa: D. Quixote.

Batista, J. (2008). *As Novidades da mudança em diferentes contexto terapêuticos* [The movelites of change in different therapeutic contexts]. Unpublished master's thesis, Universidad de Trás-os-Montes e Alto Douro, Vila Real, Portugal.

Beck, A. T., Rush, A. J., Shaw, B. F., & Emery, G. (1979). *Cognitive therapy of depression.* New York: Guilford.

Brinegar, M. G., Salvi, L. M., Stiles, W. B., & Greenberg, L. S. (2006). Building a meaning bridge: Therapeutic progress from problem formulation to understanding. *Journal of Counseling Psychology, 53,* 165-180.

Bruner, J. (1986). *Actual minds, possible worlds.* Cambridge, MA: Harvard University Press.

Castonguay, L. G., & Hill, C. E. (Eds.) (2007). *Insight in psychotherapy.* Washington, DC: American Psychological Association.

Crites, F. (1986). Story time: Recollecting the past and projecting the future. In Sarbin, T. R. (Ed.), *Narrative psychology: The storied nature of conduct* (pp. 152-173). New York: Praeger.

Cruz, G., & Gonçalves, M. M. (2008). *Mudança espontânea e momentos de inovação: Um estudo exploratório [Spontaneous change and innovative moments:A exploratory study]*. Manuscript in preparation.

Detert, N. B., Llewellyn, S., Hardy, G. E., Barkham, M., & Stiles, W. B. (2006). Assimilation in good and poor-outcome cases of very brief psychotherapy for mild depression: An initial comparison. *Psychotherapy Research, 16*, 393–407.

Fogel, A., Garvey, A., Hsu, H. C., & West-Stroming, D. (2006). *Change processes in relationships: A relational-historical approach*. New York: Cambridge University Press.

Gonçalves, M. M., & Guilfoyle, M. (2006). Therapy as a monological activity: Beliefs from therapists and their clients. *Journal of Constructivist Psychology, 19*, 251-271.

Gonçalves, M. M., Matos, M., & Santos, A. (2008). *Innovative Moments Coding System – Version 7.2*. Unpublished manuscript. University of Minho at Braga.

Gonçalves, M.M., Matos, M., & Santos, A. (2009). Narrative therapy and the nature of "innovative moments" in the construction of change. *Journal of Constructivist Psychology, 22*, 1–23.

Gonçalves, M. M., Mendes, I., Ribeiro, A., Angus, L., & Greenberg, L. (2008). *Innovative moments and change in emotional focused therapy: The case of Lisa*. Manuscript submitted for publication.

Gonçalves, M. M., Ribeiro, A., Matos, M., Santos, A., & Mendes, I. (in press). The Innovative Moments Coding System: A new coding procedure for tracking changes in psychotherapy. In S. Salvatore, J. Valsiner, S. Strout, & J. Clegg (Eds.), *YIS: Yearbook of Idiographic Science 2009 - Volume 2*. Rome: Firera Publishing Group.

Greenberg, L. S., & Watson, J. (1998). Experiential therapy of depression: Differential effects of client–centered relationship conditions and process interventions. *Psychotherapy Research, 8*, 210–224.

Gustafson, J. P. (1992). *Self-delight in a harsh world*. New York: Norton.

Hermans, H. J. M., & Dimaggio, G. (Eds.) (2004). *The dialogical self in psychotherapy*. New York: Brunneer-Routledge.

Hermans, H. J. M. (1996). Voicing the self: From information processing to dialogical interchange. *Psychological Bulletin, 119*, 31-50.

Honos-Webb, L., & Stiles, W. B. (1998). Reformulation of assimilation analysis in terms of voices. *Psychotherapy Research, 35*, 23–33.

Kelly, G. (1955). *The psychology of personal constructs*. (2 vols.). New York: Norton.

Lepper, G., & Mergenthaler, E. (2007). Therapeutic collaboration: How does it work? *Psychotherapy Research, 17*, 576-587.

Mahoney, M. (1991). *Human change processes: The scientific foundations of psychotherapy*. New York: Basic Books

Matos, M., & Gonçalves, M. M. (2004). Narratives on marital violence: The construction of change through re-authoring. In R. Abrunhosa, R. Roesch, C. Machado, C. Soeiro, & F. Winkel (Eds.), *Assessment, intervention and legal issues with offenders and victims* (pp. 137-154). Bruxelas: Politea.

Matos, M., Santos, A., Gonçalves, M. M., & Martins, C. (2009). Innovative moments and change in narrative therapy. *Psychotherapy Research, 19,* 68-80.

McAdams, D. P. (1993). *The stories we live by: Personal myths and the making of the self.* New York: William Morrow.

Meira, L., Gonçalves, M. M., Salgado, J., & Cunha, C. (2008, July). *Everyday life change: Contribution to the understanding of daily human change.* Paper presented and submitted for publication at the Proceedings of the 2nd International Conference on Psychology, Athens, Greece.

Mendes, I., Gonçalves, M. M., Ribeiro, A.P., Angus, L., & Greenberg, L. (2008). *Narrative change and innovative patterns in emotion-focused therapy.* Manuscript in preparation.

Mergenthaler, E. (1996). Emotion-abstraction patterns: A new way of describing psychotherapeutic process. *Journal of Consulting and Clinical Psychology, 64,* 1306–1315.

Minuchin, S. (1999). *Families and family therapy* (28th ed.). Cambridge, Massachusetts: Harvard University Press. (Originally work published 1974)

Neimeyer, R.A. (2000). Narrative disruptions in the construction of the self. In R. A. Neimeyer & J. D. Raskin (Eds.), *Constructions of disorder: Meaning-making frameworks for psychotherapy* (pp. 207-242). Washington: American Psychological Association.

Omer, H., & Alon, N. (1997). *Constructing therapeutic narratives.* Northvale, N. J.: Jason Aronson.

Omer, H. (1994). *Critical interventions in psychotherapy: From impasse to turning point.* New York: Norton.

Osatuke, K., & Stiles, W. B. (2006). Problematic internal voices in clients with borderline features: an elaboration of the assimilation model. *Journal of Constructivist Psychology, 19,* 287-319.

Polkinghorne, D. E. (1988). *Narrative knowing and the human sciences.* Albany: State University of New York Press.

Ribeiro, A. P., Gonçalves, M. M., & Ribeiro, E. (2009). Processos narrativos de mudança em psicoterapia: Estudo de um caso de sucesso de terapia construtivista [Narrative processes of change in psychotherapy: A good-outcome case of constructivist therapy]. *Psychologica, 50,* 181-203.

Salgado, J., & Gonçalves, M. (2007). The dialogical self: Social, personal and (un)conscious. In A. Rosa & J. Valsiner (Eds.), *The Cambridge handbook of socio-cultural psychology* (608-621). Cambridge, UK: Cambridge University Press.

Santos, A., Gonçalves, M. M., Matos, M., & Salvatore, S. (2009). Innovative moments and change pathways in a good-outcome case of narrative therapy. *Psychology and Psychotherapy: Theory, Research and Practice, 82,* 449-466.

Sarbin, T. R. (1986). The narrative and the root metaphor for psychology. In T. R. Sarbin (Ed.), *Narrative psychology: The storied nature of human conduct* (pp. 3-21). New York: Praeger.

Shoham, V., & Rohrbaugh, M. J. (2002). Brief strategic couple therapy. In A. S. Gurman & N. S. Jacobson (Eds), *Clinical handbook of couple therapy* (pp. 5-25) (3rd Ed.). New York: Guilford.

Slusky, C. E. (1998). Strange attractors and the transformation of narratives in family therapy. In M. F. Hoyt (Ed.), *The handbook of constructive therapies: Innovative approaches from leading practitioners* (pp. 159-179). San Francisco: Jossey-Bass.

Stiles, W. B. (1999). Signs and voices in psychotherapy. *Psychotherapy Research, 9,* 1-21.

Stiles, W. B., Elliot, R., Llewellyn, S. P., Firth-Cozens, J. A., Margison, F. R., Shapiro, D. A., & Hardy, G. (1990). Assimilation of problematic experiences by clients in psychotherapy. *Psychotherapy, 27,* 411-420.

Stiles, W. B., Meshot, C. M., Anderson, T. M., & Sloan, W., W., Jr., (1992). Assimilation of problematic experiences: The case of John Jones. *Psychotherapy Research, 2,* 81-101.

Valsiner, J. (2002). Forms of dialogical relations and semiotic autoregulation within the self. *Theory & Psychology, 12,* 2, 251-265.

Watzlawick, P., Bavelas, J. B., & Jackson, D. (1967). *Pragmatics of human communication: A study of interactional patterns, pathologies, and paradoxes.* New York: Norton.

Watzlawick, P., Weakland, J. & Fisch, R. (1974). *Change: Principles of problem formation and problem resolution.* New York: Norton.

White, M., & Epston, D. (1990). *Narrative means to therapeutic ends.* New York: Norton.

White, M. (2007). *Maps of narrative practice.* New York: Norton.

Wortham, S. (2001). *Narratives in action: A strategy for research and analysis.* New York: Teachers College Press.

ॐ 4 ॐ

Reconstructing the Continuing Bond: A Constructivist Approach to Grief Therapy

Robert A. Neimeyer

Kristen and Max texted each other on Friday afternoon, January 2nd, an everyday exchange about music and the boredom of a long drive through Oklahoma. Fifteen minutes after those texts, the Ford Explorer carrying Max, 19, and two of his college companions flipped three times and caught on fire along Interstate 35 near the Kansas border. Max was sitting in the back seat. A police report said he was not wearing a seatbelt, and was thrown from the car. The following morning a compassionate doctor at a hospital in Wichita confided in his distraught mother, Gayle, that Max's injury was "not a survivable event." He died in her arms and in the presence of attentive family and caregivers that afternoon.

This is what can be gleaned from newspaper accounts of the tragic accident that took Max's life. What the news failed to cover was his mother's private story that she is sharing with me in therapy some four months after his death, as she alternately attempts to integrate the trauma and quest for transcendence following the loss of her child.

A deeply spiritual person, Gayle quickly came to understand Max's early death as part of a larger spiritual journey of an "old soul," wise beyond his years, ready for release from this temporal world. But she also described "the urgency with which she sought deeper meaning and connection with Max," leading her at times to plead with God to show her a tangible sign, perhaps through an encounter with an angel, with Max, or even Jesus himself, of her son's continued existence and accessibility.

However, it is when she is least anguished that she most experiences this contact, as when she journals in a deep meditative state with her son, posing questions to him, and waiting patiently for the answer. In a recent entry that began with *"Hey, Max,"* and *"What's up, Mom?"* Gayle found herself asking, *"What work are we going to do together?"* As a bereaved parent, she feels a growing urge to invoke the story of her son's life and death to orient others with similar losses to the existential questions they raise, without suggesting easy answers. *"I know how to touch people's hearts,"* she confessed to him, *"but not how to tell this story."*

Max's reply came with clarity, and sent a shiver up my spine as I listened to her relate it: *"Your work with Bob is where the story is formulating."*

Although Gayle is still formulating that story and exploring its deeply emotional implications and most profound meanings, she senses that she "will find some lesson that can be imparted, to convey a deeper understanding of life." She is unsure at this point exactly what these lessons will be, but knows they will have to do with the conviction that "there is no death, that love lives on, and that there is no separation."

....

Journeys like Gayle's that begin in deep mourning and reach uncertainly toward equally deep meaning are only awkwardly accommodated by popular theories of grief that view it in terms of definable stages, diagnosable symptoms, or disruptive separation from the ones we love (Neimeyer, 2002). Granted, each of these perspectives offers a partial window on the experience of loss, which does indeed have its phasic aspects (Bowlby,

1980), its potentially life-vitiating complications (Prigerson & Maciejewski, 2006), and its threat to a basic sense of attachment security and relatedness (Field, Gao, & Paderna, 2005). But these approaches also draw attention away from the dialectical process of delving into the most painfully invalidating features of the loss narrative, and seeking a more coherent framework for grasping their ramifications for our ongoing lives. It is precisely this movement from symptoms to significance that a constructivist orientation to bereavement takes as its central concern, and it is the theoretical, empirical and especially the therapeutic implications of this stance that I will explore in the present chapter.

THE THEORETICAL STANCE

A constructivist theory of bereavement posits that grieving entails an active effort to reaffirm or reconstruct a world of meaning that has been challenged by loss (Neimeyer, 2001, 2006a). In this perspective, people are viewed as meaning-makers, drawing on personal and cultural resources to construct a system of beliefs that permit them to anticipate, and respond to, the essential themes and events of their lives (Kelly, 1955/1991). Across time, this "effort after meaning" confers a sense of identity and intelligibility, giving rise to a *self-narrative* that integrates the "micro-narratives" of daily life into a "macro-narrative" regarding life's purpose and direction (Neimeyer, 2006a, p. 230). The death of a loved one, however, can challenge this framework, sometimes calling into question the most basic premises that anchor one's "assumptive world" (Janoff-Bulman & Berger, 2000), necessitating efforts to integrate the discrepant experience of loss into one's autobiographical memory (Boelen, van den Hout, & van den Bout, 2006).

According to this model, *resilient survivors* who take the loss in stride without profound distress would likely be those who are able to assimilate the loss into a stable and positive meaning system, perhaps drawing on secular or spiritual beliefs that help them make sense of the loss and the life transition they are forced to undergo. *Adaptive grievers*, by comparison, may wrestle profoundly for a time with practical or existential questions concerning the death of their loved one and its implications for their sense of self, but ultimately accommodate their self narrative to the changed reality in a way that engenders renewed stability and perhaps even personal growth. In contrast to these resourceful responses, a minority of *foreclosed survivors* may assimilate the loss into a stable, but predominantly negative or pessimistic meaning system, finding in their loss yet another life experience that validates their sense of life's cruelty and meaninglessness or their own failings. Finally, *chronic grievers* may contend with an anguishing invalidation of their central assumptions about God, the universe, their loved one and other people, often experiencing an ongoing struggle to reconstruct a life narrative that accounts for their past loss, their present circumstances, and their changed future (cf. Neimeyer, 2006b).

THE EMPIRICAL WARRANT

This basic theoretical perspective accords well with a growing body of research that associates resilient and adaptive trajectories through loss with an absence of searching for meaning in the first instance and a successful quest for meaning in the second (e.g., Bonanno et al., 2004; Calhoun & Tedeschi, 2006; Davis, Wohl, & Verberg, 2007). Conversely, an ongoing attempt to search for meaning in the loss and a chronic inability to make sense of it is associated with intense and protracted grieving among such groups as bereaved young adults (Holland, Currier & Neimeyer, 2006), parents who have lost children (Keesee, Currier & Neimeyer, 2008), and older widows and widowers (Bonanno et al., 2004; Coleman & Neimeyer, in press). In fact, "sense making" is such a critical predictor of adjustment to loss that one study found it to be a near-perfect mediator of the impact of bereavement by violent death. That is, although loss through suicide, homicide and fatal accident was indeed associated with higher levels of complicated grief symptoms than loss through natural death, nearly all of the difference could be attributed to a failure to find meaning in the loss in the former instance (Currier, Holland & Neimeyer, 2006). More suggestively, recent evidence also accords with the conceptualization of a group of *foreclosed survivors* whose world assumptions are pessimistic, fragile and self-critical, and whose distress is exacerbated by the loss of a loved one (Currier, Holland, & Neimeyer, 2009).

THERAPEUTIC PRINCIPLES

If these issues of meaning do play a key role in bereavement adaptation, then therapies that foster engagement with the life narratives of the bereaved in a way that facilitates the integration, rather than avoidance, of the loss should prove useful in helping people surmount bereavement complications. Indeed, several recent therapies for complicated grief, which are demonstrably effective, make extensive use of just such procedures (Boelen et al., 2007; Shear et al., 2005; Wagner et al., 2006). Common components of these evidence-based interventions include (a) the selection of grievers who display intense and prolonged separation distress and related complications in the aftermath of loss (Currier, Neimeyer, & Berman, 2008), (b) repeated and experientially intense "retelling" of the circumstances of the death with associated feelings and reactions, often coupled with prompts for the client to take perspective on it in a healing way (Rynearson, 2006), (c) some form of guided encounter with the memory or symbolic "presence" of the loved one, as in an empty chair encounter or through drafting letters to the deceased (Neimeyer, 2001a), and (d) attempts to promote "restoration-oriented" coping (Stroebe & Schut, 1999) such as attending to current relationships and responsibilities and projecting new goals that better fit with one's new post-loss reality. In the remainder of this chapter I will build on these foundations and on the broader grounding provided by constructivist psychology (Neimeyer & Mahoney, 1995; Neimeyer & Raskin, 2000) by exploring the relevance of three overarching principles that carry practical implications for the conduct of grief therapy, illustrating each through aspects of my work with Deborah in the dark aftermath of her mother's death.

Principle 1: Use Narrative Methods, as well as Concepts, in Re-authoring Lives Disrupted by Loss

As narrative psychologists of many orientations recognize, people live their lives in stories (Bruner, 1990; Hermans, 2002; McAdams, 2006). At the most obvious level, we seem "wired," even neurologically (D. C. Rubin & Greenberg, 2003), to organize experience in narrative form, and accordingly are drawn to media—spoken, written or performed—that "package" human experience as stories that have a meaningful beginning, middle, and end, and that retain a workable degree of continuity and coherence (Neimeyer, 2000). Perhaps more compellingly, we formulate our own experience in similar terms, giving meaning to simple daily events or poignant life passages by relating them as stories to an audience of friends and loved ones, or perhaps only to ourselves in a private journal. And when the stories of our lives are too anguished to be held by these conventional witnesses, we sometimes turn to psychotherapists who we hope can hear what others cannot, and who can help us find a way forward through a life narrative that has become unlivable.

Across the course of many years of practice as a psychotherapist, I have come to view stories of loss in these terms. Because our very sense of security and identity is braided together with others to whom we are intimately attached (Bowlby, 1980), separation from the key figures in our life stories through bereavement can launch a quest to reorganize our self-narrative to accommodate the hard reality of our loss (Neimeyer, 2006b).

Fortunately, human beings have evolved to cope resiliently with life transitions, and evidence suggests that the majority of bereaved persons either integrate the loss without extended disruption of their existing sense of life's purpose or meaning, or begin to return to their emotional baseline after several months of distress (Bonanno, Wortman, & Nesse, 2004). For a significant minority, however, this is not the case, and a complicated course of grieving can ensue, marked by a profound and protracted separation distress, social disruption, and psychological and medical morbidity that can extend for years beyond the loss, if indeed it does not end in an early death through cardiac or other health problems, substance abuse, or suicide (Prigerson & Maciejewski, 2006).

In our own research, a good deal of evidence converges with this conceptualization of bereavement in narrative, meaning-making terms. For example, a prolonged effort to find some meaning in a senseless loss characterizes the struggle of fully 30% of bereaved parents (Keesee, Currier, & Neimeyer, 2008), as well as many of those who suffer the loss of a loved one through suicide, homicide or fatal accident (Currier, Holland, & Neimeyer, 2006). In both cases, the success of bereaved people in making sense of the loss in spiritual, secular or practical terms predicts the extent of their ability to surmount complicated, disabling grief symptomatology. Conversely, grievers with weaker beliefs in the meaningfulness of the world and lower perceptions of self-worth report greater distress symptoms than those who perceive the world and self in more positive terms (Currier et al., 2009), even when the losses are anticipated and normative ones through natural causes. It therefore makes sense to join our clients in sorting out the shattered or somber meanings with which they struggle in the wake of loss, in an attempt to help them integrate the reality of the death into their changed life story. In this, I have found a broad range of narrative procedures to be valuable aids in therapy (Neimeyer, 2002; Neimeyer, van Dyke, & Pennebaker, 2009), as I will illustrate in the case of Deborah below.

Principle 2: Reconstruct, Rather than Relinquish, the Relationship to the Deceased

Based largely on early psychodynamic understandings of grieving as a process of "decathexis" or "breaking emotional bonds" that tie the living to the dead (Freud, 1957), twentieth century grief theorists and therapists were mesmerized by a model of mourning as a form of "letting go of" or "saying goodbye to" the lost loved one. In the past fifteen years, however, such models have come under scrutiny, with growing numbers of scholars arguing that continuing, rather than breaking, bonds with the deceased can be a part of healthy grieving (Attig, 2000; Klass, Silverman, & Nickman, 1996). Nonetheless, recent research has suggested that reorganizing an ongoing sense of attachment to the deceased can be an effortful process, one that requires time (Field & Friedrichs, 2004) and that can meet with all manner of clinical complexities (S. S. Rubin, Malkinson, & Witztum, 2003). In general, it appears that forms of attachment that do not rely primarily on physical reminders of the loved one, that are uncontaminated by guilt and self-blame, and that are accompanied by high degrees of meaning-making regarding the loss are associated with better bereavement outcomes, permitting survivors to retain a sense of connection to the deceased but nonetheless move forward with their lives (Neimeyer, Baldwin, & Gillies, 2006). Working with clients to reformulate their continuing bonds to their loved ones in these terms can therefore play a central role in grief therapy, as illustrated in my work with Deborah below.

Principle 3: Give Voice to the Unspeakable to Track Evolving Meanings

Although constructivist therapists place a high premium on how clients attribute meaning to their experience in language, they also recognize that not only the core but also the "growing edges" of our meaning systems are difficult to formulate in public speech (Neimeyer, 2009). This implies that the deepest meanings with which our clients struggle, as well as fresh new possibilities for construing and doing life differently are typically elusive, and call for articulation in figurative rather than literal terms. In keeping with this argument, research has documented that client-therapist exchanges that are high in the use of imagery and metaphor are far better recalled by clients several months later than are more "rational," prosaic conversations, and that these same images play a pivotal role in the construction of therapeutic change (Martin, 1994). Accordingly, like their humanistic colleagues, constructivist therapists draw on a range of procedures for exploring the "felt sense" of evolving understanding, often first registered as a bodily, rather than cognitive awareness (Gendlin, 1996). A keen attention to evolving meanings of this imagistic sort played an important role in my work with Deborah, the case to which I will now turn.

A Case Observed

A Study in Complication

My first few seconds of contact with Deborah conveyed to me poignantly the severity of her suffering. Haggard and downtrodden, Deborah glanced at me with eyes that were swollen from crying, her hair disheveled, her clothing dark and rumpled, and her monotonic voice and downcast gaze reflecting the desolate mood her words soon enough confirmed. Deborah was seeking therapy with me at the advice of a friend after the death of her mother, aged 70, some 26 months earlier from complications arising from her 10 year history of diabetes. In many respects it seemed that this 45 year-old single woman was entering her third *day* of bereavement, rather than her third *year*. Indeed, she struck me as a "poster case" for complicated grief, as she recounted an unrelenting inability to accept that her mother's death was real, leading her unconsciously to check the mother's empty bedroom in their family home each morning as if to disconfirm an event she could not integrate emotionally. Unable to continue in her work as a nursing assistant to the elderly and infirm, she now found herself struggling to function in daily life. As she explained, tears and mucus streaming down her face to be periodically wiped away,

> Mostly the reason that I'm here . . . is that since her death, my mind goes blank. I'm not able to speak up for myself, [and] it seems like it gets worse, not better. It's difficult. Things don't connect up the way they used to. . . . I have to make an extra effort, and then it's all gone.

Prompting her with a question of what the hardest times were like for her, I learned that she "couldn't even fold clothes and put them in a drawer properly." Deborah elaborated,

> My mental's not good. . . . I go to bed, or to the store, and just cry and cry. I knew I needed some kind of help. I just blow up at things. . . . I feel defeated. It's just overwhelming for me. I just want to stay in bed and close the door.

I asked her, "What would you be closing the door on?", and she continued,

> I just don't like to function without her. . . . I don't have that person that gave me unconditional acceptance, the courage to go on. My brothers and sisters just get sick of hearing about it. I guess I'm just needier than they are. I just can't accept that she's gone. There's no end to the spiral. I just can't get past this overwhelmed feeling that I feel.

Listening to Deborah's labored and anguished account, I could not escape the feeling that it was as if her life effectively ended with her mother's, after four intensive years of caregiving to her mother that Deborah described as "lovely," because they permitted her to return some of the love that she felt she had received from the older woman. Now, the meaning of her own life seemed to slip out of focus, along with her life-sustaining bond with the person with whom she had always shared a home. How we could integrate the loss into the larger story of her life and reconstruct the attachment to mother that was sundered by her death became compelling therapeutic priorities.

A Narrative Intervention

As we moved toward the end of our first session, a spark of hope leaped up with Deborah's spontaneous comment, "I try to open whatever doors I can, and [try to] accept that she's gone. I *can* make decisions." Giving more tinder to the spark, I observed that there were indeed two parts to the story, and two parts of her, one of which wanted to close the door on life and withdraw, while another wanted to get some footing back in life, and make it more as she wanted it to be. Getting her nonverbal assent, I therefore wondered aloud "whether there was some small and specific step that we could take in the direction of that hope," and sketched the idea of a narrative intervention: her writing a letter *to* Mom, just as she had often written letters *for* Mom to other family members since her death as a continuation of her mother's role as the "family center point." Deborah showed a muted sign of interest, but noted, "We'd have to write that down, because it was already lost" to her impaired concentration and "blankness." I therefore picked up a pen and paper, and prompted her by asking what she called her mother, gradually eliciting the first few lines of a heartfelt letter that came haltingly through a torrent of tears. Converting Deborah's third-person statements (e.g., "I miss her," "She always listened.") into first-person affirmations (e.g., "I miss you," "You always listened."), I handed her the letter we had begun, and inquired how it would be to continue it as therapeutic homework. Her response, "It would be scary, painful," alerted me to the importance of structuring self-soothing activities (such as listening to music, taking a walk, or arranging social contact) that would give a temporary reprieve from the writing, something she felt could be accomplished by physical activity. We closed with her noting hopefully that the letter might be a way to "reconnect" with Mom and with "her positive thoughts," something she realized tearfully that she greatly needed.

Deborah's appearance for the second session immediately caught my attention: Dressed in bright "business casual" attire with a smart pair of glasses and hair that clearly benefited from her attention, she seemed to step more lightly, meeting my gaze and taking a seat eagerly for our conversation to begin. In response to my inquiry about her reaction to our first meeting in the ensuing week, Deborah permitted the flicker of a smile, and noted that "I feel that I have gotten through some of the 'yuck' I was feeling. I liked the idea of writing a letter, and wrote it 3 or 4 times," although she confessed that doing so was accompanied by "a lot of anxiety." The writing, she informed me, had helped her realize that her mother "was in a better place," as well as to recognize that "her presence was within." Elaborating in response to my signs of interest and curiosity, she also noted that she was seeing signs of Mom's presence for the first time in the dishwashing gestures of her sister, and laughingly related a story about how she blamed a recent stoppage of the sink on her mother, who often experienced a similar problem. In these and other commonplace ways, I noted, "it was almost as if she were rediscovering her mother in the course of the week," something Deborah thoughtfully affirmed.

Turning to a direct discussion of the writing, Deborah informed me that through it she "had some negativity that she dispelled from her youth, because she was the sixth of seven [children]" and hence "tended to get bound in the resentment" of having been neglected by her hard-working farming parents during her formative years. Later, however, with the birth of her own daughter, Deborah reported that her mother had "been there" for her in important ways, and she was filled with "a new feeling of gratitude" for the belated but very welcome mothering she had received. Touched, I responded, "I'm just impressed with this, and have a little shiver of appreciation up my spine as you talk about this because it seems these kinds of resentments that you had held and that had held you for decades, you began to release a little bit, in part through your writing."

Deborah smiled and nodded her assent, and at my invitation, slowly read aloud the letter she had drafted and printed on elegant stationary, addressed to her mother by her pet name:

Dear Mom, my Dearest Bertle:

I miss you. It's hard without your guidance and encouragement, but I'm doing what you told me to do almost 26 years ago. I'm completing my Associate's degree. I've been writing your son, John, [although] it's very hard for me to function.... I pray to God I'm doing what I'm meant to do in this lifetime. How I miss your words of wisdom, and how you always told me to "keep up the good work." I know you're in a better place and I will see you again. I send you the biggest hug, and I'm trying to be the person you raised me to be. I pray that the blankness of thought goes, and I am able to concentrate on the gift God gave me of having a mother like you for 43 years. I know you're keeping track of us, as your love lives in us all. I just wish that others in our family would have some of the faith, grace and love you so patiently taught us.

Until we meet again, hugs and kisses, from your daughter and friend,
Deborah

Smiling broadly, I shared my appreciation of her "loving letter, filled with such gratitude in relation to Mom." It seemed to us both that some important kind of reconnection had begun.

Returning a Mother's Legacy to Her

Exploring a bit more the family issues hinted at toward the end of Deborah's letter, I soon learned that Deborah's identification with her mother's role was not limited to writing letters on her behalf. Indeed, as she candidly acknowledged, "Since my mother's been gone I've been trying to be her piece. And I don't think that's a good place for me to be, and it's something my family doesn't have acceptance of anyway. So I need to let that go, and let *them* be *them*." "Let them be them," I echoed, adding, "and let *you* be *you*, and not just Mom's placeholder in the family. . . . Do you think that Mom would approve of that, your relinquishing her role a little bit?" Deborah's response, "I don't know how my mother would feel about that," suggested that this necessary shift required more relational renegotiation with her mother to allow it to move forward. I therefore paused and wondered aloud whether there was "another step" that Deborah might be willing to take on the heels of her liberating initial attempt at writing to Mom. She again displayed intrigue, but also hesitation, noting that "it sounds hard. . . . That's one of my greatest fears—if I stop being her portion [of the family], if everything's going to be okay, if *I'm* going to be okay. In some ways, that's where my self-esteem is." Alerted to the essential question, I picked up my writing tablet and pen, and asked, "So if we were to think of this as a psychological assignment, what kind of assignment would it be?" Deborah's response suggested the heading I wrote on the paper: "Returning my Mother's Legacy to Her." Deborah then readily accepted my suggestion that she write to that theme as therapeutic homework, seeking Mom's permission to relinquish some of the over-identification with her advice-giving presence that had helped her maintain a (problematic) continuing bond with Mom, but that clearly had been resisted by her adult siblings. We closed the session with her noting, "This sounds neat. I think I'm going to enjoy it. It's going to be a big milestone in my life." I ended our second session with real curiosity about how she would fare with the assignment in the week ahead.

Our third session of therapy took place two weeks later, following the "monthly anniversary" of Deborah's mother's death. Interestingly, Deborah opened by noting that she began "feeling down" on that day, but that when she started writing, "it was a kind of release." "What was released with that writing?" I asked. "Just the identification," she responded, "that I was trying to be my mother, and wasn't identifying with myself, doing what I wanted to do or needed to do. It was this *obsession*." She went on to explain that she compulsively tried to perceive and meet the needs of everyone in the family, just as mother had, but got a chilly reception in response. The writing, it seemed, led to an insight: "That's something I identified in the writing, that I was becoming this worry-wart of a person, and it was a very negative thing for me ... because people didn't want it. I was trying to become Mom's replacement, and you really can't do that." "It's almost like I was playing hide-and-seek with myself," she added thoughtfully, to which I inquired, "What an extraordinary image, playing hide-and-seek with yourself! What were you hiding, and what were you seeking?" Responding, she noted that she was creating an identity that wasn't her own, and one that wasn't being asked for by others. She then accepted my invitation to read the remarkable letter in which so much had become clear:

Dear Mom,

You were always the key-holder for our family's problems. You had an instinct about what to do in every situation, always made sure we felt loved and special. Since you've been gone from this world I've tried to be you within our family. I am returning your legacy to you. Our family has no acceptance, nor have they asked me to fill the hole that was made by your departure. You had one bad characteristic, and that was that you worried about us a lot. I picked up that characteristic, and this is something I've gone overboard with.... Most of all, I need to recognize that people are who they are, and I cannot make them into the person I want them to be. Mom, I am asking your permission to be me. I'm going to allow myself to be okay with who I am. I need to practice on my own individuality, and have faith that I'll be okay with myself. I have all the wonderful wisdom you taught me, and one of those things is the power of prayer.

Love, your daughter and friend,
Deborah

Finishing the letter and commenting on her growing success in relinquishing her mother's role to the relief of her siblings, Deborah then shared with me a remarkable revelation: she had learned of a job at a foundation that provided toys to seriously ill children, and with uncharacteristic self-assurance approached the prospective employer to ask that they consider her. As she observed, laughing, "For that to come out of my mouth is really new!" She was offered an interview on the spot, and was enthusiastic about the prospect of meaningful work that would let her "give back to society and to children who really need it." I affirmed this sign of growth and openness to possibility, suggesting that, "In letting go of being Mom, you made room to become Deborah again, reaching back to who you had been, and reaching forward to who you want to become." She readily agreed, noting, "The door is starting to open. . . . [Before] I felt like I was hitting my head on the wall, but I couldn't stop; it only grew greater and greater." Curious, I asked her what helped her break that pattern. She replied,

> I really think it was that first letter, and then the other one. For the longest time, it's crazy, but it was like I was still expecting my mother to walk back through that door. . . . [Writing to her] helped me to face that reality, and I realized what I was doing . . . all this crazy stuff, and see it clearly. . . . And I could see there was a reason [to her mother's death]. . . . People go on, and do different things. She's gone from this world, and doesn't need to be replaced, because I wasn't born to be her. I was born to be myself.

It seemed that Deborah, through her narrative work and its consolidation in our sessions, had begun to reorganize but not relinquish her continuing bond with her mother, in a way that no longer required her to unconsciously attempt to "be" Mom in the context of her family. Instead, in ways that were keenly felt and clearly observable, she was winning back her sense of self, and finding validation of this shift in the responses of others in the family and beyond it. Simultaneously, her mother's death seemed to be taking on a different meaning, one that did not require her physical presence in the world to leave a lasting legacy of love. As a result, Deborah noted, she wasn't "so much feeling *sad* about her death [now], it was more *nostalgic*." This was a significant emotional shift for her away from the "doom and gloom" that characterized her earlier.

Dialogue with a Dead Mother

In part to explore any relational impediment that could block Deborah's reconstruction of her bond with her mother, and in part to shore up this very move, I then suggested a novel intervention: "As we were talking about this notion of getting Mom's permission for the changes you want to make... I wondered if we could have a conversation in here, in which I interviewed your mother, briefly, about the person her daughter, Deborah, is becoming. Would that be interesting to you?" Deborah chuckled a little nervously, but agreed, and so I immediately suggested that we switch chairs "to allow us to be someone else," and began to interview her as her mother by her "public" name, Pat: "I've been having some conversations, Pat, with your daughter Deborah.... They've been interesting conversations. And one of the things she's been talking about is that she's looking for a way to let your legacy be yours, and for her to step back into being Deborah. And she's been a little bit worried as to how you feel about that.... What do you think of this move your daughter is trying to make... to make room for who she is as a person?" Deborah, as Pat, affirmed that her daughter should be who she is, and especially should "erase" any negative traits she might have given her. Alerted to this incipient metaphor, I introduced the image of a "magic pencil with lead on one end, and an eraser on the other," and asked "Pat" alternately about "what traits you would write out for Deborah to carry forward in her life," and what she would give her daughter permission to erase or relinquish. I picked up my note pad and took dictation as she pensively formulated the list of the qualities she hoped Deborah would cultivate (e.g., a loving understanding of herself, the courage to stand up for herself, a passion for life, a great love of people), those she regarded as "precious" in her daughter (e.g., that she thinks before she speaks, she's not harsh, is confident in what she knows), and those features she would encourage her to let go of (e.g., being the family caregiver, needless worry). Invited to share some "final words for this part of the conversation," "Pat" concluded that she hoped her daughter "would find total joy." After we ended the conversation with "Pat's" permission and took our former chairs, I reread her "mother's" words slowly and evocatively, as Pat brushed away a tear. "I'm crying," she said, "but it feels good. It's encouraging. I get caught up in the fact that she's not here, and I don't think she would want that." She paused and smiled. "Of course not," I replied, "she wouldn't want to be banished because she *is* here with you. When you invite her, she steps right back in." Accepting the paper with my interview notes, Deborah remarked, "This is something I may type up, because they are words of wisdom. These are like words she could have said, and when I need her words, I can have them." She continued, unprompted: "Typing them will keep me in the positive swing that has been transforming in my life the last couple of weeks... It's funny when things start to roll in the right direction."

Encounter with the Unspeakable

Deborah returned for our fourth session in a positive mood, having typed out her mother's words of wisdom, and offered me a copy as well. She had "been trying hard to apply what we were doing," at school, at her new job, and in her family. Elaborating on this theme of change, she acknowledged the need to "watch for the telltale signs" of sleep disruption, unwarranted anxiety, performance problems, or most significantly, the "blankness" that she had experienced so frequently and disruptively over the last two years. Cuing on this term, I asked her what she now understood about what this blankness meant. Her answer—that it was like a "void around her heart that wasn't filled," alerted me to the possible relevance of a "body scan" now to check on this feeling, in the wake of medical tests that had yielded no cause for concern.

> *Bob*: As you were talking about that void feeling, and doing a scan, I wondered if we could do an inward scan now on how you are doing inside.
> *Deborah*: Sure.
> *Bob*: *(closing my eyes, and slowing my rate of speech)* Just close your eyes, and find a comfortable way of sitting in the chair, putting your arms in a relaxed position, allowing the chair to support you. And allow your attention to almost in a way walk through your body, looking for any tension, any sense, any feeling that feels significant, or related to the way you are holding the grief for your mother now. When you sense something, whether it's a variation on that void or something different, just leave your eyes closed, and give me an indication of where that is and how that is for you.
> *Deborah*: *(pause)* It almost starts out of my body. It's here, it's here, it's over my head and over my shoulders *(gesturing to define the shape of the "dome")*. And it feels like a beacon,

a beacon of light, like a warmth, that understanding will come, over time.

Bob: A beacon, warmth, that understanding will come over time. . . . So it is a comforting, reassuring feeling?

Deborah: Almost like it's embracing me. . . . I always thought of heaven being upward, like a radiation, an element.

Bob: Embracing you.

Deborah: Yeah *(moving hands and fingers to show "shower" of warmth)*.

Bob: Embraced by light, around your head, around your shoulders. . . . Now, it has a pattern of movement for you?

Deborah: Yeah . . . it's kind of encompassing, coming down. It's right here now *(at shoulders)*. It might embrace the whole, but it's just kind of right here right now.

Bob: If you were just to allow it to move forward, continue its pattern of motion, whatever that might be, where would it go, how would it hold you or contact you?

Deborah: It would come around, just stop at the floor *(gesturing to define the shape of the shroud around her body)*. It would give more comfort, more understanding.

Bob: Now in this kind of image, how do you imagine yourself relating to this warmth, this beacon-like radiation around you?

Deborah: It brings me comfort, it brings me courage.

Bob: This almost resonates with some of those "spiritual principles" that you were voicing for your mother last time.

Deborah: It's just a relief. It almost feels like an exhale, that even though it's something around me, it's going to take out any negativity and absorb it and turn it into something wonderful.

Bob: I wonder if you can allow your lungs to fill, releasing with slow, rhythmic breaths *(breathing slowly with Deborah)* . . . then just allow the exhale to come, maybe feeling some of that comfort coming with that, just as you describe. . . . *(noting Deborah's emerging smile)* and a little smile?

Deborah: It's hard to explain, almost like a wisdom, and understanding, a faith that this process will continue. That it's okay to miss my mother, as long as I don't injure myself mentally or physically because of the whole sleep thing.

Bob: As you speak of that wisdom, I was feeling these tingles up my spine, down my back, down my legs. It felt like an affirmation in my body of some of what you've been describing in your body.

Deborah: It's almost like a peace is being brought to me, though I don't think the void can ever be completely.... Like there's a key that at least has opened the door *(puts hand over heart)* to that void that I feel.

Bob: The key to that void.... In this moment of peace, just allow that void to open a little bit, just to kind of glance inside and feel inside and note what's there. What would you see or feel in that space?

Deborah: The first thing is the physical, and that's the part that I could never get used to, her not being around, her body, her outline, her structure. Her voice—her voice would be something separate, her speaking, reading, singing voice. I could hear her sing sometimes to comfort herself. And in a form of praise and worship too, what she believed was God. And then it would be her laughter. I loved the way she laughed.

Bob: All of these separate voices that were all one.

Deborah: That's the things I miss most, the things that can never be. I've received all the kindness and gestures she's given throughout life. But there will never be another laughter, another smile, another reading. And just her spirituality. She had a definite thought of who God was to her. She experienced that so fully.

Bob: Almost as you now experience, in a bodily way, something that also has the feeling of the sacred. And you say it feels like a kind of warmth, a radiation, coming from heaven as well as in an emotional way, holding you, enveloping you, embracing you more. . . . Is she a part of that embrace in your image?

Deborah: I'm not sure if it's a part of her spirit, or if it's just the power that she called God radiating down. I'm not sure how that works. But I know that I could feel that tenderness, that sweetness that was just so engrained in her. So certainly, if it's not her spirit, it's one of similarity. . . .

Bob: So that tenderness, that sweetness, is not lost. It might be lost as a physical voice, but in a moment like this it is not lost as a physical experience. You can feel it around you and feel it in you. And you can speak to that, and share it with me.

Deborah: *(eyes still closed, smiling broadly)* Yeah. It's almost massaging, like, you know, when kids used to poke each other in the stomach to chuckle or whatever, like I can feel the needles and pins right now on my hands.

Bob: You know, I'm feeling them too. You're really sharing them with me!

Deborah: It's delightful.

Bob: It's the joy piece, huh?

Deborah: Yeah.

Bob: Isn't it interesting that, as we move into that void, what we get is not only grief, but also joy. In this very physical, almost childlike way, that's there right alongside the other, alongside the sadness.

Deborah: Well, yeah. I have a lot to be grateful for. A lot of people didn't have good moms, moms that embraced them and loved them. . . .

Bob: Yes. . . . If you feel ready to do so, let me invite you to take another deep breath or so, pause, and release slowly. And then open your eyes, and re-enter this little space with me again, and we can talk a little bit.

Deborah: *(smiling and gradually opening her eyes)* That was neat! *(wipes eyes with a tissue)* That was like a little hug from heaven! *(laughs)*

Bob: Wow! That's the tag line on this: A hug from heaven. I feel like I got a little pat on the shoulder myself! *(both laugh)*
Deborah: Yeah, my mom wouldn't have left anyone out!
Bob: She'd even dole out a little bit to a stranger, huh? So what was that like for you, to accept my invitation to do this inward scan, and go right to that?

In our processing of the experience, Deborah affirmed, "It was really wonderful. You asked about my mom's presence, and I really didn't feel it until I felt that tickling. It was an electrical, staticky thing. I was reaching out for that humanistic feeling, but it was an energy thing. And that makes sense, because she's spirit now." We closed the session with a shared sense of Mom's accessible presence in Deborah's life, on the level of her words, captured in typed documents; her validation of Deborah's uniqueness, delivered in our dialogue with Pat; and her ongoing impact on the family, observable in myriad contexts of everyday life. Perhaps most vividly, as we moved beyond the tangible realm of public speech to invite and engage Deborah's most private meanings of the "void" she carried throughout her bereavement, we also encountered her mother's warmth and spiritual presence, rediscovered in imagery and bodily feeling. Significantly, the reconstruction of Deborah's continuing bond with mother found strong expression in language, symbol and lived experience, and was consolidated in an exploration of her unconventional spirituality and a celebration of her revitalized life narrative in our remaining two sessions.

Concluding Remarks

Like a jazz improvisation, each "performance" of therapy is unique, as both (or in the case of couples, family or group work, all) participants "riff" off of the offerings of the other(s) in ways that cannot be specified in advance (Neimeyer, 2009). Constructivists recognize this innovative quality of all relationally responsive therapy, and accordingly view therapy as a process by which we join clients in articulating, symbolizing and renegotiating those deeply personal meanings on which they rely to formulate their experience and action (Neimeyer, 1995). Nonetheless, certain abiding principles, if not strict rules (Levitt, Neimeyer, & Williams, 2005), can be discerned in constructivist practice, and my distillation and illustration of a few such principles in this brief chapter represents one attempt to do so.

Although constructivism offers orientation to a vast range of human problems for which people seek therapy, I have focused here and elsewhere (Neimeyer, 2005, 2006a, 2001b) on its special implications for grief counseling. I do so to emphasize its usefulness as a perspective from which to view the universal problem of loss—perhaps the only psychosocial/existential challenge that will be faced by every client we consult, and of course by every therapist as well. Often, as I have acknowledged, people cope with the death of those they love with remarkable, and sometimes inspiring resilience—except when they don't, in which case they risk becoming immobilized in a world seemingly devoid of that one, compellingly essential attachment figure, unable to assimilate the apparent impossibility of the death into a life story now bleached of meaning by bereavement. Working with these impeded, shattered or vitiated life stories using a variety of narrative concepts and methods has frequently helped me join clients in identifying the strands of continuity in their lives and in their relationship to the deceased, and in weaving a new fabric of connection that also accommodates threads of new possibility. Drawing on the rich vocabulary of words, meanings, emotions and images with which each client engages this task allows me to partner intimately with them in reconstructing life out of loss, often reinventing themselves in the process. I hope that some of the ideas and illustrations I have offered in these pages provide encouragement for readers to undertake something similar in their own practice.

REFERENCES

Attig, T. (2000). *The heart of grief.* New York: Oxford.
Boelen, P., van den Hout, M., & van den Bout, J. (2006). A cognitive-behavioral conceptualization of complicated grief. *Clinical Psychology: Science and Practice, 13,* 109-128.
Bonanno, G. A., Wortman, C. B., & Nesse, R. M. (2004). Prospective patterns of resilience and maladjustment during widowhood. *Psychology and Aging, 19,* 260-271.
Bowlby, J. (1980). *Attachment and loss: Loss, sadness and depression* (Vol. 3). New York: Basic.
Bruner, J. (1990). *Acts of meaning.* Cambridge, MA: Harvard University Press.
Calhoun, L., & Tedeschi, R. G. (2006). (Eds.). *Handbook of posttraumatic growth: Research and practice.* Mahwah, NJ: Lawrence Erlbaum
Coleman, R. A., & Neimeyer, R. A. (in press). Measuring meaning: Searching for and making sense of loss in late-life spousal bereavement. *Death Studies.*
Currier, J. M., Holland, J., & Neimeyer, R. A. (2006). Sense making, grief and the experience of violent loss: Toward a mediational model. *Death Studies, 30,* 403-428.
Currier, J. M., Holland, J., & Neimeyer, R. A. (2009). Assumptive worldviews and problematic reactions to bereavement. *Journal of Loss and Trauma, 14,* 181-195.
Currier, J. M., Neimeyer, R. A., & Berman, J. S. (2008). The effectiveness of psychotherapeutic interventions for the bereaved: A comprehensive quantitative review. *Psychological Bulletin, 134,* 648-661.
Davis, C. G., Wohl, M. J. A., & Verberg, N. (2007). Profiles of posttraumatic growth following an unjust loss. *Death Studies, 31,* 693-712.
Field, N. P., & Friedrichs, M. (2004). Continuing bonds in coping with the death of a husband. *Death Studies, 28,* 597-620.
Field, N. P., Gao, B., & Paderna, L. (2005). Continuing bonds in bereavement: An attachment theory based perspective. *Death Studies, 29,* 277-299.
Freud, S. (1957). Mourning and melancholia. In J. Strachey (Ed.), *The Complete Psychological Works of Sigmund Freud* (pp. 152-170). London: Hogarth Press.
Gendlin, E. T. (1996). *Focusing-oriented psychotherapy.* New York: Guilford.
Hermans, H. (2002). The person as a motivated storyteller. In R. A. Neimeyer & G. J. Neimeyer (Eds.), *Advances in personal construct psychology* (Vol. 5, pp. 3-38). Westport, CN: Praeger.

Janoff-Bulman, R., & Berger, A. R. (2000). The other side of trauma: Towards a psychology of appreciation. In J. H. Harvey & E. D. Miller (Eds.), *Loss and trauma: General and close relationship perspectives* (pp. 29-44). Philadelphia: Brunner Mazel.

Keesee, N. J., Currier, J. M., & Neimeyer, R. A. (2008). Predictors of grief following the death of one's child: The contribution of finding meaning. *Journal of Clinical Psychology, 64,* 1145-1163.

Klass, D., Silverman, P. R., & Nickman, S. (1996). *Continuing bonds: New understandings of grief.* Washington: Taylor & Francis.

Levitt, H. M., Neimeyer, R. A., & Williams, D. C. (2005). Rules versus principles in psychotherapy: Implications of the quest for universal guidelines in the movement for empirically supported treatments. *Journal of Contemporary Psychotherapy, 35,* 117-129.

Martin, J. (1994). *The construction and understanding of psychotherapeutic change.* New York: Teachers College Press.

McAdams, D. P. (2006). The problem of narrative coherence. *Journal of Constructivist Psychology, 19,* 109-125.

Neimeyer, R. A. (1995). An invitation to constructivist psychotherapies. In R. A. Neimeyer & M. J. Mahoney (Eds.), *Constructivism in psychotherapy* (pp. 1-8). Washington, DC: American Psychological Association.

Neimeyer, R. A. (2000). Narrative disruptions in the construction of self. In R. A. Neimeyer & J. D. Raskin (Eds.), *Constructions of disorder: Meaning making frameworks for psychotherapy* (pp. 207-241). Washington, DC: American Psychological Association.

Neimeyer, R. A. (2001a). The language of loss. In R. A. Neimeyer (Ed.), *Meaning reconstruction and the experience of loss* (pp. 261-292). Washington, DC: American Psychological Association.

Neimeyer, R. A. (2002). *Lessons of loss: A guide to coping* (2nd ed.). New York: Brunner Routledge.

Neimeyer, R. A. (2005). Growing through grief: Constructing coherence in accounts of loss. In D. Winter & L. L. Viney (Eds.), *Personal construct psychotherapy: Advances in theory, practice and research* (pp. 111-126). London: Whurr.

Neimeyer, R. A. (2006a). Re-storying loss: Fostering growth in the posttraumatic narrative. In L. Calhoun & R. G. Tedeschi (Eds.), *Handbook of posttraumatic growth: Research and practice* (pp. 68-80). Mahwah, NJ: Lawrence Erlbaum.

Neimeyer, R. A. (2006b). Widowhood, grief and the quest for meaning: A narrative perspective on resilience. In D. Carr, R. M. Nesse & C. B. Wortman (Eds.), *Spousal bereavement in late life* (pp. 227-252). New York: Springer.

Neimeyer, R. A. (2009). *Constructivist psychotherapy: Distinctive features.* New York: Routledge.
Neimeyer, R. A. (Ed.). (2001b). *Meaning reconstruction and the experience of loss.* Washington, DC: American Psychological Association.
Neimeyer, R. A., Baldwin, S. A., & Gillies, J. (2006). Continuing bonds and reconstructing meaning: Mitigating complications in bereavement. *Death Studies, 30,* 715-738.
Neimeyer, R. A., & Mahoney, M. J. (1995). *Constructivism in psychotherapy.* Washington, DC: American Psychological Association.
Neimeyer, R. A., & Raskin, J. D. (Eds.). (2000). *Constructions of disorder: Meaning-making frameworks for psychotherapy.* Washington, DC: American Psychological Association.
Neimeyer, R. A., van Dyke, J. G., & Pennebaker, J. W. (2009). Narrative medicine: Writing through bereavement. In H. Chochinov & W. Breitbart (Eds.), *Handbook of psychiatry in palliative medicine* (pp. 454-469). New York: Oxford.
Prigerson, H. G., & Maciejewski, P. K. (2006). A call for sound empirical testing and evaluation of criteria for complicated grief proposed by the DSM V. *Omega, 52,* 9-19.
Rubin, D. C., & Greenberg, D. L. (2003). The role of narrative in recollection: A view from cognitive psychology and neuropsychology. In G. D. Fireman, T. E. McVay & O. J. Flanagan (Eds.), *Narrative and consciousness* (pp. 53-85). New York: Oxford.
Rubin, S. S., Malkinson, R., & Witztum, E. (2003). Trauma and bereavement: Conceptual and clinical issues revolving around relationships. *Death Studies, 27,* 667-690.
Rynearson, E. K. (Ed.). (2006). *Violent death.* New York: Routledge.
Shear, K., Frank, E., Houch, P. R., & Reynolds, C. F. (2005). Treatment of complicated grief: A randomized controlled trial. *Journal of the American Medical Association, 293,* 2601-2608.
Stroebe, M., & Schut, H. (1999). The Dual Process Model of coping with bereavement: Rationale and description. *Death Studies, 23,* 197-224.
Wagner, B., Knaevelsrud, C., & Maercker, A. (2006). Internet-based cognitive-behavioral therapy for complicated grief: A randomized controlled trial. *Death Studies, 30,* 429-453.

⋙ 5 ⋘

The Dynamic Features of Love: Changes in Self and Motivation

*Agnieszka Hermans-Konopka and
Hubert J.M. Hermans*

> *Love has been known to seize a philosopher by the heels and shake him until his categories rattle and his postulates spill out upon the floor.*
>
> Norton & Kille, 1989, p. 1

In the psychological literature two general aspects of love have been emphasized: its complexity and its transforming features. Although the complexity makes the phenomenon of love challenging to explore, its transformative features paradoxically generate possibilities for understanding its nature. Some authors conclude that love has an especially strong influence on self-organization. It can lead to a significant transformation of the self (Magai & McFadden, 1995; Person, 1988), but the mechanisms by which it produces this change are insufficiently explained. Lack of dynamic conceptualizations of emotions within theory and research can be a significant obstacle for further exploration of changes provoked by feelings in human life. We argue that for a better understanding of transformative features of love we need to develop a more dynamic concept of feelings.

We have been working to develop a more dynamic conceptualization of feelings, which can be the basis for further exploration of love's transformative features and its interpretation in terms of self theory. In our proposed model we introduce the following dynamic aspects of emotional experience: change in self and change in motivation. This chapter reports a study in which 120 Polish students rated changes induced in their self-concepts in response to fourteen different feelings, presented as two lists of emotional verbs. Compared with thirteen other feelings, love provoked the highest level of general change in self, the most general action tendencies, and the greatest positive change in self and positive action tendencies. We also note that the dynamic aspects of love can be further articulated by a comparison with inferiority and anger. These findings contribute to the dynamic conceptualization of love in terms of dialogical self theory, with special emphasis on the process of self-innovation. Results of our study can be a step towards better understanding of change evoked by love in terms of innovation processes (Hermans, 2004).

Overview of the Literature

The Complexity of Love

Love is probably the most complex and transforming human experience. Strongman (1996) concluded that if love is an emotion, it is probably the most complex of all. Love, according to this author, can have many diverse forms (e.g. romantic, companionship), which complicate further the representation of the phenomenon. Similarly, following Averill's (1985) point of view, love can be understood as a syndrome, composed of many varied components, ranging from simple responses to a full emotional syndrome. Both authors would agree that love cannot be treated as a simple process. At the same time we can easily observe that even the most basic aspects of emotional experience (e.g., positive versus negative feelings) are often difficult to explore (Barrett and Russell, 1998), traditionally defying scientific analysis. One could say that love is a challenge both for human life and for scientific interpretation. Nonetheless, the profound role of love in human life does not allow researchers to exempt this phenomenon from psychological analysis. It seems that the issue is as complicated as attractive for research. The complexity of love makes it especially difficult to study and, as Averill (1985) pointed out, this creates the danger of emphasizing only one component and, as a result, equating the whole with its part. Reducing the complexity of love to one of its components and studying such a component as an isolated phenomenon would neglect its motivational dynamics and its meaning as part of a changing self. Thus, another way of approaching the phenomenon of love is possible and even necessary. In the present article we will study love in a contextual and dynamic way by approaching it as a constituent of the self and as an instigator of actions in social relationships. We will do so by comparing changes provoked in self and motivation by feelings of love with analogical changes provoked by a series of other feelings.

Transformative Features of Love

Although the complexity of love seems to be an obstacle for the scientific understanding of love, its transformative features paradoxically can open the door for empirical exploration of this feeling. We suggest that a useful way of studying the phenomenon of love is an exploration of its implications understood as dynamic changes provoked in different psychological processes (e.g., motivation). Until now many authors underscored the significance of changes provoked by love, but little has been said about the character of these changes and their mechanisms. Person (1988) wrote that love can be treated as an agent of transformation, creating "the possibility for dramatic change. It is in fact an agent of change" (p. 23). Magai and McFadden (1995) stated that personality can be organized according to the specific emotions and at the same time change in personality is often connected with significant experiences that occur in interpersonal relationships, in which love and surprise play important roles. These authors also concluded that such changes have not yet been sufficiently explored. Person presents the point of view that love "creates some flux in personality and it opens the possibility of change and beginning of new phases of life" (p. 23). We could ask a further question: what is going on within the self while the person experiences love that it becomes more open for change? Doan (1998, p. 229) describes the dynamic nature of love as one that "encourage[s] people to be all they are, to identify their highest choices and preferences, and to live with the notion they are in the process of becoming." To further understand this process of personal growth we need to explore more the character of changes provoked by love in self. There is a clear gap between the observation that love triggers important changes in human life and the explanation of the mechanisms underlying these changes. A first step in filling this gap would require the development of more dynamic conceptualization of feelings.

Dynamic Understanding of Feelings

The majority of psychological approaches and methodologies implicitly presume that psychological concepts are static. This pervasive tendency in the field corresponds to a characteristically Western way of thinking that reifies processes as static concepts (Salgado & Gonçalves, 2007). This tendency is equally evident in the psychology of emotion, which is more focused on identifying characteristics of relatively stable factors, dimensions and structures than those of dynamic processes. Even grammatical forms used for the description of emotional experience fail to capture their dynamism, referring instead to simple adjectives and states (e.g., Feldman, Barrett & Russell, 1998; Osgood, 1966). Furthermore, the majority of investigators analyze the structure of emotions understood as factors and dimensions. One prominent example is the well-known Circumplex Model of Affect proposed by Schlosberg (1941, 1952) and developed further by Russell (1980). This model was a starting point for many methodologies in research on emotions (e.g., Larsen and Diener, 1992; Russell, 1980; Watson & Tellegen, 1985) and treats emotional experience as a static structure build up by particular factors. In another model Smith and Ellsworth (1985) proposed several dimensions of cognitive arousal that are regarded as characteristic of emotional experience (e.g., attention, pleasure, control, certainty, responsibility). These factors can differentiate specific categories of emotions in a useful way but they are not enough to describe the dynamic nature of emotions.

The domination of the psychology of emotions by static concepts may constrain the possibility of understanding their dynamic nature. The central characteristic of emotions, their processual character, has been underestimated. By studying only factors and structures, emotions are treated like architectural objects rather than highly dynamic processes. In our study we consider feelings, metaphorically speaking, more as an ever-changing stream that also adapts to its surrounding. A key step in the development of a dynamic conceptualization of feelings is to study a variety of changes provoked by feelings in different psychological processes.

Emotions and Change in Self

Averill (1992, p. 227), referring to Jamesian conceptions of emotions, emphasized that "emotions necessarily involve the self. In fear, the self is perceived as threatened, in anger as affronted, in grief as dimished and in love as reaching out to another." This accords with Greenberg (2004, p. 3), who argued, "emotion is foundational in the construction of the self and is a key determinant of self-organization." According to Morgan (1992) and Averill (1992), connections between emotions and self are bidirectional: a change in emotional life is always followed by the change in the self and vice versa. Assessment of these connections can begin with the study of the relation between feelings and observed changes in the self, as we will demonstrate in the empirical research to follow. This mode of investigation can add to the interpretation of emotion in terms of self theory. Solomon (1994) proposed to treat a theory of love as a theory of the self, which holds promise as a way of understanding the transformative features of love. We need to understand what is occurring in the self when the person experiences love and how this experience changes the self. By describing these changes we can say something more about love itself.

Hermans (2003) describes self-innovation in dynamic and spatial terms. Drawing on Dialogical Self Theory (Hermans, 2002, 2001, 2005), the self can be conceptualized as a dynamic spatial organization of "I" positions. "I" positions can be understood as interrelated and dynamic parts of self and function as field-like relationships between internal (e.g., I as active, I as friend) and external (e.g., my wife, my sister) domains of the self. Innovation of the self entails reorganization of these "I" positions, which leads to some significant change in the life of a person. There are at least three possible ways in which the self can be innovated. The first is when a new position is introduced in the organization of the self. In this theory openness to a new "I" position depends on the organization of the repertoire. We suppose that feelings can help the self be more open to new "I" positions (e.g., love), whereas other feelings (e.g., fear) will close the self for the possibility of introducing new positions. The second means of self-innovation entails a change in the organization of existing "I" positions, as when "positions move from the background of the system to the foreground" (Hermans, 2003, p. 110). The third possible mode of innovation is forming coalitions of "I" positions, in which two or more "I" positions support each other and cooperate as parts of the self.

The notion of innovation of the self is useful for the interpretation of changes provoked by feelings because it allows for thinking of the self in dynamic categories. It also helps conceptualize feelings in connection with the organization of the self. These considerations are basic points for understanding the dynamic changes in the self provoked by feelings.

Emotions and Change of Motivation

Another dynamic aspect of emotion is its action readiness. We suppose that each particular category of emotions can be characterized by a more or less specific action tendency. This allows a comparison of different specific categories of feelings in a relatively clear way. Action tendencies provoked by emotions can be explored from different theoretical perspectives. Some authors who present an evolutionary perspective (Obuchowski, 1982; Plutchic, 1980) talk about action tendencies as patterns shaped across years of evolution and help individuals adapt and survive. Other authors (Arnold, 1960; Lazarus, 1991) tend to highlight cognitive processes as a basis of emotional experience. Arnold (1960) and Lazarus (1991a) have proposed that action tendencies result from cognitive apraisals made in the context of basic concerns of the individual. Arnold (1960) also pointed out the relevance of relational aspects of action tendencies, concluding that they can be understood as changes in readiness for particular interactions with others. Motivational aspects of emotions are basically connected with their relational nature. In agreement with Arnold (1960), we explore action tendencies as readiness for particular relational behaviors.

Many theoretical models attribute various action tendencies to specific categories of emotion (Lazarus, 1991; Izard, 1991). Lazarus (1991), besides emphasizing the cognitive level of affective processes, proposed a complex model to link specific emotions with action tendencies (e.g., anger with an impulse to fight and attack, fear and anxiety with tendencies to avoid, guilt with a tendency to repair or look for punishment). At the same time he also concluded that, while some emotions are clearly associated with specific action tendencies, other emotions (e.g., sadness, happiness) do not imply particular actions.

According to Lazarus, in the case of some emotions, we may not only link categories but also subcategories of emotions with particular action tendencies. For example, he connected romantic love with a tendency toward social and physical intimacy, expression of warmth, tenderness, interest and sexual contact. In the case of "compassionate love, the same applies with respect to social and personal intimacy, but although this kind of love is overtly nonsexual or at least desexualized, it still draws on expressions . . . of physical warmth, tenderness, interest, and concern for the other" (Lazarus, 1991, p. 279).

In his Differential Emotion Theory, Izard (1991) pays special attention to the description of particular categories of emotions in terms of action tendencies. For example, interest motivates people to test reality, try new behaviors and seek to know people. Shame is linked with change in behavior, motivating self-reflection and correction of one's attitude and behaviors, while anger motivates defense, and joy evokes creativity. Sadness, on the other hand, reduces intensity of actions and motivates self-reflection (Izard, 1991).

The importance of action tendencies within emotional experience has been especially underscored by Frijda (1986, 2001). In his model, emotions can be defined as temporary changes in action readiness and awareness of these changes is described as the core of emotional experience. Action tendencies should be understood in relational terms, as readiness for initiation, maintenance or dissolution of relations with the environment. Like Friijda, we pay treat action tendencies as basic aspects of emotional experience.

Finally, Greenberg and Johnson (1988) included self-organization in their model as a central element, determining the relation between emotions and actions. This is a particularly relevant statement for our study, because we take into account both change in self and in motivation. We propose that change in self and change in motivation are aspects of the same process and that studying them in combination can explain more than either analyzed separately.

Changes in Self and Changes in Motivation: Empirical Research

Our empirical contribution is based on a dynamic conception of feelings as a necessary step in understanding their transformative features. Specifically, we explored changes in self and in motivation provoked by fourteen feelings (including love). Change in self means changes in self-experience under the influence of particular feelings. The person who is feeling sadness experiences him—or herself in a very different way in comparison to a situation in which he or she is feeling joy or love and we assume that such differences have immediate implications for changes of self-organization.

Action tendencies reflect the motivational aspects of emotions and refer to changes in readiness for particular types of behaviors. They are treated as a second dynamic aspect of emotional experience. For example, the person who is feeling positive emotions is more likely to explore new ways of behaving toward the environment than the person who is feeling negative emotions (Fredrickson, 2000). Whereas the first dynamic aspect is change in self-experience, the second can be described as a tendency to change the situation. Both aspects are connected to a change of self-organization, and may be significant factors in creating novelty, a crucial component of the transformative aspects of emotions.

METHOD

Participants

A total of 120 Polish university students, aged 21-27, participated in the study. Students were enrolled in the study of education, history and psychology at the University of Cardinal

Stefan Wyszynsky in Warsaw. As men and women may differ in their emotionality (see Brebner, 2003; Brody & Hall, 1993), the two genders were analyzed separately.

Measures

A central aspect of our methodology was the use of verbs for an exploration of feelings. The majority of methodologies use adjectives and nouns which implicitly describe emotional experience in terms of state or structure. In agreement with our preceding discussion of the literature, we are convinced that verbs can better express the change provoked by feelings than adjectives and nouns. Love, for example, may fulfill or involve, anger may disintegrate. In a sentence "joy is warming me" we can see important dynamic characteristics of emotional experience and clear connections between feelings and the self. Application of verbs for research on feelings can help to answer the question of what the feeling does to the person and how it changes the self. The two dynamic aspects of emotional experience described above were explored by using lists of verbs: the List of Emotional Verbs (Konopka, 2006) for the exploration of change in self, and the list of verbs from Self Confrontation Method (Hermans, 1986) for the exploration of action tendencies.

The *List of Emotional Verbs* includes 54 verbs found to be frequently used for the description of emotional experience (Konopka, 2006). In a previous investigation participants were instructed to select verbs that fit their experience of particular emotions (Konopka, 2006). For example, a person could choose the following verbs for the description of anxiety: anxiety is blocking me, weakening me, imprisoning me, terrorizing me, and hurting me. In the same study participants were asked to assess verbs from the list as positive or negative. Some verbs were not classified in either category. In this way we constructed three categories of verbs: positive, negative and unclassified. Table 1 gives an overview of the different categories of verbs for studying changes in the self.

The list of verbs from the Self Confrontation Method (Hermans, 1986) includes 30 terms referring to behavior in social relationships. They were not conceived as objective behaviors but as action tendencies subjectively experienced by the client. They can be used for analysis of behaviors toward another person, toward oneself or of two persons toward each other (Hermans, 1986). This list can also be used for an exploration of action tendencies evoked by particular emotions, divided analogously to the previous list into positive, negative and unclassified categories. See Table 1.

TABLE 1. VARIABLES OF THE STUDY

Dynamic aspects of emotional experience
General change in self, total number of all verbs (positive, negative and unclassified) selected by the respondent for description of change in self experience.
Positive change in self, total number of positive verbs selected by the respondent for description of change in self.
Negative change in self, total number of negative verbs selected by the respondent for description of change in self.
General action tendencies, total number of verbs (positive, negative and not classified) selected by the respondent for description of action tendencies provoked by the feeling.
Positive action tendencies, total number of positive verbs selected by the respondent for description of action dencendies provoked by the feeling.
Negative action tendencies, total number of negative verbs selected by the respondent for description of action tendencies provoked by the feeling.

Procedure

The following feelings from the Self Confrontation Method (Hermans, 1986) were explored: self-esteem, love, loneliness, strength, inferiority, anxiety, guilt, safety, tenderness, weakness, joy, anger, internal calm, and coldness. These feelings were used because they were found to be relevant to the characterization of significant experiences in the lives of a variety of clients and research subjects who applied the Self Confrontation Method to themselves (Hermans & Hermans-Jansen, 1995).

Participants were tested in groups of 20 to 30 in classroom settings. They were asked to consider each of the fourteen emotion terms, thinking of a situation in which they experienced that feeling, and then to indicate each of the verbs from the other two lists that reflected the influence of this feeling on (a) their sense of themselves, and (b) their impulses or actions, respectively. Instructions emphasized that there were not right or wrong answers, but that the important thing was to reflect their emotional experience, quickly and spontaneously. For the calculation of differences between the state of love and the other categories of feelings the Wilcoxon test was applied, comparing the number of verbs attributed to particular emotions; significant results therefore indicate that love was associated with more or less self change or change in action tendency relative to the other emotions. Gender differences were checked by the Man Whitney test.

Results

General Changes in the Self

Figures 1 and 2 show that the general change in self provoked by a feeling of love (19.61 for males and 21.22 for females) was higher than changes in self provoked by the rest of analyzed feelings ($p < .01$).

FIGURE 1. THE LEVEL OF GENERAL CHANGE IN THE SELF PROVOKED BY LOVE IN CONTEXT OF OTHER 13 FEELINGS IN A GROUP OF MALES ($N = 60$)

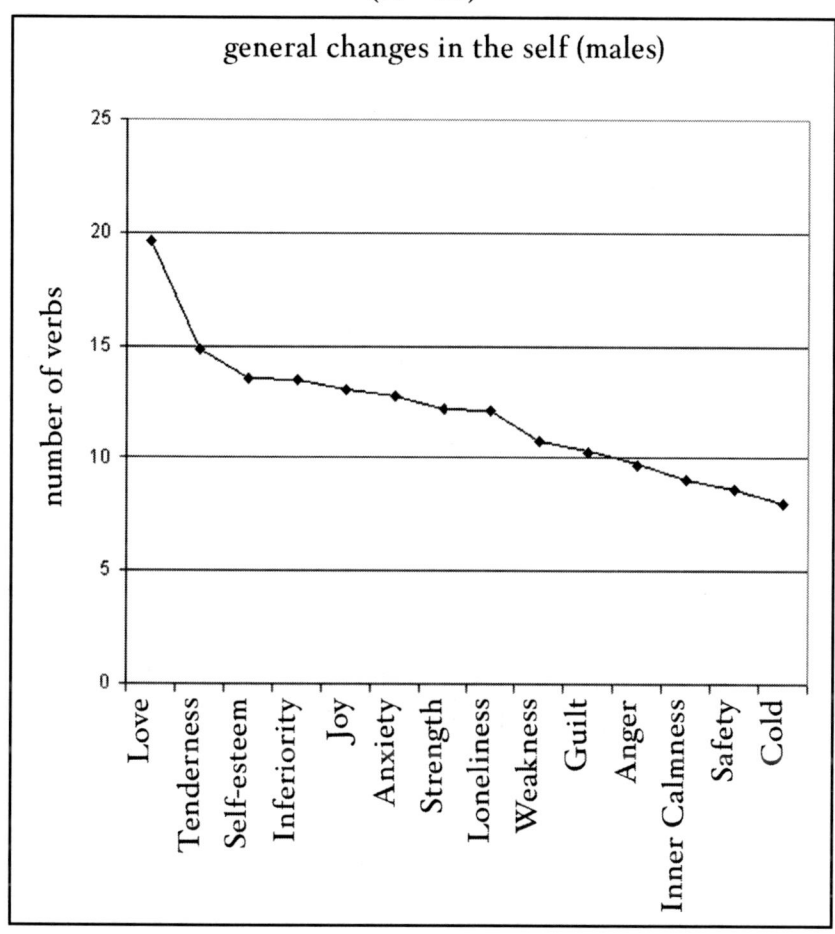

FIGURE 2. THE LEVEL OF GENERAL CHANGE IN THE SELF PROVOKED BY LOVE IN CONTEXT OF 13 OTHER FEELINGS, IN A GROUP OF FEMALES ($N = 60$)

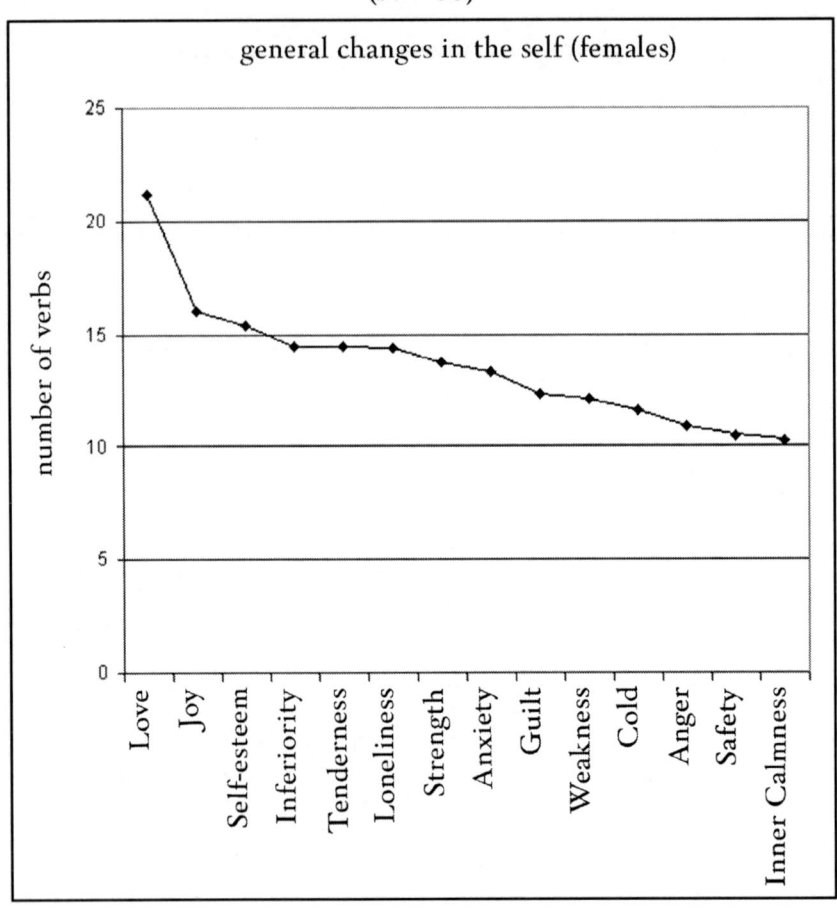

Positive Changes in the Self

Figures 3 and 4 show that love is associated with the highest level of positive change in self for both men and women (14.28 for males and 11.75 for females, $p < 0.01$).

FIGURE 3. POSITIVE CHANGE IN SELF PROVOKED BY LOVE IN A CONTEXT OF 13 OTHER FEELINGS, IN A GROUP OF MALES ($N = 60$)

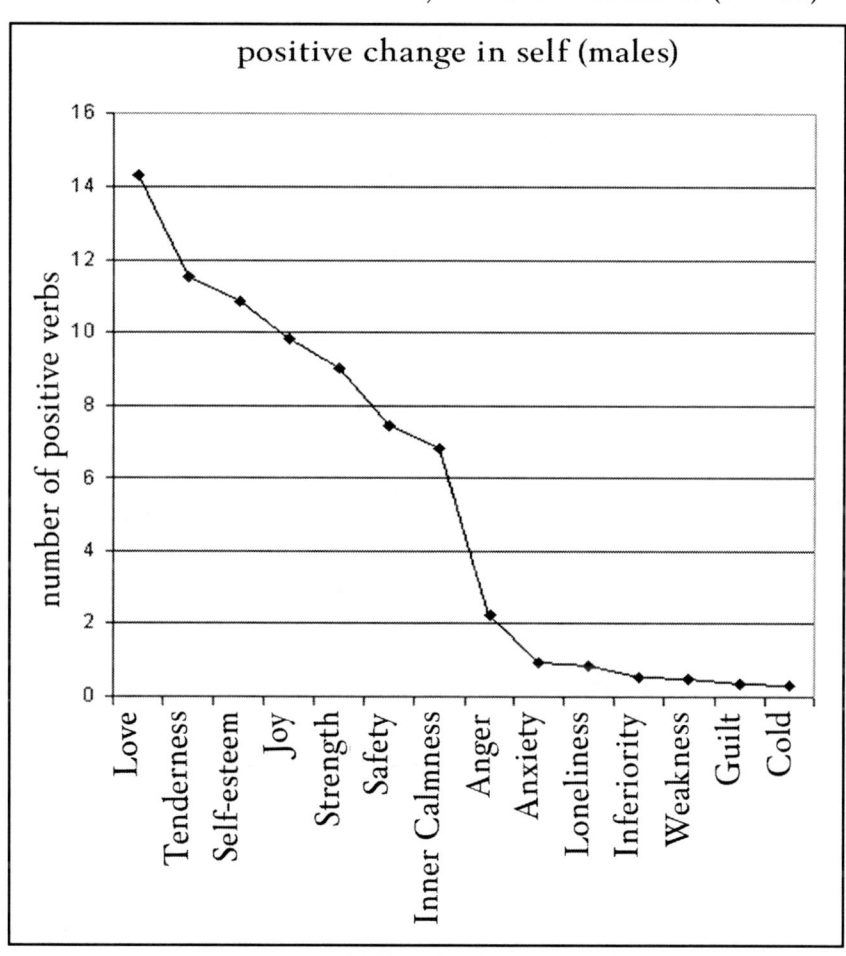

FIGURE 4. POSITIVE CHANGE IN SELF PROVOKED BY LOVE IN A CONTEXT OF 13 OTHER FEELINGS, IN A GROUP OF FEMALES ($N = 60$)

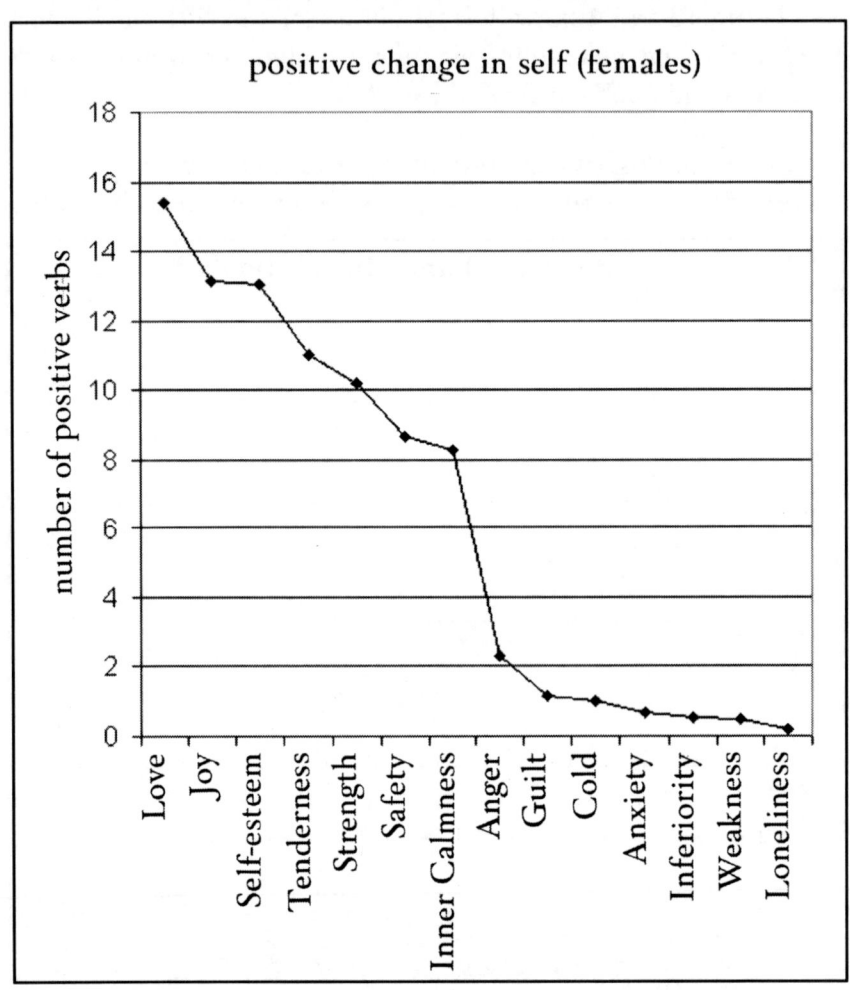

Negative Changes in the Self

Figures 5 and 6 show that negative changes in self provoked by love occurred with low frequency (1.03 for males and 1.38 for females), but that there were feelings that provoked even fewer negative changes in self: self-esteem, safety, tenderness, inner calm and joy ($p < 0.01$).

FIGURE 5. THE LEVEL OF NEGATIVE CHANGE IN SELF FOR 14 CATEGORIES OF FEELINGS FOR MALES ($N = 60$)

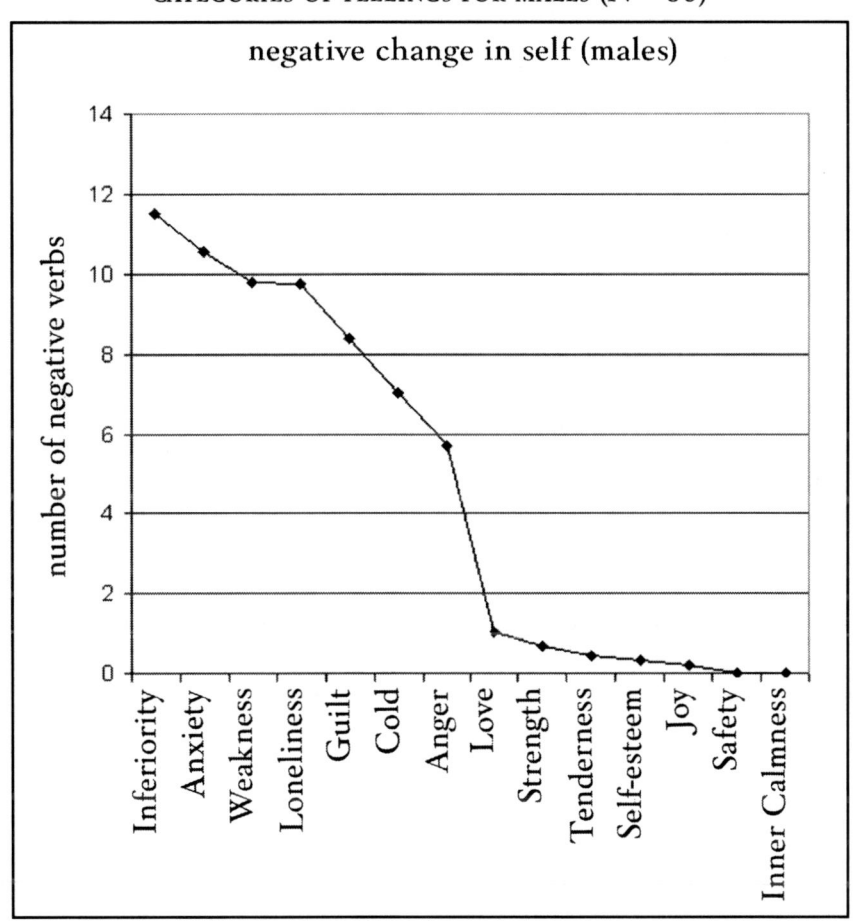

FIGURE 6. THE LEVEL OF NEGATIVE CHANGE IN SELF FOR 14 CATEGORIES OF FEELINGS IN A GROUP OF FEMALES ($N = 60$)

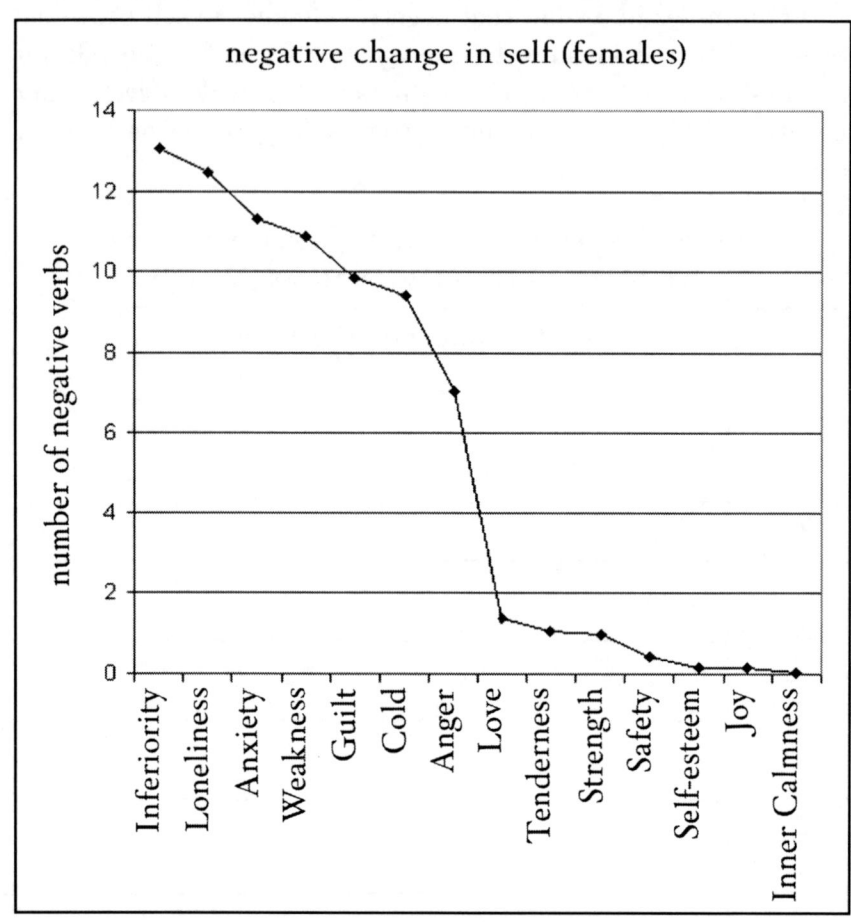

General Action Tendencies

The highest level of general action tendencies was observed for love in both samples (see Figures 7 and 8). For males the average level of action tendencies of love was 12.28 and for females it was 12.18 ($p < 0.01$).

FIGURE 7. GENERAL ACTION TENDENCIES PROVOKED BY LOVE IN A CONTEXT OF 13 OTHER FEELINGS IN A GROUP OF MALES ($N = 60$)

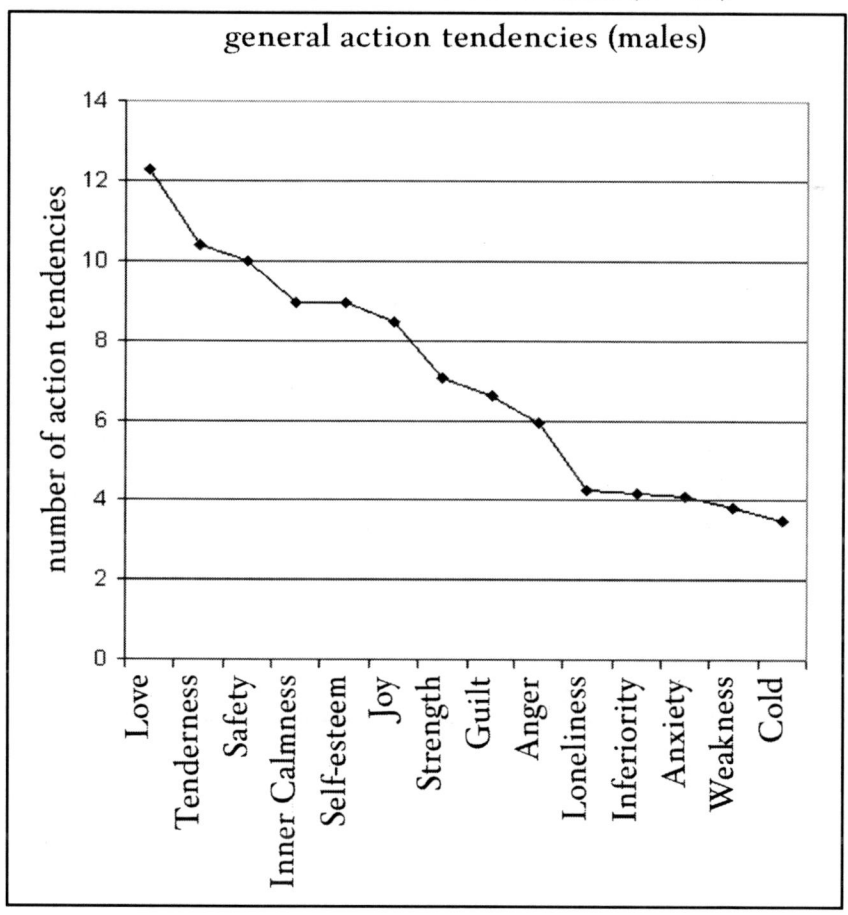

FIGURE 8. GENERAL ACTION TENDENCIES PROVOKED BY LOVE IN A CONTEXT OF 13 OTHER FEELINGS IN A GROUP OF FEMALES ($N = 60$)

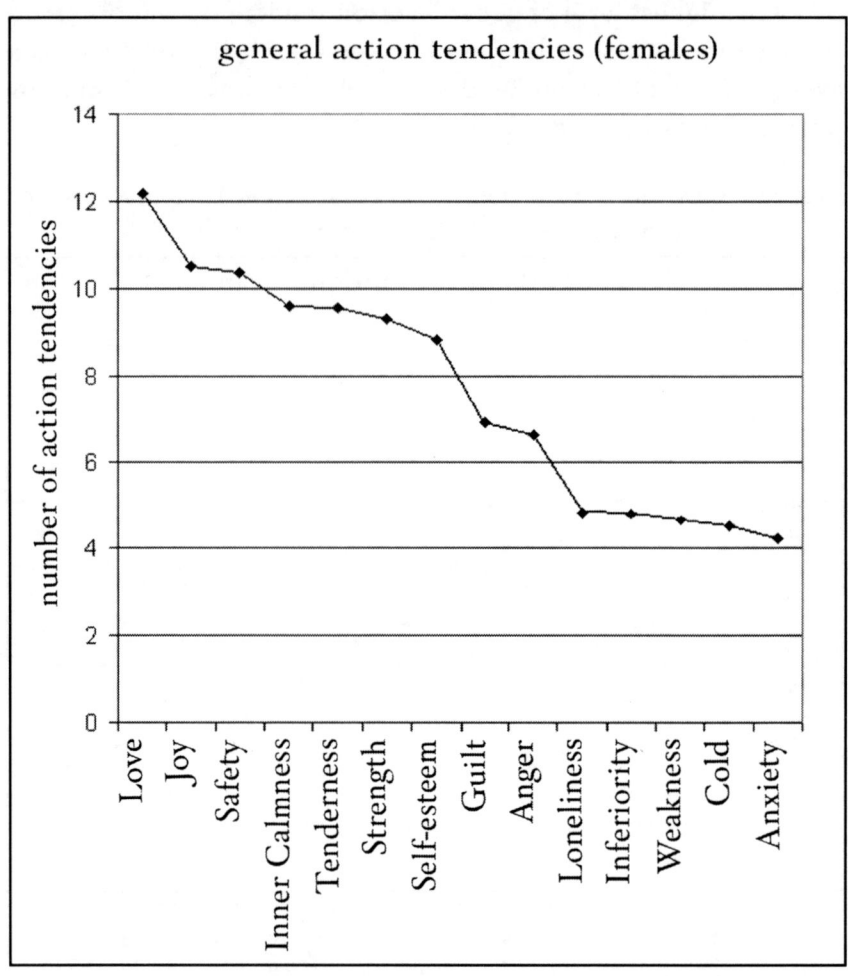

Positive Action Tendencies

The highest level of positive action tendencies was observed for love, in both samples (see Figures 9 and 10). For positive action tendencies provoked by love achieved value 11.75 ($p < 0.01$). By comparison, in females positive action tendencies provoked by love achieved a value of 12. 28 ($p < 0.01$).

FIGURE 9. POSITIVE ACTION TENDENCIES PROVOKED BY LOVE IN A CONTEXT OF 13 OTHER FEELINGS IN A GROUP OF MALES (N = 60)

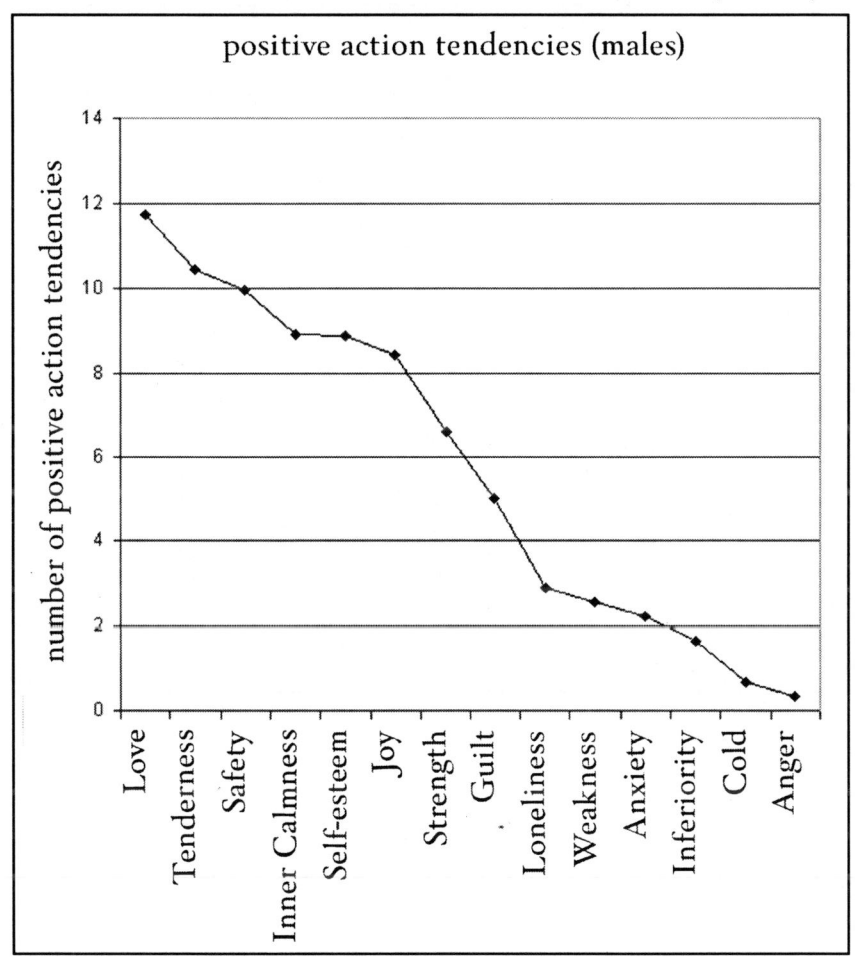

FIGURE 10. POSITIVE ACTION TENDENCIES PROVOKED BY LOVE IN A CONTEXT OF 13 OTHER FEELINGS IN A GROUP OF FEMALES ($N = 60$)

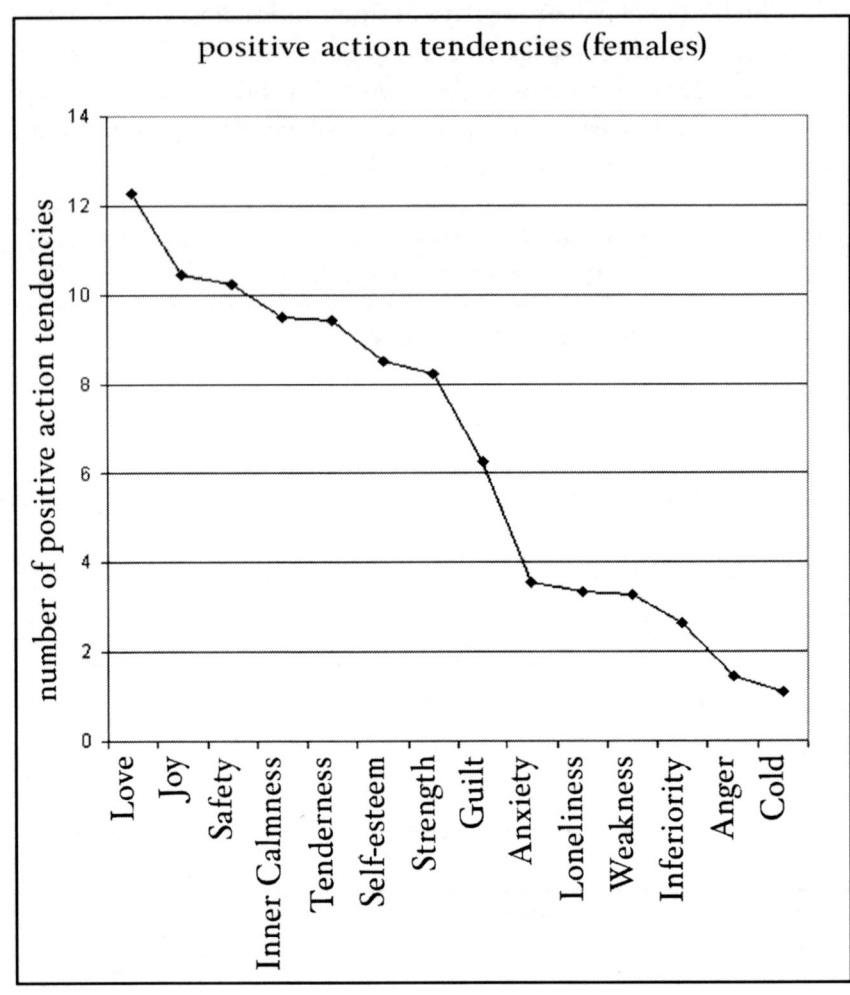

Negative Action Tendencies

Figures 11 and 12 show that love provoked few negative action tendencies together with the following feelings: tenderness, inner calm, safety and joy in both groups, as did self-esteem and strength for men. The highest level of negative action tendencies was observed for anger in both samples.

FIGURE 11. NEGATIVE ACTION TENDENCIES PROVOKED BY LOVE IN A CONTEXT OF 13 OTHER FEELINGS IN A GROUP OF MALES ($N = 60$)

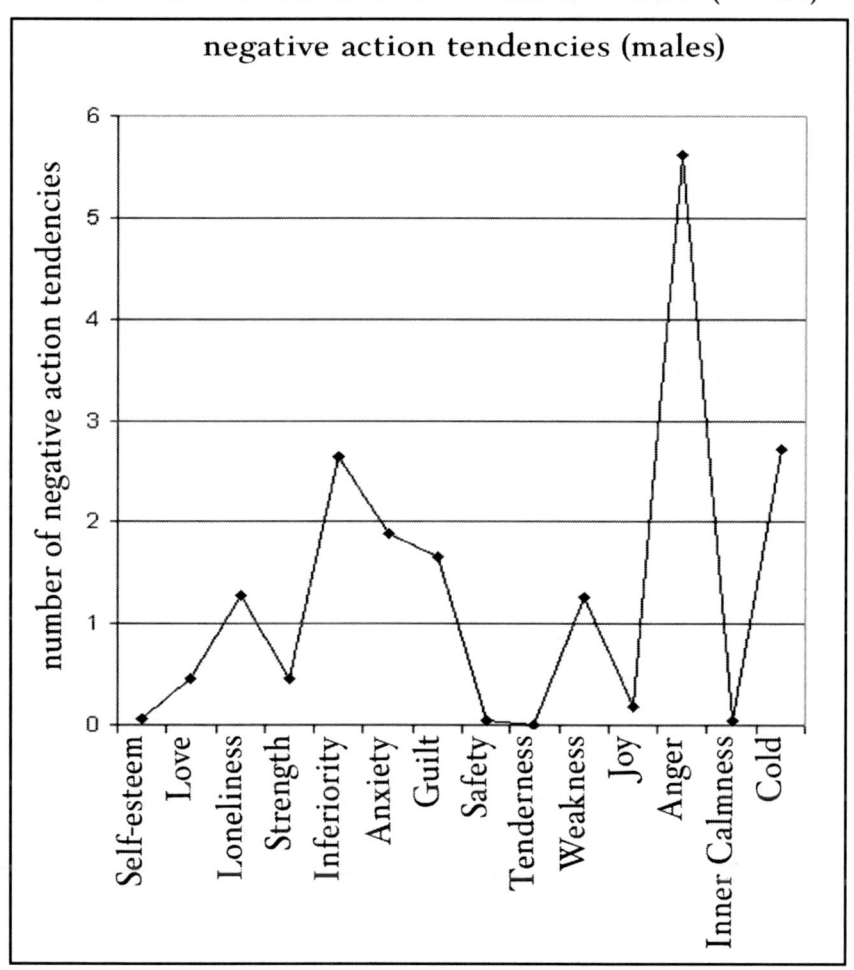

FIGURE 12. NEGATIVE ACTION TENDENCIES PROVOKED BY LOVE IN A CONTEXT OF 13 OTHER FEELINGS IN A GROUP OF FEMALES ($N = 60$)

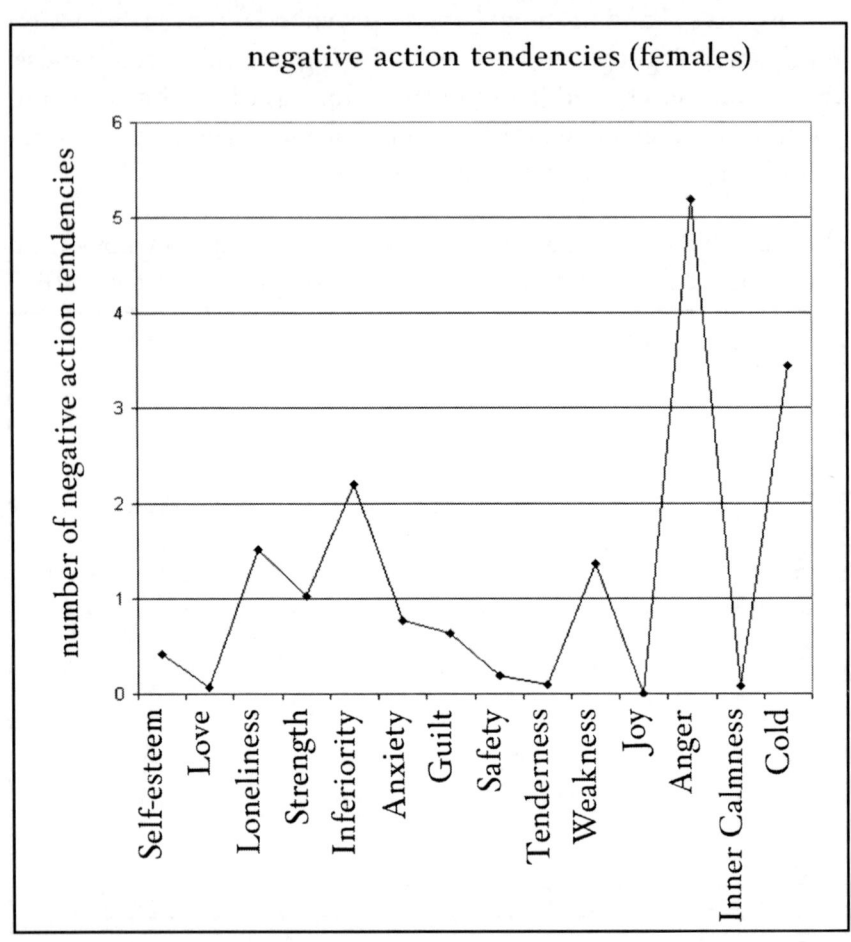

Gender Differences

No gender differences provoked by feelings of love were observed for general, positive and negative changes in either self or action tendencies.

Discussion

As the results of our empirical study show, love provoked the broadest and the most positive change in self-experience and in motivation, an effect that was evident in all categories of verbs (positive, negative and unclassified verbs). This suggests that love can be treated as the most significant factor of change in self-experience (compared with 13 other feelings). These findings are in agreement with Person (1988) who treats love as a crucial factor in inducing self-change. Our results suggest that the self is experienced in a different mode under the influence of love. They confirm the views of several authors who underscore the connections between feelings and the self (e.g. Averill, 1992; Greenberg, 2004; Morgan & Averill, 1992).

Our results strongly implicate love in the process of self-innovation (Hermans, 2003). Averill (1992) stated that love is "reaching out for another" (p. 227), implying that it evokes a metaphorical movement that goes beyond someone's perspective and into the psychological world of the other. Similarly, Buber (1947) noted that "the basic movement of the life of dialogue is turning towards the other" (p.25). The notion of dialogue and love meet each other in the movement towards the other. Basically, real contact with the other requires openness to a different perspective, which potentially provokes new ways of understanding and allows novelty to enter into the dialogue.

The observed changes point to the transformative features of emotions, especially the relevance of the close connection between feelings and self-organization. We suppose that love creates the possibility of innovation of the self as a result of the introduction of new "I" positions (e.g. I as loving, I as loved, the person I love, etc.) and for strengthening other "I" positions (e.g. I as tender, I as a dreamer), each of which could change the organization of the system. Taking into account the positive character of changes provoked by love, such innovation has a very positive meaning for the person. Similarly, Doan (1998) associated love with other positive experiences like joy, peace and contentment and self-development, claiming that love allows people to become "all they are" (Doan, 1998, p. 229).

The observed changes can be also interpreted as changes in self-organization in context of Valuation Theory (Hermans, 1986; Hermans-Jansen, 1995). If we were to treat love as an expression of motive O (longing for union), described by Hermans and Hermans-Jansen (1995), love can evoke a tendency toward unifying not only two persons but also the self.

We further observed that love contrasted with anger, inferiority and fear. According to Ellis and Malamuth (2000), anger and love in close relationships function as a system provoking contrasting behaviors. In our research love evokes the highest number of positive action tendencies and fewest negative ones, anger evokes the opposite, replicating the findings presented by Ellis and Malamuth. At the same time love and anger are not strongly polarized when we consider the changes in the self. Love achieved the highest level of positive change in self while anger did not achieve any extreme value within changes in the self. Remarkably, the feeling of anger provoked more positive change in self than all negative feelings, although it remained more negative than all positive feelings. Thus, we could conclude that in terms of action tendencies love and anger are opposite feelings, but in terms of change in self they are not. Anger provokes some changes in self-experience that were positively evaluated. This is noteworthy because in the psychological literature this feeling has been typically classified as negative. Strongman (1996) concludes that the reason for this classification is that anger is an integral part of aggression, which is negative and undesirable for society. Yet, the subjective experience of anger is not always negative. According to Izard (1991), anger has energizing functions important for fight and can be experienced as positive and adaptive. The results of our research confirm Izard's view showing that the experience of anger has positive aspects in terms of the way the person experiences change in the self following from anger.

An important finding in our study refers to the relationship between love and inferiority. These feelings show opposite features in terms of the change in the self. Whereas the highest positive change in self was observed for love, inferiority was characterized by the lowest level of positive change and highest negative change in the self. An important difference between love and inferiority also was found on the level of action tendencies. Love provoked the highest number of action tendencies while inferiority provoked the fewest. Taking these results together, we assume that positive changes in the self connected with love can increase the motivation of the person, evoking an action readiness to behave in positive ways. People experience themselves in more positive ways and this can be a foundation for increased motivation. Positive change in self-experience reflects a movement in the direction of a more positive self-image, including more self-esteem. In this way love provides a basis for positive self-esteem and self-acceptance.

More speculatively, we might reason that through love, increased self-esteem and self-acceptance serves as a basis for self-love. On the other hand, inferiority is linked with a reverse change in the self, a change in a negative direction. Under the influence of inferiority the self is experienced in more negative way. This negative change in the self decreases motivation. This opposition requires attention to the specific relation between love and inferiority. Doan wrote that people who experience love "realize they are worthy of self-love." (Doan, p. 229). Taking into account the results of our investigation, we conclude that love can be seen as a highly influential change in the self which contrasts with the experience of inferiority. Whereas love promotes positive experience of the self, inferiority implies negative self-experience and self-devaluation. Similarly, the two feelings have an opposite impact on motivation. Whereas love intensifies motivation, inferiority decreases it.

Conclusions

The results of the present study show that two dynamic aspects of emotional experience proposed in our model (change of self and motivation) can be useful for the comparison of love with other feelings. Love has been found to be the factor of the broadest and most positive change in self and motivation. We also noticed that some important aspects of its nature can be further articulated by its comparison with the feelings of inferiority and anger. These feelings, love on the one side, and inferiority and anger on the other, showed the most visible opposite dynamic characteristics. While love seems to function as a movement in the direction of self-innovation and development, leading to increased and positive motivation, inferiority can be seen as a movement into the direction of self-depreciation with a disruptive impact on motivation. At the same time anger can be described as opposite to the motivation provoked by love, as described by the greatest amount of negative action tendencies.

Our investigation can be seen as a first step in the direction of a dialogical conceptualization of love. Dynamic understanding of feelings is a proper basis for further interpretation of transformative features of love in terms of self-theory. Dialogical Self Theory (Hermans, 2000, 2001, 2004), and the concept of self-innovation based on this theory, allow for progress on that path of interpretation. The dialogical self opens the door for an interpretation of feelings as dynamic processes that can be the basis for future empirical studies on the innovative forces emerging from the affective domains of the self. In further investigations the relation between the organization of the system of "I" positions and feelings can be explored. Such a step could contribute significantly to the study of love in terms of dialogical self-theory. We agree with Solomon (1994) who approaches love via self-theory, because love and self seem to be intensely interconnected. For a better understanding of the transformative features of love, we need to look at it from the perspective of a dialogical self theory, because, in order to understand the changes provoked by that universal feeling, we need to study what is going on in the self of a person in relation to the self of another person and vice versa.

REFERENCES

Arnold, M. B. (1960). *Emotion and personality.* New York: Columbia University Press.
Averill, J. R. (1985). The social construction of emotion: With special reference to love. In K. J. Gergen & K. E. Davis (Eds.), *The social construction of the person* (pp. 89-109). New York: Springer.
Averill, J. R. (1992). William James's Other Theory of Emotion. In M. E. Donnelly (Ed.), *Reinterpreting the legacy of William James* (pp. 221-229). Washington, DC: American Psychological Association.
Buber, M. (1947). *Between man and man.* New York: Routledge Classics.
Barrett, L. F., & Russel, J. A. (1998). Independence and bipolarity in the structure of current affect. *Journal of Personality and Social Psychology, 74,* 967-984.
Brebner, J. (2003). Gender and emotions. *Personality and Individual differences, 34,* 387-394.
Brody, L. R., & Hall, J. A. (1993). Gender, emotion and expression. In M. Levis & M. J. Haviland-Jones (Eds.), *Handbook of emotions* (pp. 338-349). New York: Guilford Press.
Doan, R. E. (1998). Interviewing fear and love. Implication for narrative therapy. In M. F., Hyout (Ed.), *The handbook of constructive therapies. Innovative approaches from leading practitioners* (pp. 219-240). San Francisco: Jossey-Bass.
Ellis, B. J., & Malamuth, N. M. (2000). Love and anger in romantic relationships: A discrete systems model. *Journal of Personality, 68,* 525-556.
Feldman, L. A., Barret, L., Russell, J. A. (1998). Independence and bipolarity in the structure of current affect. *Journal of Personality and Social Psychology, 74,* 967-984.
Fredrickson, B. L. (2001). The role of positive emotions in positive psychology: The broaden-and-build theory of positive emotions, *American Psychologist, 56,* 218-226.
Frijda, N. H. (1986). *The emotions.* Cambridge: Cambridge University Press.
Frijda, N. H. (2001). The self and emotions: In H. A. Bosma, & E. S. Kunnen (Eds.), *Identity and emotion. Development through self organization. Studies in emotion and social interaction* (pp. 151-176). New York: Cambridge University Press.

Greenberg, L. S. (2004). Emotion-focused therapy. *Clinical Psychology and Psychotherapy, 11,* 3-16.

Greenberg, L. S., & Johnson, S. M. (1988). Relating process to outcome in marital therapy. *Journal of Marital and Family Therapy, 14,* 175-183.

Hermans, H. J. M. (2001). The dialogical self: Toward a theory of personal and cultural positioning. *Culture & Psychology, 7,* 243-281.

Hermans, H. J. M. (2002). The dialogical self as a society of mind: Introduction. *Theory & Psychology, 12,* 147-160.

Hermans, H. J. M. (2003). The construction and reconstruction of a dialogical self. *Journal of Constructivist Psychology, 16,* 89-130.

Hermans, H. J. M. (2004). The innovation of self narratives. A dialogical approach. In L. E. Angus, & J. McLeod (Eds.), *The Handbook of Narrative and Psychotherapy. Practice, Theory and Research* (pp. 175-191). London: Sage.

Hermans, H. J. M., & Hermans-Jansen, E. (1995). *Self-Narratives: The construction of meaning in psychotherapy.* New York: Guilford Press.

Izard, C. E. (1991). *The psychology of emotions.* New York: Plenum.

Konopka, A. (2006). *Dynamiczne aspekty doświadczenia emocjonalnego i ich osobowościowe uwarunkowania.[Dynamic aspects of emotional experience and their personality determinants]* Unpublished dissertation. University of Cardinal Stephan Wyszyński, Warsaw, Poland.

Larsen, R. J., & Diener, E. (1992). Promises and problems with the circumplex model of emotion. In M. S. Clark (Ed.), *Review of personality and social psychology: Vol. 14. Emotion and social behavior* (pp. 25-59). Newbury Park, CA: Sage.

Lazarus, R. S. (1991). *Emotion and adaptation.* New York: Oxford University.

Magai, C., & McFadden, S. H. (1995). *The role of emotions in social and personality development: History, theory and research.* New York: Plenum Press.

Morgan, C., & Averill, J. R. (1992). True feelings, the self, and authenticity: A psychosocial perspective. In D. D. Franks & V. Gecas (Eds.), *Social perspectives on emotion* (Vol. 1, pp. 95-124). Greenwich, CT: JAI Press.

Norton, D. L., & Kille, M. F. (Eds.). (1989). *Philosophies of love.* Totowa, NJ: Rowman and Allanheld.

Obuchowski, K. (1982). *Kody orientacji i struktura procesów emocjonalnych.[Codes of orientation and the structure of emotional processes].* Warsaw: PWN.

Osgood, C. E. (1966). Dimensionality of the semantic space for comunication via facial expressions. *Scandinavian Journal of Psychology, 7,* 1-30.

Person, E. S. (1988). *Dreams of love and fateful encounters: The power of romantic passion.* New York: W. W. Norton.

Plutchic, R. (1980). *Emotion: A psychoevolutionary synthesis.* New York: Harper & Row.

Plutchic, R. (1997). The Circumplex as a general model of the structure of emotions and personality. In: R. Plutchic & H. R. Conte (Eds.), *Circumplex models of personality and emotions* (pp. 17-46). Washington, DC: American Psychological Association.

Russell, J. A. (1978). Evidence of convergent validity on the dimensions of affect. *Journal of Personality and Social Psychology, 36,* 1152–1168.

Russell, J. A. (1980). A circumplex model of affect. *Journal of Personality and Social Psychology, 39,* 1161-1178.

Salgado, J., & Gonçalves, M. (2007). The dialogical self: Social, personal and (un)conscious. In A. Rosa & J. Valsiner (Eds.), *The Cambridge handbook of socio-cultural psychology* (pp. 608-621). Cambridge, UK: Cambridge University Press.

Solomon, R. C. (1994). *About love.* Lanham, MD: Rowman and Littlefield.

Schlosberg, H. (1954). Three dimensions of emotion. *Psychological Review, 61,* 81-88.

Smith, C. A., & Ellsworth, C. P., (1985). Patterns of cognitive appraisal in emotion. *Journal of Personality and Social Psychology, 48,* 813-838.

Strongman, K. T. (1996). *The psychology of emotion. Theories of emotions in perspective* (4th ed.). New York: Academic Press.

Watson, D., & Tellegen, A. (1985). Toward a consensual structure of mood. *Psychological Bulletin, 98,* 219-235.

⋘ 6 ⋙

Asking and Answering Deconstruction Questions from Within Counseling Dialogues

Tom Strong and Lara Schultz

> *The world does not speak. Only we do. The world can, once we have programmed ourselves with a language, cause us to hold beliefs. But it cannot propose a language for us to speak. Only other human beings can do that.*
>
> Rorty, 1989, p. 6

Well over a generation has passed since the deconstructionists shook academe, highbrow culture, and counseling. Deconstruction even worked its way into the title of a Woody Allen (1997) film. In counseling, narrative therapy (e.g., White & Epston, 1990) and some approaches to psychoanalysis (Spence, 1982), have embraced the linguistic insight that descriptions of reality are not the same as reality itself, nor can they ever be. At odds with centuries of modern science and philosophy (Toulmin, 1990) social constructionism (e.g., Berger & Luckmann, 1967; Gergen, 1999) grew as a critical movement in the later part of the twentieth century. The philosophic footwork for deconstructionists (who see understanding as socially constructed) came with assaults on modernity's notion of universal truth and, for many, put to rest the concept that one could correctly understand experience as it was. Here we shall refer to deconstruction as a practice where linguistic understandings brought to counseling can be temporarily suspended and reflected upon for their aptness (Norris, 1982). Our interest, in this chapter, is to explore how deconstructive practice occurs in consultations between clients and counselors.

Arguably, deconstructive practice in counseling is not new. It refers to how counselors work with clients to contextualize their linguistic understandings so as to specify the origins, examine the effects, and invite reflection on using their understandings. Counselors often ask clients about the understandings they live by as a step toward arriving at more helpful understandings. But, this often also meant counselors offering clients "correct" or "better" understandings from their theoretical and clinical wisdom (e.g., Freud, 1924/1975; Watzlawick, Weakland & Fisch, 1974).

Contemporary deconstructionists differ with others over whether meaning can be correctly put into language. They have not been alone in seeing language as both a resource and a potential problem. Predating social constructionism, Buddhists (e.g., Suzuki, 1956) saw human meaning as mental impositions on the flow of lived experience. Wittgenstein (1958) felt our use of language is tied to *particular* "language games"—as contextualized meanings. Kelly (1955) and subsequent constructivists view meaning as ultimately arising from personal and social attempts to organize experience in terms of personal constructs, whose validation relies at least as much on social consensus as on extralinguistic "reality" (Neimeyer, 1995; 1998, 2008). Bakhtin (1984) saw meaning as "heteroglossic," in how speakers create understandings specific to time and place when trying to be understood. For post-structuralists, like Foucault (1972), language use invokes political loyalties to particular versions of the real and the good competing for cultural and relational acceptance or dominance. Collectively, these thinkers question the taken-for-granted role language plays in constructing any understanding as "real" or "best."

What makes deconstructive conversations particularly interesting as a research phenomenon is that they show counselors and clients actively using language to reflect on understandings possibly modified through their conversational interaction. The presumption is that this is no mere exercise in semantics, as clients' "realities" are at stake as assumed linguistic understandings of experience and unquestioned beliefs are invited for scrutiny. Since this is often a new and possibly challenging experience for clients, looking more closely at how counselors invite and engage clients in deconstructive conversations offers a unique window on how aspects of meaning-making (see Strong, 2003) in counseling occur. What follows are our discursive and retrospective accounts of how some deconstructive conversations took place in single-session lifestyle consultations between social constructionist counselors and clients.

BACKGROUND

Recent forms of "deconstructionist" counseling (e.g., White, 1992) have sparked controversies. Advocating for deconstructionist practice implies that no linguistic account of experience can be considered absolutely *correct*. Such correctness, in discourse terms, relates to how particular communities of speakers use and evaluate language, as is the case for different forms counseling discourse (Danziger, 1997). The discursive issue deconstructionist critiques brought to a head was how *ultimate* descriptions (Habermas, 1988) should be decided.

What might seem a semantic issue takes on a different gravity given concerns raised by Foucault (1972, 2006). Specifically, Foucault equated language use with relationships of power, particularly over what dominates as linguistic representations. Behind different descriptions are different cultural assemblages of understanding, action and human relatedness (Bourdieu, 2003, Deleuze & Guattari, 1987) informing people in their relational projects. For example, how one defines and then acts on a definition of poverty can have widely different consequences. At one Canadian conservative think tank, children's glasses were defined as a "luxury" and thus argued against as a permissible government expense for families receiving government assistance (Williamson & Reutter, 1999). If warranted in policy and community discourse such a definition clearly becomes more than a position in a political argument; it becomes an organizing, if not governing, feature in the lives of those participating in such a discourse.

Why all this matters when considering deconstructive conversations in counseling relates to seeing words and language use as more than a neutral activity. For example, naming a client's problem in moral, medical, legal, or even counseling theoretical terms (e.g., Freudian versus behavioral) invokes more than a description; systematized ways of understanding and acting are mobilized. Of greatest concern for a deconstructionist approach to research or counseling is how some ways of understanding and action dominate or obscure others (Fairclough, 1989; White, 1992). Thus, a "politics of making meaning" (Kogan, 1998) is exemplified in how their meanings are regarded and possibly modified. Witness the difficult conversations families can have over how things are described, understood and talked about (Bar-On, 1999; Ochs & Taylor, 1992). Similarly, deconstructive conversations in counseling have implications beyond the meanings used by clients and counselors in the consulting room.

Deconstructive conversations have as their primary critical thrust the question: why "this" understanding or practice over others? Counseling is often the first opportunity for clients to reflect upon the role that words and language play in articulating problems and solutions. Usually, the word-reality hook-up is an unquestioned matter, and this is also why deconstructive questions can seem so challenging to ask and answer. Such questions invite suspending judgment regarding what people take for granted in using language (Norris, 1982). But such questions also help to identify the particular discourses people use in making sense of experience and acting on "it" (Winslade, 2005). Counselors inviting clients to reflect upon any discursive construction challenge not only clients' senses of reality, but the collective grasp of (or for Rorty, 1989, "solidarity" with) those with whom they share such a discourse.

A colleague (Chris Kinman, personal communication, December 27, 2006) described Jacques Derrida as a Jewish mystic for some of what we have been relating. Like the earlier mentioned Buddhists, the flow and wholeness of life is beyond language for Derrida (1976, 1995), so any contending description of reality achieves the solidity of a word-reality hook-up at the expense of other competing, yet inescapably incomplete, descriptions. Words for Derrida are what humans audaciously impose on experience to make it understandable to themselves and others. But, this comes with huge costs should we commit, knowingly or unknowingly to any description. Leaving things undescribed can also be a problem—words give us "handles" on experience, or "linguistic prostheses" as John Shotter (1993) once described them. Deconstructive questioning can in this sense seem conversationally akin to kicking away a person's crutches. Derrrida's point was not to push people into an abyss of unknowing; it was to see them critically engage with the meanings shaping their experiences and life options.

Little has been written about deconstructive practice in counseling, save for its mention in White and Epston's (1990) approach to narrative therapy. White wrote something close to what we have been saying: "persons' lives are shaped by the meaning that they ascribe to their experience, by their situation in social structures, and by the language practices and cultural practices of self and of relationship that these lives are recruited into" (White, 1992, p. 122). This notion of "recruitment into" suggests interesting conversational "footing" (Goffman, 1979) from which to initiate deconstructive conversations with clients. It implies an unintended and usually unaware process of taking up particular discourses and practices. Given that one's most important language development experiences occur as young children in interaction with adults using *their* language unquestioningly (Vygotsky, 1978), such linguistic recruitment is understandable. Being asked to reflect on "being recruited" into a previously unquestioned language can seem odd at first. Deconstructive conversations try to initiate another recruitment process, but one made more explicitly in how questions are put about language use, and one from which new linguistic alternatives can be considered.

Most descriptions in the counseling literature on deconstruction paint a more benign picture of deconstructive practice than what we have been describing. Clients are depicted as being invited into conversations that expand meanings (Gottlieb & Gottlieb, 1997), or involve poetic processes of meaning-making with counselors (Speedy, 2005; Strong, 2003). Elsewhere the descriptions are more procedural (Freedman & Combs, 1996; White, 1992), or pedagogical as they relate to training counselors (Boston, 2005). But, being a counselor or client inside a dialogue where deconstruction is being proposed, or where the plausibility of such a way of talking is being tested between them, presents pragmatic and other considerations. It is to these considerations, how deconstructive conversations actually occur in single session consultations analogous to counseling, and how they are remembered that we will now turn our attention.

WHERE COUNSELING AND RESEARCH METHODS CAN OVERLAP

Counseling can be seen as a quintessentially social constructionist, or discursive, activity given how understandable realities are discussed, constructed, upheld, or deconstructed within it (McNamee & Gergen, 1992; Miller, 1997). Counseling is also anything but a neutral activity (Eaton, 1998; Parker, 1999). Social constructionist counselors, recognizing this, are mindful not only of the theoretical and other positions they bring to talking with clients (Griffith, & Griffith, 1992; Winslade, 2005) but of how speaking from any position plays out as they talk with clients (Strong, Busch, & Couture, 2008). It is on this latter point that our view and analyses of counseling depart from common depictions in the clinical and research literatures.

Some might see reference to counseling as an activity as a call for process research where particular activities (what Greenberg, 1999, has referred to as little "o" outcomes) can be understood thematically or measured in terms of efficacy (Greeenberg & Pinsof, 1986; Rennie, 1998). This kind of research falls short in accounting for conversational interaction, when contrasted with the methods of discourse analysis (e.g., Wooffitt, 2005) where the focus is on language use in interaction—turn-by-conversational-turn. Bringing this point together with our earlier comments, we see such discursive methods of research as useful in helping to show how the linguistic work of social construction and deconstruction is undertaken and accomplished.

Thus, we join discursive psychologists (e.g., Edwards & Potter, 1992) and discourse analysts (e.g., Ferrara, 1994; ten Have, 1999) to focus on how conversational interactions occur between people, and what results from these interactions. Literally, *what* clients and counselors use and *how* they take their respective turns as they talk and listen can shape their understandings and actions (Heritage, 1984). Too often missing in the clinical or research literature, for us, is the important conversational work that goes on in the seemingly innocuous immediacies of counselor-client interactions. Our social constructionism is microdynamic in focus, finding theoretical compatibilities with the microsociological views of Goffman and Garfinkel. Goffman (1967) would see clients and counselors talking and listening so as to "manage" the course and personal stakes in their dialogues, while Garfinkel (1967) would see both client and counselor practically interpreting each other, to conversationally work out how they will go forward.

Question and answer sequences offer one such juncture to observe how this kind of conversational work occurs—on what Garfinkel (2002) described as "conversation's shop floor." Sequences where deconstructive questions are posed and answers are elaborated should show what counselors and clients use and do, but more importantly should show what results from what they use and do, as they are talking. Discourse analysis in this sense shows what is conversationally accomplished as evidenced in what speakers do with each other's talk. Discourse analysts, heuristically and analytically, take up a point from Wittgenstein (1958); that "nothing is hidden" in what develops between people. In this regard, discourse analysis looks micro-analytically at social interaction for what speakers show each other; or, to borrow again from Garfinkel (2002), to what they make "instructably observable." It is a research method, par excellence, for showing the little "o" outcomes of micro-processes in counseling (Greenberg & Pinsof, 1986; Strong et al, 2007). We turn now to micro-analyzing how deconstructive questions were asked and answered in client-counselor consultations, to shed some light on the conversational pragmatics involved. By also asking clients and counselors to comment on their participation in the same passages our hope is to thicken our understanding of those pragmatics.

Our Research

Six counselors, with graduate training and supervision in social constructionist approaches to counseling, participated in single one-hour consultations that took place at the University of Calgary with twelve volunteer "clients" who sought the hour to discuss lifestyle issues. These *consultations* and follow-ups (referred to by Elliott, 1989, as comprehensive process analyses) were advertised as non-therapeutic in intent, and counselors and clients volunteered knowing they would be asked to review their videotaped participation later with a research assistant. The client participants were a mix of university employees, senior undergraduate or graduate students and members of the general public. Where "clients" raised concerns beyond the scope of the consultation, referrals were made to mental health services. Clients chose the consultation topics (e.g., career contemplation and reflection on relationships) and the counselors brought mutually agreeable closure to their consultations.

As part of a larger study, the videotaped consultations were reviewed for particular passages where, in this case, deconstruction questions were asked or attempted between counselors and "clients." Fifteen videotaped passages met the following criteria:
- The passage demonstrated an effort by the therapist to invite the client to reflect upon the language the client had used in describing some aspect of "the problem."
- The passages usually showed a client responding to such a question in some way.
- The passages showed various ways these question and answer sequences were (or in some cases were not) brought to some kind of resolution between client and counselor.

The selected videotaped passages were analyzed using discourse analyses primarily informed by conversation analysis (CA, ten Have, 1999), a method that focuses on the turn-by-turn words, actions and accomplishments of participants in conversation. CA permits a microanalysis of what transpired in these question-and-answer sequences. To assist with these microanalyses we used the software program "Transana" (Version 2.20) developed for discourse analysts by researchers at the University of Wisconsin, Madison (for website information, see Woods, 2006). This program uses a split-screen format, permitting simultaneous transcription and analyses of digitized audiovisual passages of conversation.

The transcribed micro-details permit an almost slow-motion (to tenths of a second) attention to developments as speakers initiate new courses of conversation or respond to each other. How they include or exclude each other through how they take up, contest, or ignore an immediately prior utterance is a focus of analytic interest. Thus, speakers are seen as talking across a conversational gap as they take turns talking—a fundamental juncture where conversation takes on preferred or "dispreferred" developments for those speaking (Pomerantz, 1984). Client-preferred developments matter to narrative therapists (Freedman & Combs, 1996) for whom collaborative interaction is a primary concern. So, discursive micro-analyses can help account for how posing and answering questions is handled as a collaborative activity.

The Conversations

We microanalyzed fifteen passages where deconstruction questions were asked and answered. The wording and presentation of these questions varied dramatically, but the asking and answering of deconstructive questions generally involved some or all of the following:

1. Counselors welcomed clients' meanings with curiosity. This welcoming curiosity, referred to elsewhere as "not knowing" (Anderson, 1997), involved a deconstructive attitude of suspended judgments and commitments regarding meaning (Norris, 1982). Operationalized, this curiosity was evident in how counselors inquired frequently

about the meanings and understandings clients presented. Some describe this practice as "ethnographic listening" (Hoffman, 2001) for how answers to such questions contextualize understandings for counselors and clients.
2. Building on the previous point, deconstructive questions often asked clients to *locate* particular understandings and meanings to a time and place where the understanding or meaning was considered and accepted as the best account of experience.
3. Deconstructive questions also helped to "unpack" meaning by requesting specific descriptions that invite reflection upon how problems were linguistically constructed (Monk, Winslade, Crockett, & Epston, 1997).
4. First time deconstructive questions were typically asked tentatively, often with a prefacing comment to orient clients to the intent of the question they were to be asked. For example, a counselor might say, "I'd like to get a better understanding of how you came to understand things the way you have" before asking a deconstructive question.
5. First-time answers from clients usually involved more conversational work as clients attempted to show how they had made sense of the questions and how they could speak from within the questions' frames of reference.
6. Once clients and therapists successfully initiated a common deconstructive conversation from asking and answering the first deconstructive question, further deconstructive questioning often occurred to invite clients to critically evaluate prior meanings or actions in light of alternatives passed over.

For us, how deconstructive questions are "packaged" by the counselor is a matter of considerable analytic and clinical interest. Not only are there considerations of what to say, and in what manner, but there are also issues of timing or appropriateness—all of which are based on the counselor's sense of how the client might receive such a question. In a sense, asking a first deconstructive question can be an unusual rhetorical move, an unexpected departure from prior ways of conversing. What goes into a counselor's question packaging, and a client's subsequent response, shows how they manage such rhetorical developments in taking their turns at talking, and how they negotiate their relationship *as they talk* (Roy-Chowdhury, 2006; Sacks, Schegloff, & Jefferson, 1974). To speak of rhetorical moves and packaging might seem unsavory to some counselors. But to discourse analysts these are features of everyday dialogue, things speakers naturally do to stay relevant, respectfully responsive, and understood as they take turns in talking with each other (Sacks, et al, 1974; Pomerantz, 1984). It is precisely for this reason that we see discourse analysis as useful for showing the rhetorical and packaging features of question-and-answer sequences that might otherwise slip under most counselors' conversational radar.

Seen as analyzable dialogic performances, such sequences have much to teach us (Madill, Widdicombe & Barkham, 2001). Most textbooks leave out these relevant performative features of counseling, as if counselors and clients spoke in steady monotones of perfectly grammatical prose. Actual dialogues occur much differently. *How* speakers take their turns at talk, including the ways words are put, where silences occur, and how the conversational floor is shared is quite relevant to those engaged in the immediacies of dialogue. To paraphrase Wittgenstein (1974), sometimes spoken words are places to hang our intentions. Along with discourse analysts and discursive psychologists (e.g., Edwards & Potter, 1992) we consider talk as actions occurring in relationally responsive ways. Questions themselves can be seen as interventions which elicit particular kinds of responses from clients (Tomm, 1988). What matters, from the perspective we have been relating, is how counselors and clients work out their use of words and other features of communication, after the counselor introduces a question. We now turn to see how a deconstructive question was asked and answered. As in all the exemplars to follow, "C" is the client and "T" is the counselor.

Exemplar 1. How does stress come into your life?

```
 1  C  those things
 2  T  Ok {leans back away from client} So why don't you tell me (.) a
 3        little bit more about how stressss (.hhh) {moves hands in a
 4        sideways motion at chest level and then back down to lap} sort of
 5        comes into your life (.3) n wha - what {raises hands and moves
 6        them in an up and down motion at chest level and then lowers them
 7        back to lap} stress ↓causes you (.7) {Head tilt to the left and back
 8        to centre}
 9  C  Umm (.8) Well (.4) jisst genrally I find that(.)like um (.7) come to
10        school an then when I go home
11  T  {nods head forward}
12  C  get really tired (.5) and then I'll try nd sorta ↓u know like eat and
13        whatever
14  T  {nods head forward}
15  C  an play the piano or something then get ↓bac get down to doin
16        work n then (.5 ) as soon as I ↓like (.2) start workin
17  T  {nods head forward and smiles slightly}
18  C  (.3) I'll be like ↑uh {laughs} ↑WELL I DONT WANNA WORK
19        so then {raises hands and moves them in sideways motion at
20        stomach level then lowers them back to lap} I'll jus try n (.2 )do
21        something to get focused again *but I find that I can never like*
22        (1.2) umm (.8) well I eventually do get down to it
23  T  {nods head forward}
24  C  but I think thats juss (1.0) {raises hands and moves them in a
25        sideways motion at stomach level and then lowers them back to
26        lap} th - the timing issue its sort of (.7) like {moves right hand to
27        the right and then back to body} (.7) you *still have a bunch
28        of time* n then (.4) then left with nnn-not as much time and >it
29        becomes more stressful >cuz theress (0.3)<less time to do
30        everything> that I(0.5) wannt to get donnn< (.)sso↓
31  T  Ok{head nod downward}↓ So it: sounds like um stress{raises
32        hands in sideways motions from hips to chest level then back down
33        to hip level} sort of comes into your life and sort of runs
34        interference n: you deal
35        with stress and that eventually↑ [
36  C                                     [Yeah
```

The passage shows an unusual deconstructive invitation, or question, from a counselor to a client to locate a meaning for a phenomenon (stress) and to describe its occurrence, as it relates to the client. When T begins on line 2 to ask his question it is clear he does not simply launch into the question in a straightforward manner. He, instead, shows a departure from prior talk using what are termed "discourse markers" (Schiffrin, 1987); in this case using a verbal ("Ok") and nonverbal marker (leaning back) as ways of signaling that he is about to introduce something new to the flow of their conversation. This gets back to an aspect of "packaging" or recipient design discussed earlier, in this case so that new developments are not responded to as irrelevant or disrespectful non sequiturs. A discourse marker is used to ready a listener for something new; here, to keep T's question from seeming like a blurt from nowhere. Looking at lines 2 through 8 it is clear that T is putting a lot of further effort into packaging his question. Significant gestures are used, and the words spoken have what others have referred to as a "turbulent delivery" (Silverman, 2001). The notion of "use" here generally refers to what the analyst observes, and does not ascribe intentions to the counselor, as in a consciously used "turbulent delivery." Indeed, one of the most useful things about discourse analysis is how it makes evident taken-for-granted features of discourse. One might think T is tongue-tied or effusive until they put themselves in T's position facing C asking a quite unusual question. A downside of the transcription shown is that it looks extraordinarily busy and does not capture adequately the simultaneity of talking and listening. As T is putting his unusual question to C, C is attentively responding to each of T's sequence of utterances that make up the 7 lines shown as constituting the question. How speakers are received as they talk influences what they eventually say, however well formulated the question may have been prior to being posed.

Moving on, what next matters is what C does with T's unusual question on line 9. C's response similarly shows a struggle to find adequate words. This should not be surprising. C has been asked to talk from somewhere that is perhaps new for C to speak from. His full response initially reads like a car sputtering to a start. It should also be noted that the "only" thing T does for the next 22 lines is nod using an acknowledgment token (ten Have, 1999), a form of what some counselors refer to as "encouragers" (Ivey & Bradford Ivey, 1999). We have put inverted commas around "only" because research has clearly shown that narration is a collaborative activity easily derailed in the absence of such encouragers (Bavelas, Coates, & Johnson, 2000). While it takes a bit before C can locate the words and context for how "stress comes into" his life, by line 18 he underscores a potentially key part of his answer by marking what he is about to say with laughter and by then giving added emphasis to some words (WELL I DONT WANNA WORK). This emphasized phrase, a complaint, seems to function as a digression within his account after which the words are more tentative about managing time better, but culminate in line 30 with a phrase similar to the previously emphasized one—this time without such emphasis ("less time to do everything>that I(0.5) wannt to get donnn<").

T and C returned independently to review their participation in the videotaped passage above. C found being asked this question "hard to answer…because it makes you think a lot" at a time when he was mostly focused on having his counselor understand his concern. T was surprised this question was identified by us as a deconstructive question, when he thought of it as an externalizing question. Externalizing questions are used in narrative therapy (e.g., Freedman & Combs, 1996; Strong, 2008) to help elicit a description of concerns as being outside the person. An example in this case might be to shift the problem description from C's concern about "being stressed" to a description of stressors he could be addressing. While we agree that T may have intended to ask an externalizing question, and the question asked may have helped to have seed a later externalizing discussion, from our dialogical (Linell, 2001) perspective what C does with T's question is to locate and unpack "stress." The distinction we make is important both analytically and clinically: what matters with counselor intentions as articulated in particular questions and comments is how clients respond. This is how they show they are practically interpreting counselors' questions and utterances, irrespective of counselor intentions.

Let us now move on to a second deconstructive question and answer sequence.

Exemplar 2: Unpacking "uncertainty"

```
1   C   ...that (.3) {opens clasped hands on lap and then clasps them again} this
2       feeling will influence (.7) my {opens clasped hands on lap and then
3       clasps them again} decisionsss around school
4   T   {nods head forward} OK {raises left hand to shoulder and back down
5       to lap} You sait uncertainty
6   C   {nods head}
7   T   I'mm wondering if {raises right hand to shoulder and moving towards
8       body} you could tell me a bit more about (.6) ↓th-thhat.
9   C   {nods head} Um I guess I find it really scary to be (.6) in debt
10  T   {writes on notepad on lap}
11  C   (1.0) umm {raises eye gaze upwards towards the ceiling} (5.9) I don't
12      know {shakes head slightly} I guess p-pr-probably its like something I
13      learned from my ↑parents
14  T   {nods head forward}
15  C   (.3) you know you just really {unclasps hands and moves them in a
16      downward motion at lap and then reclasps hands} try not to have debt
17      an you know
18      I-I'm {unclasps hands and moves them in a sideways and then
19      downward motion at lap level and then reclasps hands} ok with a
20  T   mortgage but (.2) I think
21  C   and I'm even ok with student loans
22      {nods head forward}
23  T   but {moves left hand up and down side at chest level} this line of credit
24  C   is
25      what has me gettin really nervous an
26      {scratches head} Mmhmm
27      cause A there's aaa top outt {moves left hand in a sideways motion at
28  T   chest level} and how long - I don't know how long I'm going to be able
29  C   to go {moves
```

```
30  T  left hand up and down at chest level then back to lap} before I max that
31  C  outt
32  T  but (.3) I guess just that sense of (2.1)
33  C  {writes on notepad on lap}
       *↓what happens next.* {looks at therapist}
       (hh)
       *↓and then what.* {nods head}
       Mmhmm[
            [yeah{nods head}
```

The passage sees C completing a turn at talk (about "decisions around school"), to which T responds with what in CA is referred to as a "repeat" (Mellinger, 1995). The "repeat" in this case is about "uncertainty" and after acknowledging receipt of C's previous utterance, and marking the start of a new line of talk ("Ok"), T uses the repeat to request C to build on something C has already said—in this case, to unpack "uncertainty." But it is clear that some effort goes into posing and responding to this line of inquiry given the tentativeness involved in T's asking the question (see wording lines 7 and 8) and, more importantly in C's emotional ("really scary") and hesitating (line 11's 5.9 second pause can seem like an eternity when counseling) response. Silverman (2001) described such passages as showing speakers "constructing delicate objects" between them, and that some of this had to do with the moral nature of the topic discussed (in this case, C's contemplating going further into debt). Once C gets a start on this topic, however, she needs only a few strategically placed acknowledgments from T (note the specific words preceding T's head nods) to elaborate in ways that feature embedded rhetorical questions (e.g., line 11's "I don't know"). Rhetorical questions of this nature have been described by Koshik (2005) as useful in implicitly informing others about complaints about or challenges faced with absent parties (e.g., C's parents). These can be seen as invitations for T to join her in different lines of inquiry; for example, about how long C will be able to go before she "maxes out," or about "then what?" The passage concludes with C's "yeah," a decision we made in presenting this passage to you given that T followed up with a somewhat unrelated question.

In asking C to later review this passage, she commented that T's asking the question made her feel "very heard" for helping her explore "more about where I am getting those messages about debt." C sounds like a deconstructionist for saying this. Narrative therapists see locating social and cultural messages—those informing understandings constructed to describe any problem—as important in creating conversational space for alternative understandings (Freedman & Combs, 1996). C continued, "it was really useful in terms of deepening the meaning for me and yeh, I really felt like I was gaining ... little ways of thinking about the issue that I hadn't thought about before." For T, what stood out was that, not only was the question about "uncertainty" but that both of them, prior to and during the initial phase of talking about "uncertainty," spoke in quite uncertain ways. This kind of synchrony of what is talked about, semantic subject (uncertainty) and how the subject is talked about (uncertainly) can be an interesting feature of dialogue as it is *performed* by speakers. Speakers need not only coordinate their semantic understandings but their ways of talking as well, and in some respects T's question joined C's uncertainty by inquiring about it. This notion of counselors joining *how* clients talk as part of the conversational change process was recently reviewed in an examination of the conversational practices of renowned family therapist, Karl Tomm (Strong & Tomm, 2007). T sounded a lot like C when he responded that deconstructive questions "really increase the chance of... making some understanding, shared understanding."

The final exemplar looks anything but the kind of deconstructive question one associates with narrative therapy (e.g., White, 1992). For the sake of space, we will not report on the retrospective comments from the client and counselor involved. We chose the passage mainly because the counselor explores with the client cultural and social messages as they pertain to client's concerns. But this passage features good therapeutic discourse as Ferrara (1994) identified it: it shows an "interweave" of client and counselor words and ways of talking.

EXEMPLAR 3: SEPARATING WHAT "YOU" THINK FROM WHAT OTHERS THINK ABOUT BEING ALONE

1	T	{moves left hand from back of neck to hip level} (hhh)um {raises right hand to
2		chest level and moves hand slightly toward F} to you *alone* means something
3		very different (.2) to uh your sister and maybe
4	C	{nods head}
5	T	to (.) uh {moves hands in a circular motion} I think our culture sort of talks
6		about um::↓ (.6) you know social
7	C	{clasps hands on lap}
8	T	(.6) butterflies as the normal *thin* to aspire to right↑ [
9	C	[Mmhmm {nods head}
10	T	[when theres a lots of people in our society who value (.5) in-inn {moves hands
11		in up and down motion at chest level} *that alone [time*[
12	C	[mmhmm[{nods head}
13	T	[and think itz (.9) um [
14	C	[oh yeah {nods head}
15	T	a very positive thing↑ and you {gestures with open right hand towards R} might
16		be one of those people↑
17	C	{nods head and upper body forward}I know I am {laughs}
18		Yeah↑ {looks upward towards the ceiling} I-I {unclasps hands on lap and fidgets
19		with hands} think I am↑, I just (1.8) I don I-I mean I know {looks upward
20		towards the ceiling} therez other issues related to that↓ theres theres not wanting
21		{moves upper body and hands to the right and back to centre} to be hurt↑ an *so
22		you know I kinda isolated {moves open hands down towards lap} [myself from
23		people and*↑[
24	T	[well you know I wonder
25	C	{nods head and shifts body in chair}
26	T	I wonder about (.4) um that's kind of whatz fueling your sisters thinking about
27		al[
28	C	[mmhmm {nods head}
29	T	it-its you um (.6) not wanting to be hurt {moves right hand towards R and back}
30	C	{nods head}(hh)
31	T	or you um not wanting to reach out {moves right hand towards R at chest level}
32		but thats not true because you tol {moves right hand back to lap} jus told me you
33		wan to reach out an stay connected but you wan to balance
34	C	{nods head}
35	T	that with alone time becuz you value it *for yourself*↓
36	C	(hhh) {looks up towards the ceiling} yeah
37	T	mmkay
38	C	an-an-an but my { moves hands in an alternating up and down motion} balance I

```
39        mean whats (.) whats comfortable=my comfort zone is probably (.4) quite a
40        different um:: (.6) level than (.2) maybe somebody else {moves hands to lap}
41   T    mmhm
42   C    and-an I think as I get older (1.3) I don't (2.3) I don't know that I cou=I don't
43        know that I could {places open hands on clavicle} um be as {lowers
44        hands to chest level} she would like me to be and just an go out {moves hands
45        away to the right} with them once a week to the to the pub an listen to music
46        {moves right hand up and down and then reclasps hands at chest level} and drink
47        an-and an then go off {moves left hand in a jerky downward motion and then
48        back to lap} and do other things (.) every night I-I just (.6) {shakes head} I-I just
49   T    are you ok with that↑
50   C    yeah↑
51   T    great {smiles and laughs and nods head}
52   C    {nods head slightly} yeah↑ I mean {looks towards ceiling and puts hands
53        underneath her legs on the chair} the little bit when I go out with the girls↑ its
54   T    its {looks down towards the floor} enough right now↑
55   C    right
56   T    an its littler,(.2) yeah[
57   C                         [yeah[
58   T                              [yeah
59   C    (.2)So its smaller and[
60   T                          [(head nod)mm-hmmm
61   C    and ah(.3) you already were buffered↓ you knew it was there and if it wasn't
62        going to go away but[
63   T                        [mm-hmm[
64   C                               [That's when I got this curio:s thing abut (.) God
65        >Iwonder if this will become actually useful to you some day<[
66   T                                                                [yeah () yeah,
67   C    and I think what was really useful tooo was that tha::t buffer that I have (.4)
68   T    Tha::t↑ hasn't gone[
69   C                       [Right↓ (nodding head)
```

Looking at this lengthy passage closely, what launches it is T's (the counselor's) "*alone* means something very different" comment. This is expanded on in later T's comments regarding cultural messages that one must aspire to be a "social butterfly." C gives her the go ahead with acknowledgment tokens up to where T, on lines 15 and 16, asks teasingly, "you might be one of those people" (note that transcription shows upward arrows to denote the normal rising inflection ↑ associated with asking questions). As with earlier passages we have examined, the invitation implicit in C's question, while "taken up" by T, is responded to in ways that denote some effort in putting words to the line 17-23 initial answer. Such "uptake" (ten Have, 1999) is important to discourse analysts who see this as evidence that conversational partners are staying collaborative (Clark, 1996) in how they take their turns at talking. C could, for example, have changed to an entirely different topic. C's answer itself offers potentially rich material worthy of further discussion ("therez other issues related to that ↓ theres theres not wanting ...to be hurt ↑ an *so you know I kinda isolated ...myself from people"). T, on line 26, joins C's answer but narrows down the focus by "wondering" about what C's sister might think on the topic, another example of Koshik's (2005) rhetorical questions that solicit one's conversational partner's views of what absent (but relevant) parties might think. T uses "repeats" (Mellinger, 1995) here as well to link what C earlier said to how her sister might regard what is said. This relates to a common narrative therapy practice known as "audiencing" (Monk et al, 1997) where clients are invited to imaginatively place what is being discussed in relational context. This is to gauge how the discussion topic would be received and how it also can be used as a step toward inviting clients to contest or negotiate others' possible negative receipt of the topic. The effect of C's focus on the sister is evident in how T differentiates her own views from those of her sister (see line 54: "its enough right now"), again in somewhat halting language. This is partly what we meant earlier when we indicated that a second phase of deconstructive questioning can help clients choose preferred meanings—a topic worthy of further examination itself. Lines 56 through 64 show a rapid fire synchrony between C and T with their latching ("[") "yeahs." Of particular interest are the lines 65 through 69 where T uses another "wondering" question related to the position just elicited from C. C's response is a quick "yeah, yeah," followed by her citing the usefulness of her "buffer"—a word introduced earlier by T. This illustrates Ferrara's (1994) notion of discursive interweave (use of shared words) and "uptake." T further checks in on the usability of the "buffer" ("that hasn't gone"), to which C responds with an affirmative head nod and "right."

CONCLUSIONS

When there is no access to one's own personal "ultimate" word, then every thought, feeling, experience must be refracted through the medium of someone else's discourse, someone else's style, someone else's manner, with which it cannot immediately be merged without reservation, without distance, without refraction. (Bakhtin, 1984, p. 202)

Our focus has been to show deconstruction as a dialogic practice that could occur in many aspects of counseling, as conversational work by counselors in initiating back and forth dialogue with clients to bring resolution to problem understandings. So, our aim here has been to show deconstructive dialogues as they actually occurred between counselors and clients and, in a couple of cases, to hear back from them about what being engaged in such dialogues was like. The Bakhtin quote above fits our view that deconstructive conversations are about locating one's understandings in others' words and discourses that can never ultimately capture experience.

Three passages of deconstructive dialogue can scarcely capture the diverse ways counselors and clients take part in such dialogues. This was not our intent. Instead, our aim has been to invite readers to "step inside" a few of these dialogues to gain a sense of some of the pragmatic and conceptual issues involved when engaging in deconstructive dialogues. The passages shown offered variations on the kinds of deconstructive questions identified in books explicating narrative therapy (e.g., Freedman & Combs, 1996, White & Epston, 1990). This brings us back to a point made in the first exemplar, about how counselors may intend and even accurately ask questions as depicted in such books. What matters, however, is how clients answer their questions—sometime clients might answer an externalizing question with a deconstructive answer. It would be interesting to micro-analyze questions master counselors, like Michael White, ask for what clients do with what they ask (see Kogan & Gale, 1997 for this kind of analysis). We chose instead to focus on how some deconstructive dialogues—via questions and answers—took place in single-hour consultations between counselors and clients who discussed concerns that were intentionally not of clinical severity (for more discourse analyses of this kind check out Ferrara, 1994; Couture, 2005, or Hutchby, 2007).

We have similarly not tried to be exhaustive in our discourse analyses (Wooffitt, 2005). Discourse analysis is a well established and diverse research tradition where one finds a rich literature examining many facets of dialogue we had no space to get into here. What we bring from discourse analysis is a sense of how the largely taken for granted conversational work of counseling occurs around a specific practice (here, deconstruction). We see deconstructive questions as invitations counselors make to clients to join a particular style of discourse.

The clients we spoke to in this research noted that being asked to locate or unpack (our words) their understandings was useful in coming up with other ways of understanding, but that the questions could be very hard to answer. In each of the three exemplars shown, deconstructive dialogues elicited rich material and it was clear that more was involved than simply answering a crisp deconstructive question. Counselors played an important role, through acknowledgments and further questions, in helping clients deconstruct prior understandings and elaborate new understandings in their place. Sometimes the new understandings offered improvements that clients could use in fashioning new evaluations or courses of actions. But each dialogue also achieved what Norris (1982) described as suspending one's prior understandings so to reflect upon them and consider alternatives. Going into such conversational places of unknowing requires something akin to midwifery skills (i.e., giving dialogic birth to new language), except as this applies to being a good discursively informed listener: ready to invite and join clients in contesting prior inadequate language and beliefs while putting language to previously unarticulated experiences (Weingarten, 1995). Doing all this inside a dialogue that is unfolding partly as a result of one's participation is part of the conversational work we have tried to make more evident here.

REFERENCES

Allen, W. (1997). *Deconstructing Harry* (film). New York: Jean Doumanian Productions.

Anderson, H. (1997). *Conversation, language and possibilities.* New York: Basic Books.

Bakhtin, M. (1984). *Problems of Dostoevsky's poetics.* (C. Emerson, Trans. & Ed.) Minneapolis, MN: University of Minnesota Press.

Bar-On, D. (1999). *The indescribable and the undiscussable: Reconstructing human discourse after trauma.* Budapest: Central European University Press.

Bavelas, J. B., Coates, L., & Johnston, T. (2000). Listeners as co-narrators. *Journal of Personality and Social Psychology, 79,* 941-952.

Berger, P., & Luckmann, T. (1967). *The social construction of reality.* New York: Doubleday.

Boston, P. (2005). Doing deconstruction. *Journal of Family Therapy, 27,* 272-275.

Bourdieu, P. (2003). *Language and symbolic power* (J. B. Thompson, Ed; G. Raymond & M. Adamson, Trans.). Cambridge, MA: Harvard University Press.

Clark, H. H. (1996). *Using language.* Cambridge, UK: Cambridge University Press.

Couture, S. (2005). *Moving forward: Therapy with an adolescent and his family.* Unpublished doctoral dissertation, University of Calgary, Alberta.

Danziger, K. (1997). *Naming the mind: How psychology found its language.* London: Sage.

Deleuze, G., & Guattari, F. (1987). *A thousand plateaus: Capitalism and schizophrenia* (B. Massumi, Trans.). Minneapolis, MN: University of Minnesota Press.

Derrida, J. (1976). *Of grammatology.* (G. C. Spivak, Trans.). Baltimore: Johns Hopkins Press.

Derrida, J. (1995). *Points...: Interviews, 1974-1994* (E. Weber, Ed.; P. Kamuf, Trans.). Stanford, CA: Stanford University Press.

Eaton, J. (2002). Psychotherapy and moral inquiry. *Theory & Psychology, 12,* 367-386.

Edwards, D., & Potter, J. (1992). *Discursive psychology.* London: Sage.

Elliott, R. (1989). Comprehensive Process Analysis: Understanding the change process in significant therapy events. In: M. Packer. & R. B. Addison (Eds.), *Entering the circle: Hermeneutic investigation in psychology* (pp. 165-184). Albany, NY: SUNY Press.

Epston, D. (1993). Internalizing discourses versus externalizing discourses. In: S. Gilligan & R. Price (Eds.). *Therapeutic conversations* (pp. 161-177). New York: Norton.

Ferrara, K. (1994). *Therapeutic ways with words.* New York: Oxford University Press.

Fairclough, N. (1989). *Language and power.* New York: Longman.

Foucault, M. (1972). *The archaeology of knowledge and the discourse on language* (A. M. Sheridan, Trans.). New York: Pantheon.

Foucault, M. (2000). *Power* (J. D. Faubion, Ed.; R. Hurley, Trans.). New York: The New Press.

Freedman, J., & Combs, G. (1996). *Narrative therapy: The social construction of preferred realities.* New York: Norton.

Freud, S. (1975). *A general introduction to psychoanalysis* (J. Riviere, Ed. & Trans.). New York: Pocket Books. (Original work published in 1924).

Garfinkel, H. (2002). *Ethnomethodology's program: Working out Durkheim's aphorism* (A. Rawls, Ed.). Lanham, MD: Rowan & Littlefield.

Gergen, K. J. (1999). *An invitation to social construction.* London: Sage.

Goffman, E. (1967). *The interaction order.* New York: Pantheon.

Goffman, E. (1979). Footing. *Semiotica, 25,* 1-25.

Gottlieb, D. T., & Gottlieb, C. D. (1996). The narrative/collaborative process in couples therapy: A postmodern perspective. *Women and Therapy, 19*(3), 37-47.

Greenberg, L. S. (1999). Ideal psychotherapy research: A study of significant change processes. *Journal of Clinical Psychology, 55,* 1467–1480.

Greenberg, L. S., & Pinsof, W. M. (1986). Process research: Current trends and future perspectives. In: L. S. Greenberg & W. M. Pinsof (Eds.), *The psychotherapeutic process: A research handbook* (pp. 3-20). New York: Guilford.

Griffith, J., & Griffith, M. E. (1992). Owning one's epistemological stance in therapy. *Dulwich Centre Newsletter, 1,* 11-20.

Habermas, J. (1988). *Legitimation crisis.* Oxford: Polity.

Have, P. ten (1999). *Doing conversation analysis.* Thousand Oaks, CA: Sage.

Heritage, J. (1984). *Garfinkel and ethnomethodology.* New York: Polity.

Hoffman, L. (2001). *Family therapy: An intimate history.* New York: Norton.

Hutchby, I. (2007). *The discourse of child counseling.* Philadelphia: John Benjamins.

Ivey, A. E., & Bradford Ivey, M. (1999). *Intentional interviewing and counseling: Facilitating client development in a multicultural society* (4th ed.). Pacific Grove, CA: Brooks/Cole.

Kelly, G. A. (1955). *The psychology of personal constructs.* New York: Norton.

Kogan, S. (1998). The politics of making meaning: Discourse analysis of a "postmodern" interview. *Journal of Family Therapy, 20,* 229-251.

Kogan, S. M., & Gale, J. E. (1997). Decentering therapy: Textual analysis of a narrative therapy session. *Family Process, 36,* 101-126.

Koshik, I. (2005). *Rhetorical questions: Assertive questions in everyday interactions.* Philadelphia: John Benjamins.

Linell, P. (2001). *Approaching dialogue.* Philadelphia: John Benjamins.

Madill, A., Widdicombe, S., & Barkham, M. (2001). The potential of conversation analysis for psychotherapy research. *The Counseling Psychologist, 29,* 413-434.

McNamee, S., & Gergen, K. J. (Eds.) (1992). *Therapy as social construction.* London: Sage.

Miller, G. (1997). *Becoming miracle workers: Language and meaning in brief therapy.* New Brunswick, NJ: Transaction Publishers.

Mellinger, W. M. (1995). Talk, power and professionals: Partial repeats as challenges in the psychiatric interview. In J. Siegfried (Ed.), *Therapeutic and everyday discourse as behavior change: Toward a microanalysis in psychotherapy process research* (pp. 391-418). Norwood, NJ: Ablex:

Monk, G., Winslade, J., Crockett, K., & Epston, D. (Eds.) (1997). *Narrative therapy in practice: The archaeology of hope.* San Francisco: Jossey-Bass.

Neimeyer, R. A. (1995). Constructivist psychotherapies: Features, foundations, and future directions. In R. A. Neimeyer & M. J. Mahoney (Eds.), *Constructivism in psychotherapy.* (pp. 11-38). Washington: American Psychological Association.

Neimeyer, R. A. (1998). Social constructionism in the counseling context. *Counseling Psychology Quarterly, 11,* 135-149.

Neimeyer, R. A. (2008). *Constructivist psychotherapy: Distinctive features.* London: Routledge.

Norris, C. (1982). *Deconstruction: Theory and practice.* New York: Methuen and Company.

Ochs, E, & Taylor, C. (1992). Family narrative as political activity. *Discourse & Society, 3,* 301-340.

Parker, I. (Ed.) (1999). *Deconstructing psychotherapy.* New York: Routledge.

Pomerantz, A. M. (1984). Agreeing and disagreeing with assessments: Some features of preferred/dispreferred turn shapes. In: J. M. Atkinson & J. Heritage (Eds.), *Structures of social action: Studies in conversation analysis* (pp. 57-101). Cambridge: Cambridge University Press.

Rennie, D. (1998). *Person-centered counseling: An experiential approach.* London: Sage.

Rorty, R. (1989). *Contingency, irony, and solidarity.* New York: Cambridge University Press.

Roy-Chowdhury, S. (2006). How is the therapeutic relationship talked into being? *Journal of Family Therapy, 28,* 153-174.

Sacks, H., Schegloff, E., & Jefferson, G. (1974). A simplest systematics for the organization of turn-taking for conversation. *Language, 50,* 696-735.

Schiffrin, D. (1987). *Discourse markers.* New York: Cambridge University Press.

Silverman, D. (2001). The construction of "delicate" objects in therapy. In: M. Wetherell, S. Taylor, & S. J. Yates (Eds.). *Discourse theory and practice:A reader* (pp. 119-137). London: Sage.

Speedy, J. (2005). Using poetic documents: An exploration of poststructuralist ideas and poetic practices in narrative therapy. *British Journal of Guidance and Counseling, 33,* 283-298.

Spence, D. (1982). *Narrative truth and historical truth. Meaning and interpretation in psychoanalysis.* New York: Norton.

Strong, T. (2008). Externalizing questions: A microanalytic look at their use in narrative therapy. International *Journal of Narrative Therapy and Community Work,* (Issue 3), 59-71.

Strong, T. (2003). Getting curious about meaning-making in counseling. *British Journal of Guidance and Counseling, 31,* 259-273.

Strong, T., Busch, R. S., & Couture, S. (2008). Conversational evidence in therapeutic dialogue. *Journal of Marital and Family Therapy, 34,* 388-405.

Strong, T., & Tomm, K. (2007). Family therapy as re-coordinating and moving on together. *Journal of Systemic Therapies, 26*(2), 42-54.

Suzuki, D. T. (1956). *Zen Buddhism: Selected writings of D. T. Suzuki* (W. Barrett, Ed.). New York: Doubleday Anchor.

Tomm, K. (1988) Interventive interviewing. Part III. Intending to ask lineal, circular, strategic or reflexive questions. *Family Process, 27,* 1-15.

Toulmin, S. (1990). *Cosmopolis: The hidden agenda of modernity.* Chicago: University of Chicago Press.

Vygotsky, L. S. (1978). *Mind in society: The development of higher psychological processes.* (M. Cole, Ed.) Cambridge, MA: Harvard University Press.

Watzlawick, P., Weakland, J., & Fisch, R. (1974). *Change: Principles of problem formation and problem resolution.* New York: Norton.

Weingarten, K. (1995). Radical listening: Challenging cultural beliefs for and about mothers. *Journal of Feminist Family Therapy, 7*(1/2), 7-22.

White, M. (1992). Deconstruction and therapy. In D. Epston & M. White (Eds.), *Experience, contradiction, narrative & imagination: Selected papers of David Epston & Michael White* (pp. 109-151). Adelaide, South Australia: Dulwich Centre Publications.

White, M., & Epston, D. (1990). *Narrative means to therapeutic ends.* New York: Norton.

Williamson, D. L., & Reutter, L. (1999). Defining and measuring poverty: Implications for the health of Canadians. *Health Promotion International, 14,* 355-364.

Winslade, J. M. (2005). Utilising discursive positioning in counselling. *British Journal of Guidance and Counseling, 33*(3), 351-364.

Wittgenstein, L. (1958). *Philosophical Investigations* (3rd ed., G.E.M. Anscombe, Trans.). New York: Macmillan.

Wittgenstein, L. (1974). *Philosophical grammar* (R. Rhees, Ed.; A. Kenny, Trans.). Los Angeles: University of California Press.

Woods, D. (2007). Transana (Version 2.20). Retrieved from: http://www.transana.org/

Wooffitt, R. (2005). *Conversation analysis and discourse analysis.* London: Sage.

APPENDIX

Transcription Notation

Symbol	Indicates
(.)	A pause which is noticeable but too short to measure.
(.5)	A pause timed in tenths of a second.
=	There is no discernible pause between the end of a speaker's utterance and the start of the next utterance
:	One or more colons indicate an extension of the preceding vowel sound.
Underline	Underlining indicates words that were uttered with added emphasis.
CAPITAL	Words in capitals are uttered louder than surrounding talk.
(.hhh)	Exhalation of breath; number of h's indicate length.
(hhh)	Inhalation of breath; number of h's indicates length.
( )	Indicates a back-channel comment or sound from previous speaker that does not interrupt the present turn.
[	Overlap of talk.
(( ))	Double parenthesis indicate clarificatory information, e.g. ((laughter)).
?	Indicates rising inflection.
!	Indicates animated tone.
.	Indicates a stopping fall in tone.
**	Talk between * * is quieter than surrounding talk.
> <	Talk between > < is spoken more quickly than surrounding talk.
{ }	Non-verbals, choreographic elements.

Source: Kogan, (1998)

PART III

SOCIAL JUSTICE

෬ 7 ෭

Doing Justice: A Witnessing Stance in Therapeutic Work alongside Survivors of Torture and Political Violence

Vikki Reynolds

Davoud is facing a refugee hearing that will decide whether he can remain in Canada, or be forcibly returned to Iran, where he was tortured for eight years in prison, and survived the executions of his comrades. His lawyer thinks a letter from a counselor will help him to prove that he has a mental illness, which would strengthen the argument that he was actually subjected to political violence. That is if the marks on his body are not enough, but his lawyer tells him they haven't been for other claimants. Therapy is not something that makes sense politically to Davoud, a committed Marxist, and he is adamant that he is not mentally ill. In fact Davoud's profound resistance to losing his mind under torture is what continues to keep intact his picture of who he believes himself to be. In moments of torment, when paralyzed by his fear for his family still in Iran, he remembers his determined acts of resistance, which opens a space for hope. As part of a myriad of resistance strategies, Davoud played a fabricated TV talk show every night in his own mind, viewing the same segment repeatedly, in which he is being interviewed for winning a gold medal for loyalty. He holds his own counsel on all of these thoughts. Davoud has a photograph of his youngest child; it was taken long ago in the life that has been ripped away from him. In it she is wearing the knowing and faraway smile of an old woman. He thinks of her and his boys now, wondering what expressions they are wearing, and his own face softens. He drags his focus back to the work of the present, putting together a strategic plan for presenting a useful story of himself at his intake meeting at the clinic tomorrow.

My hope-filled purpose in this writing is to articulate my engagement with relational ethics and a particular *just* positioning for therapeutic work with survivors of torture and political violence. This writing is not meant as a map for therapeutic practice, but rather an invitation to back up, and consider our ethical positioning for moving into the work, from which our theories and practices flow.

I am going to define torture and my understandings of witnessing, and then outline some tentative assumptions that have been useful to me in this work. I will outline a *witnessing position* and the *witnessing principles* that provide the scaffolding for my work alongside survivors of torture and political violence. While this writing addresses therapeutic work alongside survivors of torture, I also attempt to hold these ethical positionings at the center of all of my therapeutic work in response to trauma and interpersonal violence.

TORTURE AND POLITICAL VIOLENCE

The United Nations convention against torture and other cruel, inhuman or degrading treatment and punishment describes torture as any act by which severe pain is intentionally inflicted on a person for political purposes, such as silencing dissent and police investigations. To be considered torture the violence must be condoned by the government or state agent and impunity to the violators assured (Amnesty International, 2000). It is important to discern torture from *torturous*, as many people describe surviving brutalizing families as torturous experiences. Political violence and torture are different because they are state sanctioned, meaning that the government decrees that the violence is legal, the government benefits from the violence, and most often government agents perform the violence.

Torture has become a trope in popular culture, and is used as an archaic marker of our collective histories of past atrocities. This can be a very dangerous misreading of the current practices of state sanctioned violence. At the time of this writing, the U.S. President has vetoed a bill, passed by both houses of Congress in the United States, that would limit the CIA's use of "enhanced" interrogation methods that are considered torture by various human rights organizations. President Bush rejected the bill because "it took away one of the most valuable tools in the war on terror" ("Bush vetoes," 2008). Canada has also participated in the present-day use of torture.[1] For these reasons the use of torture metaphors needs to be closely examined and never engaged in lightly in therapy, especially as we risk relegating torture to a fictitious past or a metaphorical present by doing so, and may obscure our own governments' involvement.

The most important teachers in this work are refugees who have been the survivors of torture and political violence. (I prefer the word victim to survivor, for reasons of linguistic clarity regarding responsibility for violence [Coates & Wade, 2004], but I've chosen to use the word survivor because that is what many people use to identify themselves.) While I do not think it is useful to compare false hierarchies of traumatic pain,

---

[1] The Canadian government willingly allowed a Canadian citizen of Syrian birth, Maher Arar, to be deported by the USA to Syria, where he was tortured and forced to sign a false confession that he was a member of the terrorist group Al-Qaeda. The head of the Royal Canadian Mounted Police (RCMP) resigned over the issue, and Arar was fully exonerated by the O'Connor report ("Maher Arar", 2008). There is a current investigation into the tragedy of three other Canadians also deported to be tortured, and pending lawsuits against the government, Center for Strategic and International Studies (CSIS) and the RCMP for their participation in torture ("Arar considered," December 15, 2006). Most egregiously, a young Canadian, Omar Khadr, has been detained since the age of fifteen by the U.S. government and has made serious claims that he's undergone torture at the naval base in Guantanamo Bay, where he remains ("Omar Khadr," 2007). The Canadian government has not demanded freedom of this youth despite international calls for his immediate release.

I have been informed and transformed in my work alongside survivors of torture and political violence whose experiences of isolation, deprivation, lack of safety and access to dignity are extreme. However, it is not the oppression that has transformed me, but rather witnessing the acts of resistance.

These are the people to whom I attempt to hold myself and my work accountable. This particular ethical positioning for *doing justice,* which I refer to as an *ethic of resistance* (2008), has been, in a profound sense, co-created alongside survivors of torture and the people who work with them. While certainly not a homogenous group, for many survivors of torture and political violence the torture never ends, as they continue to fear for loved ones still at risk or actually in the hands of torturers. Many are torn from their families and their children; an experience one man told me was akin to trying to live with your heart outside of your body. Some live in extreme isolation, dislocated into a culture not their own, with no one to share a meaningful greeting in their language, or touch them in kindness. Despite Canada's international legal obligations to both offer refuge and to financially support refugees, many survivors of torture live in poverty and struggle to meet their basic needs, such as housing. Most refugees would rather be home, holding their babies to their hearts, catching familiar turns of phrase or well-worn tunes, and breathing in the very particular fragrance of a family dish. However, many Canadian citizens expect them to exude gratitude in all of their interactions within systems they cannot navigate. Many are unable to trust members of their own communities because their trust was broken, their bodies tortured, by people from their culture. Fear of government informants in this faraway place of refuge is very real. Responding to the horrors they have witnessed and experienced is confounding for many survivors in these contexts.

For me the center of therapeutic supervision is the therapist's relational ethics, as opposed to an emphasis on any model or technique. By this I mean the interconnections of theory and practice in relationship with ethics. This is based on my belief that the spiritual pain that therapists often experience in work alongside survivors of torture and political violence stems from the incongruence of the therapist's theories and practices with their ethics. This spiritual pain arises from the discrepancy between what feels respectful, humane, generative, and contexts that call on us to violate the very beliefs that brought us to this field. When our work alongside exploited people seems to ask us to accommodate people to injustice and violence, we can easily become exhausted, isolated and spiritually pained. In response to this spiritual pain, which is often spoken of in prescriptive ways as burnout, I engage in dialogue with therapists to articulate their relational ethics, and to align their theory and practice with these ethics. Creating an ethical positioning for *just practice* alongside survivors of torture and political violence is important for therapists at the onset of this work, if they are to sustain their ability to be of use to clients. I understand sustainability as an ongoing aliveness, a genuine connectedness with people, and a presence of spirit.

WITNESSING

I articulate my therapeutic engagement with survivors of torture as *witnessing* (Reynolds, 1997, 2002; Radke, Kitchen, & Reynolds, 2000). This speaks to a particular ethical stance, rather than a prescribed set of tools or techniques. I embrace a witnessing metaphor as it speaks to my hope that we can do this work in communion with each other. Witnessing speaks to a hoped-for connection, a social poetics (Katz & Shotter, 1996) of *being held up* collectively, experiencing ourselves as alongside others, and having those others responsively involved in our undertakings driven by shared ethical responsibilities.

My hope in using a witnessing metaphor is to bridge the worlds of therapy and activism. A commitment to the practices of witnessing in activist cultures is tied to the responsibility and duty of the witness to move beyond the hearing of individual pain to a collective response-ability (Wade, 2007) to take action against injustices. Positioning myself in therapy and therapeutic supervision as a witness has profound ethical and practical implications for the work. The therapist is not an audience to this person's individual struggle, a positioning that could invite practices of judging, diagnosing, educating, explaining, encouraging, applauding (White, 1999). An audience position is outside of, looking in on performance. Witnessing acknowledges that we are in this together, that as therapists we participate in the relational performance (Turner, 1987).

Accommodating survivors to private lives of hell is nothing any of us wants to do, but I think if we reflect on our practice it is a possibility given the helping fields' connections to ideals and values of neutrality and objectivity (Cushman, 2007). Although the term witnessing comes from many rich cultural, spiritual and religious traditions, I connect my engagement with these practices to activist cultures, human rights defenders, and new social movements. In activist culture, the presence of the witness can be a resistance against human rights violations and the political repression of voices of dissent. Witnessing is a performance of solidarity[2] with the intent to hold governments and corporate powers accountable for abuses of power and to bring the individuals who perpetrate and benefit from the torture to justice. Where activists have been murdered, witnesses refuse to accept "disappearances," and call for justice and accountability. The presence of an international activist

---

[2] I want to acknowledge that the word solidarity is contested and problematic. Like much language from social justice movements, solidarity—in some situations—has been co-opted and used as a tool of oppression, rather than liberation. Despite this, I am loath to surrender the term, and certainly unwilling to surrender the practices and rich histories and traditions of solidarity. Here I will align myself with Wittgenstein's (1953) idea that the meaning of the word is in its use, and in this present writing I engage the term solidarity to mean that our liberation, our ways forward towards something *just*, are woven together.

community is a profound act of faith in the power of witnessing. These teachings of solidarity from activist culture have informed this witnessing work. A witnessing stance aims to open our work in hope-filled and just directions and configures therapeutic relationships as sites of belonging that can promote connections of *solidarity*.

While I am open to bearing witness to all of the details of torture if that is what the survivor finds meaningful and believes is necessary, my ethical position is an inclination to witness resistance. I'm looking for the sites of resistance against torture, and the particular practices the person created to maintain connection with humanity in contexts that are outside of human understanding. It is my therapeutic experience that witnessing conversations bring forward sites of resistance that assist the person in moving out of torture's totalizing story, and re-member (Myerhoff, 1972, Madigan, 1997) them with their most meaningful and connective ways of being.

Tentative Assumptions

My ethical positioning for work with political violence and torture is based on some assumptions that have been very useful to me. I am not offering these as truths, but rather as ethical approaches that have made a difference in the lives of survivors of torture and political violence I've worked alongside, and that have helped sustain me in this difficult work.

I have a very tentative overriding assumption about my work with survivors of torture and political violence, which helps me maintain hope in the face of terror. I personally believe that people who are tortured have many opportunities to die, and always a final choice about when torture can end. Choosing death in these situations is something I honor as resistance to torture. Given these choices, albeit limited and inhumane, I hold on to hope that the person I'm in therapeutic relationship with will not choose to die now.

This tentative assumption is not a truth, but has helped me resist the paralyzing and silencing tactics of torture on me in my role as the therapist.

Of course survivors of torture and political violence do die and their deaths are sometimes constructed as suicides within the dominant discourses of society and of therapy itself. Experience has led me to attribute these deaths to torture, to the particular people involved in the acts of torture, to the governments or political groups that sanctioned the torture, and to particular people in wider social contexts (such as owners of multinational corporations) that benefit from the torture. In this context, I see the linguistic construction of suicide as victim blaming and in a very profound sense an abdication of responsibility as a global community to address torture. A witnessing stance is upheld by taking a position for justice, holding complex understandings of the political world, and an ongoing examination of our ethical positioning.

The Witness' Positioning

1. The Witness addresses power, taking a position for justice in a social political world.

I am often identified as political, a political therapist, or a political activist. Of course all therapists are political, dealing in relationships of power. While there has been much scrutiny of politically located therapists, and concerns that we may be "doing politics" with our clients, my experience as a therapeutic supervisor has led me to believe that therapists who are co-located as activists are very aware of their power and their political positioning. The supervisory relationship of activist/therapists addresses the need for therapists to de-center their activism in the therapeutic relationship. Therapists who identify as neutral and non-political may not acknowledge their access to power or their political locations, and are perhaps more likely to unknowingly replicate both acts of power-over and status quo agendas in the therapeutic relationship. What often goes unspoken is the inherently political position of neutrality.

An *ethic of resistance* requires discernment of what is just and what is fair. Fairness, not unlike equality, is a liberal notion based on the construct of a just world with equal access and possibility. When justice is our organizing principle, all are not necessarily treated equally.

In situations where there is a scarcity of resources and abundance of need therapists are often put in positions of having to make individual decisions, such as who gets bus tickets for free, in which they are not able to be fair. Fairness is a great value in our cultures and certainly no one sought therapeutic training in order to practice unfairness. But where there is one bus ticket and three people asking, therapists are put in a position of having to decide what is *just*, and so they may find themselves telling one survivor that they do not have a bus ticket for them, when in fact they are withholding a ticket for a more-needy survivor. Of course bus tickets are a benign example. These kinds of experiences can lead to spiritual pain, and what gets called burnout. However, if we acknowledge the social structures that uphold oppression, as opposed to seeing these acts as something we are individually responsible for, then justice is not constructed as an entirely individual problem of the therapist, but something we are collectively responsible for as a society. I can better tolerate being unfair if I'm attending to an *ethic of resistance* that is centered in being just. This requires a complex analysis and practices of solidarity.

2. The Witness has complex understandings of the political world and critical engagements with language.

In work with survivors of political violence it is imperative to have understandings of the political world. People from the global South and oppressed positions spend a great deal of time in therapy educating therapists about the realities of their lives. The point is not for me to do my homework on the political situation in Somalia, for example; but to have a critical analysis of the workings of global power, a framework that is able to embrace the complexity and specificities of a person's lived experiences related to Somalia. Therapists are more likely to address power when working with survivors of torture and political violence, but a complex critical analysis is of use in all therapeutic relationships, as no relationships exist in apolitical locations. Therapists who worked alongside survivors of torture and political violence contest the construction of the sociopolitical world as a natural development, and critique the taken for granted premises that the world could not be structured in other and more *just* ways. This requires critical analysis, and ongoing questioning. Knowing that the world could be other than it is offers a great site of hope.

It is easy to get caught up in a false binary of heroes and villains in this work, but the reality of lived experience is that many people in political struggles have used some semblances of power over others, including interpersonal violence. I believe we need to take a position against torture and political violence, without entirely conflating the complexity of the person in front of us as a helpless and innocent victim. Conversely, therapists are tempted to speak of survivors as courageous, which may not fit for the person at all (Roth, 2008), as survival sometimes required acts that survivors themselves believe lack honor. These practices replicate simplistic hero worshiping of survivors, and coming from therapists these naïve platitudes can be a barrier to the person honoring their own authentic and complex identities. Placing survivors of torture on pedestals is very seductive, and a practice that situates them as *other* and not *part of.* Such naïve positioning is patronizing of the person, and allows no room for the survivors to step into accountability if there are situations for which they believe they must account. Here I think it is useful to hold ourselves to practices of witnessing and not replicate rituals of confession.

Critical understandings of language are important in all therapeutic conversations as we construct our understanding of the world through language (Wittgenstein, 1953).[3] In particular, with my work alongside survivors of political violence and torture, I am interested in what Linda Coates and Allan Wade (2007) speak of as the *four operations of language*, meaning the ways that language is used to conceal violence, obscure perpetrator responsibility, conceal victims' responses and resistance, and blame/pathologize victims. Alternatively, they suggest that in the context of therapy we engage with counter operations, using language to reveal violence, clarify perpetrator responsibility, elucidate and honor victims' responses and resistance, and contest the blaming/pathologizing of victims. Without an overt intention of utilizing language in these liberatory ways therapeutic conversation can replicate all of the operations of language, holding survivors of torture responsible for their own suffering, displacement and poverty.

Critically engaging corporate media is very useful in understanding the context of political violence. Corporate media[4] often use the same linguistic constructions and strategies as those discussed above to hide our collective resistance to corporate power and global injustices. Corporate media construct a discourse within a false binary of winners and losers. Whenever activists are represented, when we do participate in the media that are fit to print, we are the losers.

---

[3] A full description of the social construction understandings of language is beyond the scope of this ethical positioning paper, as my purpose here is to critique language used to serve or resist abuses of power.

[4] Naming what is often misleadingly referred to as mainstream media as corporate names the owners' intentions for the product of media, which is financial gain for their stockholders. Alternative media seek to widen the range of what is spoken, and provide more diverse discourse. Autonomous media are organized around anarchist principles, meaning that small groups of involved people have more of a say in how their own lives are mediated, and become the media (Langlois & Dubois, 2005).

A critical engagement with language invites us to be more ambiguous in our readings of events, and celebrate the small acts of justice, which may not make us winners, but certainly make life-saving changes in the lives of real people on the ground.[5]

3. Witnesses constantly examine their ethical positioning for work alongside survivors of torture and political violence.

There are many paths to liberation in work with survivors of torture and political violence. I've worked alongside therapists and psychiatrists who engage ethically and effectively with diverse models of therapeutic intervention in work with the trauma of torture, from Rorschach tests to Narrative Therapy. No theory or practice is harm free: As Ani Difranco (1993) says, "Any tool is a weapon if you hold it right." For me the quest is not to find the perfect therapeutic intervention, but to examine my ethical positioning for work alongside survivors of torture and political violence.

To do this work, ethically, I believe the witness greatly benefits from critical ongoing therapeutic supervision, and approaching the work collectively. Positions of solidarity are of great use for the supervisor and the therapist as well as for the survivor of torture. It is this ethical understanding that has informed the process for therapeutic supervision I have developed, which I refer to as a *supervision of solidarity*. Within the structures of this community-making supervision, the ethics of the therapist hold the center of the conversation,

---

[5] As an example, a major corporate media project is continually being engaged to frame all activist interactions and resistance against the war in Iraq as failures. Activists failed to stop the war. While that may be true in a construction of winners and losers, it is certainly not true in the material lives of many people who are not dead, because the war that was planned was stopped. The war of "shock and awe" was not able to go forward because of global resistance and solidarity, which changed much in terms of tactics and body count. Noam Chomsky says this was the most encouraging moment in human history, when global activists united to fight a war before it occurred.

and are supported and critiqued from a position within community.

Therapists hold embodied knowings of their own relationships with ethics and this is often experienced as discomforting. At times, we can talk ourselves out of our discomfort, or allow our supervisor or peers to answer to our discomfort and alleviate it. I welcome this discomfort as a resource to the therapist[6], a communication from the body which requires not a solution but an attending-to. Often our discomfort can be an invitation to revisit our ethics in the moment: Practices of smoothing over discomfort can silence this important knowing.

Resisting certainty, and continually engaging with reflexivity[7] requires constant vigilance and I think moral courage. Embracing ambiguity[8] as a resistance to certainty and an opening of possibilities also allows for multiple meanings to come forward through conversations that may be messy, take many turns, and at times appear scattered. For survivors of torture, meaning making is rarely straightforward, contexts are complex, and ambiguity may provide a potential path.

The following witnessing principles provide the scaffolding that support therapeutic work alongside survivors of torture and political violence.

---

[6] The languaging of resourcing, used here, comes from the therapeutic supervision of Johnella Bird (2006).
[7] While theoretically I can reference reflexivity to multiple sources, I was first able to articulate reflexivity in practice through Stephen Madigan's (1991) therapeutic supervision of my work alongside survivors of torture and political violence.
[8] The Fifth Province work of Nollaig Byrne and Imelda McCarthy (1998) is centered in an ethic of ambiguity, and their teachings specifically have accompanied me in these directions, as un-chartable as they may be.

Witnessing Principles in Work with Survivors of Torture and Political Violence

1. Structuring Safety

Co-creating relationships of enough safety, outside of the false binaries of safe and unsafe (Bird, 2000), is a cornerstone of this work. Practices such as continually negotiating permission can help invite safety, and contest the commodification of permission, by which I mean that a consent form is not a contract that gives the professional the fixed, concretized right to replicate interrogation practices. Developing particular structures of safety is a core competency for any therapist working alongside survivors of torture and political violence, requiring compassion, creativity and critical therapeutic supervision. Re-telling details of torture, with no transformation or liberatory negotiations of new meaning can be re-traumatizing for the survivor. As a practice of safety the witness works diligently to try to ensure that the conversation is not re-traumatizing.

- What ways of knowing yourself let you trust that you will be able to say no to me if I ask something that is not okay?
- What will it take for you to be able to say no to me if I ask you a question that's not all right?

The therapist benefits by developing a rich capacity to hear *no* in the myriad of ways in which it is conveyed by survivors. Anything short of a heartfelt yes in therapeutic conversation can be a sign to slow down, re-negotiate permission, and honor the survivor's courage in saying no to a person with power.

- This hesitation just now, is this one of the ways you have of telling me that this is not a useful question right now?
- You know, I'm thinking that that was not a very useful question. Do you agree? Thanks for letting me know that. Do you have any ideas of what a more useful question could be?

These are risky conversations, and if the therapist does not provide scaffolding for safety, a place for a tentative trust in the relationship, the consequences to the survivor may be extreme. Often, in these situations, the therapist's first clue that trust has been broken is the disappearance of the survivor. These are the people we most want to talk to in terms of accountability and teaching us how to be safe-enough. Therapists who work with survivors of torture are familiar with that cold-bellied feeling of losing connection with a survivor. Lynn Hoffman speaks to this rupture in the relationship between therapist and person as akin to cutting an artery (2002, p. 242). The survivors may go underground, try to cross another border, lose themselves in substance abuse, or prudently dismiss any further thoughts of seeking help. The consequences to survivors are enormous when trust is broken.

Trauma work with survivors of torture and political violence often exists within a landscape of refugee, immigration and legal action. Interrogation and court appearances are often required for issues of settlement. This reality problematizes safety, and the therapist seeks to differentiate conversations from interrogation. In work with survivors we borrow from the safety of others. Good allies in settlement and legal work introduce me to their clients, and I use that trust as a bridge to create relationships of enough safety with the person. In a profound way I believe this witnessing work is always communal—we do this work on the shoulders of others and we shoulder each other up.

2. Cultural and Collective Accountability

In work with survivors of torture and political violence I position myself culturally as a member of an extended Irish Catholic, English, Newfoundland family. I acknowledge that in this territory I am from colonizing culture, and I struggle to resist replicating colonization in my work with survivors of torture from diverse cultural locations, most of which are marginalized.

I hope to hold myself accountable to the survivor of torture, and to their cultural locations. I do not want to replicate dominance, most especially colonization, in this relationship. Accountability requires a complex analysis, in which the multiplicity and intersectionality (Grant, 2001) of sites of both power and oppression are acknowledged and addressed. Richard Day (2005, p. 18), a grassroots anarchist, commits to "groundless solidarity and infinite responsibility"—*groundless* meaning that our ethics are not tied to one oppression. Day refers to *infinite responsibility* where we strive always to be open to another, to the multiplicity of ways that we might be incongruent with our ethics; ways that we are not in authentic solidarity.

This means that I work to address my privileged and statused identity as a passport holding Canadian when working with refugees. Activists, such as the group No One Is Illegal (n.d.), contest government sanctioned identity attacks on the legitimacy of undocumented refugees' rights to personhood.

- What does it mean to call someone an illegal person?
- What does it mean when the state uses this language?
- What does it mean when a state having obligations to universal law uses this kind of language against a person seeking refuge from torture and political violence?

In this witnessing work cultural consultants are a great resource to me, as they hold cultural knowledges and can help invite me to accountability (Tamasese 2001, Waldegrave & Tamasese 1993, Waldegrave 1990). I invite people hired as interpreters to be present as all of who they are in these conversations, and invite their embodied reflections (Katz & Shotter, 2004; White, 1995) to what they have witnessed. Holding cultural and language knowledges qualifies the interpreter as a cultural consultant, and in my experience invites an extended positive social response (Wade, 2007) to the survivor, as well as promoting the sustainability of the cultural consultant. I am ever mindful that many interpreters carry their own repertoires of resistance (Burstow, 1992) and histories, which is different from seeing them as also pathologized by trauma.

Accountability is something that we do together in relationship. Individual accountability can be a limiting idea, especially if it constructs the responsibility for social contexts of injustice as a personal project. The contexts of deprivation and injustice, where survivors of torture live and we work, require enormous, collaborative, and resourced social responses. Torture requires responses from all global citizens, and the responsibility for this ought not to lie with individual therapists but instead reflect our socially constructed relational responsibilities (McNamee & Gergen, 1999). Collective accountability contests the individuation of responsibility, and offers hope in finding ways forward together.

When a therapist from the dominant culture—and where I live in Canada that is a white therapist—engages in racism, I can be seduced into wanting to isolate him and fabricate his identity as a racist. And I can work very hard and very publicly to construct myself as a very different white person. Collective accountability invites me to step up, lean into my white brother, and find our way forward together. This is not based on me being a good person, but on my understanding that all racism benefits me as a member of the dominant culture, whether I perform it or not. Leonard Peltier, perhaps one of the most important political prisoners in the world, speaks about the fact that he is just an ordinary person who did what his culture has taught him to do in defending his community and his elders and that he is not extraordinary.[9] "You must understand. . . . I am

---

[9] Leonard Peltier is serving two concurrent life sentences in prison in the United States of America for the killings of two FBI agents on the Pine Ridge reserve in South Dakota in June of 1975. Peltier was extradited from Canada and the United States government has admitted it used false testimony to apprehend him, as they also have admitted that much of the testimony used against him at trial was fabricated. Despite these grave concerns, he remains in prison and has served over thirty years. Governments throughout the world and human rights organizations have called for a complete commuting of his sentence, meaning that there is no evidence that convicts him of these crimes. More context to Leonard's story is revealed in Robert Redford and Michael Apted's film, *Incident at Oglala*, and the website of the Leonard Peltier Defense Committee.

ordinary. Painfully ordinary. This isn't modesty. This is fact. Maybe you're ordinary, too. If so, I honor your ordinariness, your humanness, your spirituality. I hope you will honor mine. That ordinariness is our bond, you and I. We are ordinary. We are human. The Creator made us this way. Imperfect. Inadequate. Ordinary. . . . We are not supposed to be perfect. We're supposed to be useful" (Peltier, 1999, p. 9). Collectively addressing racism or any form of oppression is not a heroic act, but is in fact a performance of our normalcy, our collective ordinary humanity.[10]

While I believe in holding ourselves collectively accountable to the intersections of our sites of privilege in all anti-oppression work as an ethical stance, I am very aware of the limitations of the theories and practices of accountability. I believe that at times accountability holds the center in our work, when justice would be better served by creating a context in which the violence does not occur. When, for example, homophobia happens, there is blood on the floor, and while accountability can offer the hope of repair to relationships and begin to create some way forward together through paralysis, it does not render the violence of homophobia undone. All conversations across difference are inherently risky conversations, and of greater risk to some than others. Therapists learn this work on the backs of clients. There is no other way forward, and I believe a hard truth is that there is no innocent position.

---

[10] Many therapists who work alongside survivors of torture and violence feel extremely uncomfortable when the exploitation of the clients' life is used to esteem us as therapists, and construct our identity as extraordinary. I believe that this construction of being put upon a pedestal is actually a position "outside of", as if our work is other than normal. I think it is important to contest this act of being put on a pedestal, as it does several things. Firstly, it exploits the experiences of clients, secondly, it engages in a hierarchy of pain that is not useful, and thirdly, it relieves *ordinary* citizens from their discomfort and obligation to do something about the contexts that have made torture possible.

3. Collaboration

Collaboration invites safety and gives more opportunities for the survivor of torture to decide what will be talked about and what will be of use. It is my ethical obligation in the role of the therapist to bring hope to the situation and to provide a structure for the work. I attempt to do this without taking a position of expertise on the life of the survivor of torture or taking prescriptive positions around what they need to do. My hope is for the relationship to be survivor centered, and this requires the de-centering of myself as the therapist. Critical therapeutic supervision has been a great resource to me in moving towards the creation of particular collaborative practices.

While I am very influential in the therapeutic relationship, as the therapist I cannot be solely responsible for it, as safety cannot be ensured by any one partner in a dialogue. The gift of collaboration invites the sharing of power and with that a concomitant sharing of responsibility. As therapists, we do not save people and we are not responsible for people dying. A collaborative stance (Anderson, 1997) requires the letting go of some power on the part of the therapist and this can be experienced as profoundly discomforting when the survivors we work with are in extreme situations and death is ever near. I believe that aiming for these collaborative positionings has sustained me, especially when torture eventually claims the life of a survivor of political violence.

Witnessing therapists attempt to attend minutely to the living collaboration with the survivor. This ethic connects with what Shotter (1984, 1993) refers to as joint action, where our dialogue together cannot be seen as an individual project but only exists responsively. It is helpful not to collapse efficacy, the marker of outcomes used in research, with effectiveness, which is what the survivors get to say about their experience of the work (Tilsen, 2008). Continual invitation for the dialogue facilitate this as a collective responsibility, but collaboration with survivors is a good enough idea in its own right as it simply makes the conversations more useful (Wade, 2005). After I have asked a long involved theoretically beautiful question a survivor may look at me with puzzlement or invite me to ask that again, both of which are invitations for me to engage more usefully in dialogue with them in that moment. Sometimes I will ask a beautifully crafted question, and the survivor will say, "Oh, did you mean to ask . . ." and then go on to ask a much more useful question. Humbling stuff, collaboration, and so useful.

4. Honoring Resistance

There are three main assumptions I make about resistance in my work with survivors of torture and political violence:
- I believe that whenever a person is tortured they resist.[11]
- Resistance ought not to be judged by its ability to stop the torture.
- Resistance is important for its ability to maintain a person's connection to humanity.

I believe that torture is, and ought to remain, outside of human understanding. In this work, as with other therapeutic work with trauma, I am interested in meaning, not truth. While I am very interested in the particularities of acts of resistance, I am working hard not to investigate or interrogate the survivor of torture for a true, legal, or binding account of the acts of torture. Without a purposeful commitment to witness resistance, it can be disappeared, or be constructed narrowly, so that only resistance that successfully stops torture is acknowledged.

---

[11] The ubiquitous nature of resistance is often referenced to Foucault (1979), for his adage that wherever there is power there is resistance. Of course, the cultural histories of resistance are harder to reference, but have been passed along within connected groups of activists since ages before the Diggers. (This group also called themselves True Levelers, and in England in the mid-1600s these folks attempted to take back the commons, their resistance taking the form of planting crops on Crown land.)

A witnessing stance can assist me in declining invitations to make sense of torture, and focus on making sense of the acts of resistance.

Often survivors of torture have had to give torture's account of their identities for immigration and refugee processes. The torture story constructs flawed and mentally-ill identities, and a witnessing stance for the work aims to invite and support the person to reclaim or create fluid and preferred storying of them. In this witnessing work I am looking for the person's own account of their sites of resistance, their resistance knowledges (Wade 1997, 1996), and the meanings these acts of resistance hold for the person.

5. Belonging, Community, Solidarity

Witnessing intends to resist the individuation and isolation of the torture survivor. Liberation psychologist Ignacio Martín-Baró, (1990) believes that torture is best understood from a perspective that is both psychosocial and sociopolitical, meaning that the path to liberation lies not in the individual psyche of the victim, but within social relations. The meanings given to the acts of torture are social, not individual. Torture dis-members, dis-connects and removes people from their sites of belonging—with refugees this happens in a very geographical and physical way (Reynolds, 1997). In resistance to this dis-location, witnessing work is situated within communities of concern (Madigan & Epston, 1995). Witnessing provides community-making conversations, which aim to connect survivors with preferred others in creative ways. Witnessing attempts to re-member (Madigan, 1997) and re-connect, with particular attention to cultural meanings (Prowell 1999), and works towards *belonging* survivors in community. I believe, along with many others across time, that culture is a site of healing (Richardson, 2004), as I believe that doing justice can promote healing.

A witnessing stance brings forward positive social responses (Wade, 2007) for the survivor of torture. These responses can be acts of resistance in their own right. For survivors of torture who must flee their own nations, positive social responses may legitimize the survivor's understandings of their right to sanctuary in the face of Canadian racism and anti-immigration rhetoric and structures. In this era of the *war on terror* these ideas have been strengthened.

As an act of solidarity the witness has an ethical responsibility to respond to the social contexts that make possible and support attacks on human dignity. To do less is to risk accommodating the person to oppressive contexts, and to tacitly participate in a continuation of torture for political and capital gain. My own response to witnessing these stories of private pain is to address the public issues in the time honored practices of social justice activists, and work for change.

My understandings of solidarity are derived from activist traditions of looking for points of connection and weaving people together through commonly held affinities and "moments of mutuality" (Schack, 2006). Activist cultures engage in solidarity by actively looking for and weaving together connecting practices of both resisting oppression and promoting social justice. Solidarity speaks to an understanding that just ways of being are most often interconnected, as are our struggles to realize social justice. This spirit of solidarity has been beautifully articulated by Lily Walker (as cited in Sinclair, n.d.), an Aboriginal women's leader: "If you come here to help me, then you are wasting your time. But if you come here because your liberation is bound up in mine, then let us begin."

6. *Witness, not Gossip*

It is an ethical obligation of the witness to decline their own curiosity, in particular, as it relates to the details of torture. These are fascinating and compelling stories. Practices of declining curiosity for its own sake are useful here. The witness resists being seduced by the torture story, and works to decline the privileging idea that the therapist has a right to know everything. I tell survivors of torture that I need to know what they think I need to know, so that I can be of use. Inviting survivors at the outset to consider the influence of speaking allows for therapeutic space to slow the re-tellings down, so that survivors may have agency about what is spoken or not spoken. This practice aims to position the therapeutic conversation as something different than the interrogation under torture. It also honors the survivor with the storytelling rights (Epston, 1998).

In therapeutic supervision, therapists often share with me their urgency to get to the *real work*, and negotiations of permission and safety can often be the victims of this urgency. I implore therapists to connect with the immediacy of the relationship with the person. Negotiating safety in this moment with this person in this context is most often the work that can be most helpful. Foregrounded against a backdrop of political violence, this permissioning of the survivor can be transformative.

- As we're sitting here now and you are considering what you're going to tell me, I would like you to travel ahead in time until after this meeting, and think about how you will be with the telling. How might you feel about the telling tomorrow? Might the telling of this get in the way of the counseling relationship? Might the not telling of this get in the way of the counseling relationship?
- As you're sitting here now, and considering what you're going to tell me, I'd like you to consider what you know about yourself, that let you trust that you can decide if you will speak or keep your own counsel. What do you know about our relationship that might help you trust your right to tell or not tell?

While I invite survivors to resist unhelpful questions, the onus is on me to not articulate them. Questions informed by a naïve curiosity can pose great threats to safety, and to the therapeutic relationship.

7. Immeasurable Outcomes

In contrast to prescriptive stories of burnout as the "effect" of this work alongside survivors of political violence and torture, my life has been immeasurably expanded and my hopes amplified in response (Coates, Todd, & Wade, 2003) to bearing witness. As therapists, I believe that we do more than survive this most difficult work: We can be transformed in the doing of it alongside survivors. What are possible to measure as outcomes often miss the most salient connections of our collective humanity.

The glass milk bottle is slipping out of my hand. As I rush for the store counter I have a near miss with a delivery guy. We pirouette around each other in the tiny aisle by the register, and although it is fluid there is an arresting moment when we really look at each other. The bottle gets safely delivered to the counter, and I put my other stuff up there, and slowly turn around to make sure I haven't caused too much trouble. The delivery guy says, "How's your day Madame?" It's an out of place greeting, a greeting not of this time.

"I'm okay, just a little uncoordinated – you?"

"Do you remember me?" he says in a softer voice, and the jovial mood between us dissipates.

I say, "Yeah, I know that I know you, but I don't recall your name."

He says "Victoria, my name is Ahmid."

In the speaking of his name my breath catches, and the space between us shortens and I don't know who has moved. "Yeah, yeah, I know you, Ahmid. You're Kurdish, yes. How are you?"

In answer he puts down his tray, reaches into his pocket, pulls out his wallet and meticulously removes a school picture. "This is my boy." We can't talk and yet it's all said in casting our eyes on the same photo of a young boy, maybe twelve, in an ordinary picture that could be from any school in Vancouver. The cashier is watching, there is another shopper behind Ahmid; nobody seems put out that we have been captured in time together. Ahmid addresses the other people, passes his son's picture around, first into the hands of the shopper behind him, who holds the picture as if she were holding his child. Ahmid says, "This woman saved my son. She got him here to Canada."

I know that this is not true, there was a team of people involved, good lawyers and determined settlement workers, and my role was primarily as his therapist. I don't correct Ahmid, because this is his story for the telling, and the present story is his son, whose open-faced smile greets us all like a blessing.[12]

REFERENCES

Amnesty International (2000). *Torture worldwide: An affront to human dignity.* New York: Amnesty International Publications.

Anderson, H. (1997). *Conversation, language, and possibilities: A postmodern approach to therapy.* New York: Basic Books.

Arar considered threat to U.S., Wilkins says. (2006, Dec. 15). *CTV.ca.* Retrieved April 25, 2008 from http://www.ctv.ca/servlet/ArticleNews/story/CTVNews/20061215/arar_layton_061215?s_name=&no_ads=

Bird, J. (2006). *Constructing the narrative in super-vision.* Auckland: Edge Press.

---

[12] The critical pedagogy teachings of Paulo Freire (1970) and the lifework and execution of liberatory psychologist Ignatio Martín-Baró (1994) have contributed much to the ethics of this work in terms of moving beyond individual pain into social and collective responsibility for oppression, and the duty of the witness to work for change and justice. I want to acknowledge the differential price extracted from people from the global South and racialized and *minoritized* people from the global North, and recognize the generosity that has enabled them to teach me and for me to benefit from their lived experiences. The survivors of torture and political violence I have worked alongside in New Zealand, Australia, Dharamsala India, Santiago Chile, Vancouver's Downtown Eastside, neighborhood centers and clinics throughout Vancouver, and the political refugees I worked and lived alongside in Botswana Africa are the heart of this work. I have had generative and supportive therapeutic supervision, which I experience as practices of solidarity, from Heather Elliott, Stephen Madigan, and Colin Sanders. Enriching collaborations with Allan Wade and Cathy Richardson have sustained and moved me in this work.

Bird, J. (2000). *The heart's narrative: Therapy and navigating life's contradictions.* Auckland: Edge Press.
Burstow, B. (1992). *Radical feminist therapy.* Newbury Park: Sage.
Bush vetoes interrogation limits. (2008, March 8). *BBC News.* Retreived March 8 2008 from http://news.bbc.co.uk/2/hi/americas/7285290.stm
Byrne, N., & McCarthy, I. (1998). Marginal illuminations: A fifth province approach to intro-cultural issues in an Irish context. In M. McGoldrick (ed.) *Re-visioning family therapy: Implications of race and culture for clinical practice.* New York: Guilford press.
Coates, L., & Wade, A. (2007). Language and violence: Analysis of four discursive Operations. *Journal of Family Violence, 22,* 511-522.
Coates, L, & Wade, A. (2004). Telling it like it isn't: Obscuring perpetrator responsibility for violence. *Discourse and Society, 15,* 499-526.
Coates, L., Todd, N., & Wade, A. (2003). Shifting terms: An interactional and discursive view of violence and resistance. *Canadian Review of Social Policy, 52,* 116-122.
Cushman, P. (2007). *Where do psychotherapy narratives come from? Avoiding the arrogance of monoculturalism and the dead-end of relativism.* Keynote address given at the Therapeutic Conversations 7 Conference, Vancouver, Canada.
Day, R. (2005). *Gramsci is dead: Anarchist currents in the newest social movements.* London: Pluto Press.
DiFranco, A. (1993). My IQ. On *Puddle dive* [CD]. Righteous Babe Records.
Epston, D. (1998). Personal communication.
Freire, P. (1970). *Pedagogy of the oppressed.* New York: Continuum.
Foucault, M. (1979). *Discipline and punish: The birth of the prison.* New York: Vintage Books.
Grant, K. (2001, March). *Realities of race.* Workshop presented at the University of British Columbia, Vancouver, Canada.
Hoffman, L. (2002). *Family therapy: An intimate history.* New York: W.W. Norton.
Katz, A., & Shotter, J. (1996). Hearing the patient's "voice." Toward a social poetics in diagnostic interviews. *Social Science and Medicine, 43,* 919-931.
Katz, A., & Shotter, J. (2004). On the way to "presence": Methods of a "social poetics." In D. Pare & G. Larner (Eds.), *Collaborative Practice in Psychology and Psychotherapy.* New York: Haworth Clinical Practice Press.
Langlois, A., & Dubois, F. (Eds.) (2005). *Autonomous media: Activating resistance and dissent.* Montréal: Cumulus Press.

Madigan, S. (1997). Re-considering memory: Remembering lost identities back towards re-membered selves. In D. Nylund & C. Smith (Eds.), *Narrative therapies with children and adolescents (pp. 338-355)*. New York: Guilford Press.

Madigan, S., & Epston, D. (1995). From "spy-chiatric gaze" to communities of concern: From professional monologue to dialogue. In S. Friedman (Ed.), *The reflecting team in action: Collaborative practice in family therapy* (pp. 257-276). New York: Guilford Press.

Madigan, S. (1991). Discursive restraints in therapeutic practice: Situating therapists' questions in the presence of the family. In *Postmodernism, deconstruction and therapy: Dulwich Centre Newsletter* (pp. 13-20) Adelaide: Dulwich Centre Publications.

Maher Arar (2008). Retreived April 25, 2008 from http://www.maherarar.ca/

Martín-Baró, I. (1994). *Writings for a liberation psychology*. Cambridge: Harvard University Press.

Martín-Baró, I. (Ed.) (1990). *Social psychology of war: Trauma and therapy*. San Salvador: UCA Editors.

McNamee, S., & Gergen, K. (1999). *Relational responsibility: Resources for sustainable dialogue*. London: Sage Publications.

Myerhoff, B. (1972). *Number our days*. New York: Simon and Schuster.

No one is illegal (n.d.). Retrieved December 30, 2008 from http://noii-van.resist.ca

Omar Khadr: Coming of age in a Guatananmo Bay jail cell. *CBC News in Depth*. (2007, June 4). Retrieved April 25, 2008 from http://www.cbc.ca/news/background/khadr/omar-khadr.html

Peltier, L. (1999). *Prison writings: My life is my Sundance*. New York: St. Martin's Griffin.

Prowell, J. (1999). Reflections on issues of culture. *Gecko, 2, 43-50*.

Radke, C., Kitchen, M., & Reynolds, V. (2000). *Witness not gossip: The gender group at Peak House*. Unpublished article.

Reynolds, V. (2008). An ethic of resistance: Frontline worker as activist. *Women Making Waves, 19*(1), 5.

Reynolds, V. (2002). Weaving threads of belonging: Cultural witnessing groups. *Journal of Child and Youth Care, 15*(3), 89-105.

Reynolds, V. (1997). Therapeutic conversations with survivors of torture. In A. Hamilton (Ed.), *BC Association of Counselors of Abusive Men Conference Proceedings* (pp. 57-60). Vancouver, BC: Association of Counselors of Abusive Men.

Richardson, C. (2004). *Becoming Métis: The relationship between the sense of Métis self and cultural stories*. University of Victoria: Unpublished Masters thesis.

Roth, S. (2008) Personal communication.
Schack, M. (2006). Personal communication.
Shotter, J. (1984). *Social accountability and selfhood.* Oxford: Blackwell.
Shotter, J. (1993) *Cultural politics of everyday life: Social constructionism, rhetoric, and knowing of the third kind.* Milton Keynes: Open University Press.
Sinclair, R. (n. d.). Participatory action research. In *Aboriginal and Indigenous Social Work.* Retrieved November 21, 2008, from http://www.aboriginalsocialwork.ca/special_topics/par/index.htm.
Tamasese, K. (2001). Talking about culture and gender. In C. White (Ed.), *Working with the stories of women's lives* (pp. 15-22). Adelaide, Australia: Dulwich Centre Publications.
Tilsen, J. (2008). Personal communication.
Turner, V. (1987). *The anthropology of performance.* New York: PAJ publications.
Wade, A. (2008). Personal communication.
Wade, A. (2007). Personal communication.
Wade, A. (2005). Personal communication.
Wade, A. (1997). Small acts of living: Everyday resistance to violence and other forms of oppression. *Journal of Contemporary Family Therapy, 19*(1), 23-40.
Wade, A. (1996). Resistance knowledges: Therapy with aboriginal persons who have experienced violence. In P.H. Stephenson, S.J. Elliott, L.T. Foster, & J. Harris (Eds.), *Canadian Western Geographical Serie:, Vol. 31.A persistent spirit: Towards understanding aboriginal health in British Columbia* (pp. 167-206). Victoria, British Columbia: Department of Geography.
Waldegrave, C., & Tamasese, K. (1993). Some central ideas in the "Just Therapy" approach. *Australian and New Zealand Journal of Family Therapy, 14,* 1-8.
Waldegrave, C. (1990). Just therapy. *Dulwich Centre Newsletter, 3,* 5-8.
White, M. (1999). Reflecting-team work as definitional ceremony revisited. *Gecko, 2,* 55-82.
White, M. (1995). Reflecting team as definitional ceremony. In M. White (Ed.), *Re-authoring lives: Interviews and essays* (pp. 172-198). Adelaide: Dulwich Centre Publications.
Wittgenstein, L. (1953). *Philosophical investigations.* Oxford: Blackwell.

~ 8 ~

Constructivist Mentoring as Social Justice

Sara K. Bridges

> *I've come to the frightening conclusion that I am the decisive element in the classroom. It's my personal approach that creates the climate. It's my daily mood that makes the weather. As a teacher, I possess tremendous power to make a student's life miserable or joyous. I can be a tool of torture or an instrument of inspiration. I can humiliate or humor, hurt or heal. In all situations, it is my response that decides whether a crisis will be escalated or de-escalated and a student humanized or de-humanized.*
>
> Haim Ginott, 1972, pp. 15-16

Since the late 1970s mentoring has been increasingly used as a term to describe the ways in which a more advanced or experienced person may guide, support, encourage and help a more junior person to succeed in life, be it in a chosen career, educational goals or simply with the tasks of daily living (Daloz, 1999). What mentoring is, how it is accomplished, and who benefits from it have all been topics of empirical and theoretical inquiry (e.g. Atkinson, Casas, & Neville, 1994; Daloz, 1999; Luna & Cullen, 1998), making a clear case for the many benefits that come from having an effective mentoring relationship. Further, there are some who suggest that mentoring is more than simply a "good idea," arguing instead that mentoring is actually an ethical or moral obligation for those more advanced in their fields (Green & Hawley, 2009; Humble, Solomon, Allen, Blaisure, & Johnson, 2006; Russel & Horne, 2009). This is especially true for those in psychology doctoral training programs, which create "colleagues" who themselves are committed to generative professional relationships with those in need (Luna & Cullen, 1998).

Clearly, having a good mentoring relationship with a faculty member as a graduate student in psychology (as well as other fields of study) is beneficial to students as they navigate their way through the many hoops required in doctoral programs (Espinoza-Herold & Gonzalez, 2007; Forehand, 2008; Johnson, 2002; Luna & Cullen, 1998). In fact, in his 2008 awards address for Distinguished Career Contributions to Education and Training at the 116th annual convention of the American Psychological Association, Forehand (2008) made a very strong argument for the necessity of high-quality mentoring relationships for graduate students in psychology. He stated that skillful mentoring is essential for graduate student development, which in turn is essential for the continuation of academic and scholarly pursuits. Thus, the need to help students through the rigorous and confusing process of becoming a psychologist was clear. Forehand's research revealed two main elements of mentoring that undoubtedly facilitate excelling in graduate school: (a) tasks and activities that are explicitly related to academic performance and completing all the required elements and (b) tasks that hold a more emotional tenor. Indeed, much of the research on mentoring has focused on the academic needs of the students (Dohm & Cummings, 2002, 2003), while the multicultural and feminist literature on mentoring points to the unique emotional and relational mentoring needs of graduate students (Atkinson, Neville, & Casas, 1991; Brown, Davis, & McClendon, 1999; Espinoza-Herold, & Gonzalez, 2007; Gilbert & Rossman, 1992). To me, the divide between the academic and emotional mentoring needs of graduate students is an artificial one based more on the comfort level of the mentor rather than the specific mentoring needs of the students. In this chapter, I (a) explore the need for mentoring graduate students, (b) connect recent emphasis on social justice advocacy in counseling psychology to the mentoring needs of graduate students in psychology, and (c) detail how a constructivist approach to mentoring is distinctive in its ability to meet the advocacy and mentoring needs of graduate students. I suggest that beyond responding to proximate needs of students as they advance toward their degrees, good mentoring can offer students a relational experience and a model that embodies a uniquely constructivist approach to mentoring—one that provides a supportive foundation for their professional careers. Finally, I offer some general recommendations for constructivist mentoring with graduate students.

MENTORING OF GRADUATE STUDENTS

For Forehand and others (e.g., Humble, Solomon, Allen, Blaisure, & Johnson, 2006; Johnson, 2002), a mentor serves as a guide into the life of academia, with all its hoops and potential pitfalls. Indeed, the term "mentor" has been defined as a trusted advisor, guide, counselor, and "interpreter of the environment" (Daloz, 1986, p. 207), with its origin believed to have come from Homer's *Odyssey*. Mentor was an Ithacan noble in the *Odyssey* and as a close friend and advisor to Ulysses, Mentor was asked to provide care and protection for Ulysses' son, Telemachus, while Ulysses was off fighting the Trojan War. Mentor was left to educate, to provide ethical guidance and to care for Telemachus, and thus the term *mentor* seems to be derived from this relationship (e.g., Forehand, 2008; Johnson, 2002). However, as we will see later, the role that Mentor was asked to play and the role that he actually did play were not exactly the same. Aside from how well Mentor of the *Odyssey* actually conducted his tasks, having a mentor as a guide and helper is often cited as one of the most important resources for students' successful advancement in graduate school and their careers (Forehand, 2008; Humble, et al., 2006; Johnson, 2002; Luna & Cullen, 1998).

Graduate study in psychology is an arduous process. There are multiple tasks that must be accomplished and roles that must be performed throughout one's program. Young adults who, as undergraduate students, had barely begun the academic study of psychology, enter a rigorous sequence of activities that lead them through advanced learning, scholarship, and practice toward becoming fully functioning as professionals and possibly even as teachers and mentors themselves. In this process, multiple relationships must be managed with teachers, advisors, supervisors, peers, research participants, and clients, not to mention their own friends, significant others, and family. For many students, entering a doctoral program means charting new territory, finding one's way on a path that has not yet been traversed by those well known to them (i.e., family or friends). Given all the unfamiliar challenges, there are many ways to stray off the path towards success. Further, being a graduate student is arguably itself a position of marginal status in a larger hierarchical academic system (Brown, Davis, & McClendon, 1999; Humble et al., 2006; Johnson, 2002; Luna & Cullen, 1998). Graduate students must struggle to figure out and fulfill the requirements and effectively ascend to the top of the hierarchy, becoming an equal and even a leader among those who were once quite powerful authorities in their lives. As Forehand (2008) emphasized, graduate students are the future of psychology and care must be taken to help them achieve their academic and professional pursuits.

Findings on graduate student success suggest that students do well in research when they work closely with an advisor or research mentor and join research teams early in their graduate studies (Love, Bahner, Jones, & Nilsson, 2007). Having an early start with a team and a mentor, students are more likely to feel efficacious in their ability to conduct research and tend to be more prolific in their research production over the course of their graduate career (Dohm & Cummings, 2002, 2003). Understanding the process and ethics of conducting meaningful research is not a skill that many graduate students obtained during their undergraduate careers. Thus mentoring graduate student research projects has been identified as not only an important means of professional socialization in the employment of scientific methods, but as a valuable approach to learning the competencies necessary for the ethical conduct of research—intellectual honesty and personal responsibility for the rights and welfare of research participants (Fischer, Wertz, & Goodman, 2008; Forehand, 2008). Additionally, graduate students who have positive relationships with their mentors report more satisfaction in their programs, more positive perceptions of the academic climate, and also report feeling that they navigated the potential pitfalls of graduate school more effectively (Alvarez, Blume, Cervantes, & Thomas, 2009; Brown, Davis, & McClendon, 1999; Daloz, 1999; Humble, Solomon, Allen, Blaisure, & Johnson, 2006; Kelly & Schweitzer, 1999; Russel & Horne, 2009).

MENTORING AND SOCIAL JUSTICE

Plainly stated, mentoring appears to be good for graduate students. But is it necessary—ethically necessary? Particularly in counseling psychology, there has been a call to consider "extrapsychic forces that adversely affect the emotional and physical well-being of people" (Kiselica & Robinson, 2001, p. 387) in addition to the interpersonal or intrapersonal factors that have traditionally been the focus of therapy. Partially this move towards considering larger societal factors in conceptualizing client difficulties is a reaction to the dissatisfaction of feminist and multicultural therapists and theorists with a psychology that has traditionally ignored the experiences of women and people of color (Goodman et al., 2004). This call for social justice advocacy and action focuses on marginalized groups in society and what counselors and counseling psychologists need to be doing to rectify the overwhelming inequality that is so widespread in Western society (Goodman et al., 2004; Kiselica & Robinson, 2001; Steele, 2008; and see Raskin, 2010 [this volume] for a critique of the social justice construct in counseling psychology). Further, Fischer et al. (2008) argue that because science is power and is never value free, ethical research practice in psychology involves forming respectful, accountable relationships with marginalized groups as equal partners whose interests are served by research topics, methods, and outcomes.

Although not specifically focused on the mentoring needs of graduate students as a form of social justice, many articles have been written on the specific mentoring needs of members of groups requiring the social justice advocacy efforts of counseling psychologists, such as ethnic minorities (e.g., Alvarez, Blume, Cervantes, & Thomas, 2009; Brown, Davis, & McClendon, 1999; Davidson & Foster-Johnson, 2001; Gasman, Hirschfeld, & Vultaggio, 2008; Walker, Hanley, & Wright, 2001), women (Gilbert & Rossman, 1992; Hollingsworth & Fassinger, 2002; Humble, Solomon, Allen, Blaisure, & Johnson, 2006; Johnson, 2002), and lesbian, gay, bisexual and transgender (LGBT) students (Lark & Croteau, 1998; Russel & Horne, 2009). Psychology, a field that has been genuinely concerned with its own contribution to the values of equal opportunity, has been hospitable to an increasing number of women and ethnic minorities. Continuing experiences of subordination and vulnerability among historically marginalized groups make them especially in need of responsive advocacy on the part of mentors who are in a position to facilitate their becoming empowered leaders through graduate school education. Articles about mentoring dysfunction and deficiencies in graduate school make clear how poor mentoring does a great disservice to students (Forehand, 2008; Johnson & Huwe, 2002). Mentors play a significant role in the support of and advocacy for individuals who are ascending in the social hierarchy, through psychology, into positions of authority and leadership.

Graduate students, like all members of subordinate social groups, feel they have few rights as they struggle to meet their own educational challenges, emotional needs, and reactions to the extrapsychic factors that adversely affect their progress through their academic programs (Humble et al., 2006; Luna & Cullen, 1998; Russell & Horne, 2009). The academic community can be very intimidating, and classroom instruction offers little in the way of lessons that teach students how to maneuver through the tasks that must be completed, the egos and relationships that must be managed, and the personal anxieties that must be displayed and dealt with in appropriate ways (Luna & Cullen, 1998).

Traditional perspectives on mentoring follow the hierarchical academic patterns where the mentor's knowledge and experience is of paramount importance in the relationship with the person being mentored (at times referred to as the *mentee*, a term Koocher calls "linguistically challenged" (2002, p. 510), or the *protégé*—the protected person, both of which come with their own unique difficulties). In these traditional mentoring relationships, the mentor has both spoken and unspoken power in the relationship, while the person being mentored (i.e., the student) is given the clear message that he or she should follow the mentor's guidance and any plans that have been established for the student's development regardless of whether or not the student agrees with these plans. Because such mentoring disallows students' input in their development, it may inadvertently reenact and reinforce the subordinate status and vulnerable position of the student. Therefore these traditional perspectives have been criticized by feminist and multicultural scholars (among others), who are cognizant of issues concerning social equality in power relations. In particular, the feminist literature on mentoring has critiqued traditional Western mentoring for ignoring the personal and relational components inherent in becoming a psychologist, as well as the unique impact of the power differential in academic settings

(Gilbert & Rossman, 1992). From a multicultural perspective, traditional theories of mentoring have been criticized for ignoring the voices and experiences of ethnic minorities and for taking a "one size fits all" approach (Davidson & Foster-Johnson, 2001). I use these criticisms as a starting point for illustrating a constructivist theoretical approach to mentoring graduate students in psychology.

CONSTRUCTIVIST MENTORING AS SOCIAL JUSTICE

How is constructivist mentoring different than other forms of mentoring? What makes constructivist mentoring unique? The constructivist emphasis on the importance of subjectivity in meaning making suggests an egalitarian model for mentor relationships, one that decenters the traditional authority of the mentor and promotes dialogue. First, the constructivist perspective takes the position that the mentor does not have a unique or privileged understanding of the experience of the student, while placing the experience of the student at the center of the student's educational and professional development. However, it is virtually impossible to have a mentoring relationship in academia that does not consist of power differentials and hierarchy. These characteristics are endemic to the structure of academic life. By explicitly calling attention to the importance of the student's own subjectivity and agency in the meanings of the educational process, a constructivist perspective provides options for maneuvering gracefully through these dynamics and structures in a way that honors and meets the needs of the student.

Similar to constructivist approaches to supervision, a constructivist approach to mentoring supports the establishment of role relationships—relationships where both parties work to construe the unique construing processes of the other (Leitner & Faidley, 1995). As with feminist and multicultural approaches to mentoring, a constructivist approach supports the open discussion of power in the relationship and the need to address hierarchical conflict when it arises. Moreover, acknowledging the constructive agency of both the mentor and the student in their relationship introduces a framework of equality and mutuality between individuals with different levels of knowledge, expertise, and social position.

Researchers have developed constructivist models of counselor supervision based on these principles (Feixas, 1992). Although such models are conceptually similar to previous models of supervision, they differ in their emphasis on the experiences and needs of the supervisee. In particular, there is no longer a simple emphasis on the needs of the supervisee's clients or on the supervisor's view of the supervisee's educational progress in the areas of theory, practice and ethics. This shift in orientation toward an emphasis on the specific needs of the supervisee is especially applicable to mentoring graduate students because it introduces a primary concern for students' unique experience and needs (both explicit and implicit) into the mentoring process. For instance, the mentor would encourage students to express their experience of their coursework and professors, their clinical work and supervisors, their research and advisors in the context of their own career dreams and aspirations as an important part of the mentoring relationship. In this way, a uniquely constructivist mentoring orientation can be developed that is distinctively able to holistically incorporate all parts of the student's life as needed.

As a postmodern theoretical position, constructivism holds the personal meaning-making systems of clients central to understanding how they interpret their world and respond to life events. According to the tenets of constructivist counseling (i.e., Bridges & Raskin, 2008; Bridges & Neimeyer, 2005; Gergen, 1999; McNamee, 1996; Neimeyer & Bridges, 2003; Neimeyer, 1995; Raskin, 2002), constructivist therapists take a non-expert stance in relation to clients, avoid the objectivist or reductionistic diagnostic methodologies common in many more traditional psychotherapies, and recognize the social embeddedness of meaning making processes (Kelly, 1955/1991). Moreover, constructivist counselors take a collaborative approach with clients and also with supervisees.

Postmodern constructive thinking in the area of research has paralleled these developments in the field of counseling. The traditional authority of the researcher and the assumption that the researcher has an exclusive privilege of objectivity and power has been questioned. Critiques of the implicit values and politics of social science research in the 1970s and the liberation movements of the 1980s have led those in the social sciences to alter their methods and views of good science, suggesting collaborative, dialogical approaches that relinquish many traditional privileges of the scientific researcher (Vidich & Lyman, 2000). Social science has undergone a crisis of authority in which researchers have become accountable to non-researcher voices regarding the purposes and directions of research, the ownership of data, the perspectives of analysis and interpretation, issues of the audience and authorship, and questions of who benefits from the research (Maracek, Fine, & Kidder, 1997). Decentering of the traditional locus of power, researchers are relinquishing authority as an ethical imperative and moving toward collaborations with non-research oriented stakeholders and research participants (see Denzin & Lincoln, 2005). Just as students of constructivist counseling are being asked to give up hierarchical priority and power in relation to their clients, students of constructivist research are being asked to more fully attend to the needs, experiences, and interests of those being researched.

Extending these same principles and practices, Feixas (1992) presented a constructivist model of counselor supervision. The model is based on the assumption that, because the supervisor can only understand the problems of the supervisee's clients through the supervisee's constructions of them during supervision, the primary focus of supervision should be on the supervisee. Feixas pointed out that although it is always important to maintain concern for the client, the supervisor's relationship with the supervisee will ultimately allow the supervisee to feel more confident in his or her work and will result in the supervisee's more competent delivery of therapeutic services. Leitner and Faidley's conceptualization of role relationships (1995) helps to explain how this process may occur. Individuals engage in "role relationships" with each other when they completely validate each other's ways of understanding their lives; this does not mean that they necessarily agree with each other's ways of meaning making, rather that they accept this meaning-making as valid and true for their partner in his or her way of understanding the world. Applied to counselor supervision, the supervisor would model for the supervisee not necessarily a complete understanding of the supervisee's ways of making meaning, but an authentic validation of them to facilitate the supervisee's development.

Similarly, in constructivist supervision, the focus of the supervision is on the supervisee's complaint, which fosters not only a change in the counseling case, but also, by forming a role relationship between the supervisee and the supervisor, there is the potential for a change in the supervisee's feelings about the case and about counseling in general. It should be noted that the role relationship identified here is slightly adapted from the original definition offered by Leitner and Faidley (1995) because the relationship is somewhat asymmetrical (the supervisor needs to validate the construing processes of the supervisee, but the opposite is less important or even less appropriate). However, the primary intent is the same. Once the creation of this adapted role relationship between the supervisor and the supervisee is accomplished, the resulting validation would hopefully encourage the supervisee to create a role relationship with his or her clients in turn.

When applied to mentoring, these concepts would translate into a focus on the mentor/student interactions within the process of navigating the journey through graduate school. In other words, instead of working simply on accomplishing the academic tasks, research projects, and clinical training, the mentor endeavors to understand and validate the student's unique ways of making meaning of these graduate school engagements and the social, institutional and academic challenges that are endemic to the process.

What I am proposing is that one of the best ways of promoting social justice for the marginalized graduate student in academia, and thereby to model the kind of ethical relationship that the student is developing with clients and research participants, is through the development of a role relationship between the mentor and the student. The purpose of this role relationship in the mentoring process is the development of the graduate student. Brown, Davis, and McClendon (1999) suggest that having a true mentoring relationship with a marginalized population requires the faculty person to enter into a process of mutual self discovery. I am suggesting that this process of mutual self-discovery be extended through mentoring relationships with all students, a process which in itself can be an enriching process for the mentor (Koocher, 2002; Russel & Horne, 2009). Moreover, regardless of whether it is the intent of the mentoring relationship or not, it is naive to think that students are not attempting to construe the construing processes of the mentor.

Thus deliberately entering into role relationships potentially helps students to develop fully into colleagues by the end of their academic program and to take the experience of a validating meaning-based relationship into their future careers. In addition, by striving to fully validate and understand students' experiences, mentors may be able to detect and address difficulties early in the graduate school process. Further, the experience of having their meaning-making deeply validated by the mentor has the potential to help students learn independently to detect and cope with problems on the parts of clients, research participants, and students they teach.

Not unlike other models of supervision, Feixas' (1992) conceptualization of constructivist supervision stresses the importance of its learning component. Likewise, it emphasizes the different types of expertise held by the supervisor and the supervisee. Although supervisors have their own expertise in supervision, the supervisees are the experts on their experiences providing counseling. Therefore, just as supervisees stand to learn from supervisors, so the supervisors also have the opportunity to learn from supervisees. Relating this concept to mentoring, the provider of the mentoring is no longer viewed as having all the answers to graduate student concerns. Instead, the mentor looks to the student's expertise to inform their generation of problem-solving strategies. Such an approach replaces the potentially hierarchical nature of the mentoring relationship with one that bears more resemblance to a mutual working alliance (Humble et al., 2006; Schlosser & Gelso, 2001). Ideally, this more collaborative relationship improves the ability of mentors and students to work together to develop methods of addressing concerns of the student while in graduate school.

Now, let's return to the story of Odysseus, Telemachus and Mentor. Interestingly, as Koocher (2002) recounts, while Mentor was in fact a trusted advisor to Odysseus, he "failed miserably at his assignment" (p. 509) of keeping Odysseus's household and belongings (and wife) safe while Odysseus was fighting the Trojan War. When Odysseus returned from war, he found suitors of his wife Penelope living in his house, eating his food and drinking his wine. Mentor had lectured the suitors, but done little else. On those several occasions when Mentor did indeed appear to give wise and sage advice to Telemachus, as Koocher points out and a careful reading of the Odyssey confirms, it was not actually Mentor at all. Instead it was the goddess Athena, who appeared to Telemachus disguised as Mentor, the person from whom Telemachus could truly "hear" the advice. Athena wisely knew how to take a form that would match Telemachus' ways of making meaning and understanding his world (not to mention the difficulties inherent in convincing someone you are a goddess and your advice should be taken seriously). Similarly, in constructivist mentoring, the mentor works to understand the needs of graduate students and how best to approach their needs for support, guidance, help and encouragement, rather than simply thinking that students should conform to independently imposed expectations of the program or mentor.

RECOMMENDATIONS AND CONCLUSIONS

While not solely under the domain of constructivist mentoring, it is clear that understanding the specific needs of the student is crucial to providing the right style of mentoring. In fact, although the possible options for mentoring behaviors can include sponsorship, protection, challenge, counseling, acceptance, etc. (Green & Bauer, 1995), not all students require or benefit from all of these behaviors—regardless of the "well meaning nature" of the mentor. Constructivist mentoring entails taking the understanding of the specific needs of the student and combining it with an attempt to understand the unique construing processes the student uses to make meaning in life. By honoring and validating students' local knowledge and meaning-making, the mentor is able to work within the students range of convenience without setting up a threatening (e.g., invalidating core meaning-making structures) experience for them. Students bring life experience and knowledge to a graduate program that can be utilized and adapted to help them to find a way through their education successfully. Graduate school is not an immediate "fit" for all students. Working with their existing meaning-making structures, as opposed to attempting to force them into a "graduate student" mold, is good for both the student and those who endeavor to work with them. Students are experts on their own experience and mentors have expertise in how to successfully navigate a graduate program, conduct research, provide clinical services etc.; together they work to explore how students can best manage their academic careers.

Although making the path to academic success a straightforward one for graduate students may successfully induct them into the "Ivory Tower" of academia, it may also have the unfortunate side effect of reinforcing a hierarchical structure that places graduate students in a marginalized position in the first place (Humble et al., 2006). Granted, there are requirements that must be met for a student to be successful in a graduate program. However, when there are options for different paths a student might take, it is the role of the constructivist mentor to offer these paths as options, not mandates or obligations. Students who are not familiar with the hierarchy of traditional academia usually benefit from being provided with a "map of the territory" of the academic department and the profession in general. Yet the choice to follow well traveled paths or strike out in different directions is one for students to make on their own, albeit in conjunction with their mentor. For example, "Shannon," a 32-year-old doctoral student was offered a graduate assistantship position teaching courses about research methods at the undergraduate level. Shannon did not know that this was a "prized" position in this very traditional department and that only the very strongest students who had been identified as "destined" for academic positions in the future were offered a chance to teach these courses. Shannon decided to take an outreach position in the student affairs office instead, and simply informed the chair of the department of her decision. The chair was surprised at her decision, decided that she must not be interested in academia, and no longer took a "special interest" in Shannon and her development as an academic. The role of a mentor in this example would not necessarily be to advise Shannon to take the teaching position, but rather to help Shannon develop a broader view of the decision she faced, including the ramifications that went well beyond the work she would be doing for the semester. Had Shannon known the ramifications, she might have chosen to strike out on her own rather than taking the expected path, but with the mentor's help she could have also engaged in "impression management" if she chose to do so.

It is difficult for students to make well informed decisions and, being a marginalized group in academia, they often don't have access to all relevant information nor a good grasp of the emotional climate of the department. Working from within students' own construct systems, mentors can help them understand the consequences of their decisions and actions in relation to those who hold a great deal of power over their progress through the program. Further, recognizing the marginalized position of students, it may be important for the mentor to serve as an advocate for them, similar to what is recommended for work with clients in the social justice literature (see Goodman et al., 2004 and Kiselica & Robinson, 2001 for reviews). Although advocacy serves to help remedy the power imbalances between students and the larger academic community, there is also the risk of undermining students' own capacities to manage their situations. Thus, it is vital that advocacy for students is undertaken with explicit permission from the students themselves. Similarly, it is important to respect the individual student's need for closeness or distance in the mentoring relationship. Entering a mentoring role relationship and understanding how students makes sense of their surroundings enables mentors to adjust to the specific needs of each student. For example, some students want frequent contact with detailed conversations about the ins and outs of their experiences in the graduate program and others might find this same type of involvement invasive or a form of micromanagement. Discovering what best fits for each student comes from explicit conversations about the nature of the mentoring relationship, including an exploration of the inherent power differences between the student and their mentor.

Finally, a word about maintaining mentoring role relationships in academic communities—expanding the role of a mentor from the traditional mentor role as primarily, if not solely, an academic or research advisor can be challenging for those most comfortable with the predominant professor/student narrative. A mentoring role relationship can come across as "too close" or "too nice" for those coming from traditional academic backgrounds and it may be necessary to have transparent conversations about the nature of constructivist mentoring relationships to help some faculty members to become accepting (or at least tolerant) of more inclusive ways of relating to students. Constructivist mentoring is theoretically and ethically based, and although it may look different from "traditional" forms of mentoring, it nevertheless strives to serve the student's best interests at all times. Similar to feminist and multicultural approaches to mentoring, being a constructivist mentor serves the whole person of the student and does not reduce the student to the roles they embody in academic settings. It is unlikely that graduate students will become less marginalized in academia anytime in the near future. Although some may argue that the marginal status of graduate students is part of the educational process and simply part of being socialized into the profession, this chapter suggests that having a constructivist mentor to provide options, validate experiences, and understand meaning making endeavors enriches the experience of being a graduate student and will generate future professionals who learn to value egalitarian role relationships and thereby promote social justice in their own professional relations to clients, research participants, colleagues, and those they eventually mentor.

References

Alvarez, A., Blume, A., Cervantes, J., & Thomas, L. (2009). Tapping the wisdom tradition: Essential elements to mentoring students of color. *Professional Psychology: Research and Practice, 40*(2), 181-188.

Atkinson, D., Casas, A., & Neville, H. (1994). Ethnic minority psychologists: Whom they mentor and benefits they derive from the process. *Journal of Multicultural Counseling and Development, 22*(1), 37-48.

Atkinson, D. R., Neville, H., & Casas, A. (1991). The mentorship of ethnic minorities in professional psychology. *Professional Psychology: Research and Practice, 22,* 336–338.

Bridges, S., & Neimeyer, R. (2005). The relationship between eroticism, gender, and interpersonal bonding: A clinical illustration of sexual holonic mapping. *Journal of Constructivist Psychology, 18*(1), 15-24.

Bridges, S. K., & Raskin, J. D. (2008). Constructivist psychotherapy in the real world. *Studies in meaning 3: Constructivist psychotherapy in the real world* (pp. 3-30). New York, NY: Pace University Press.

Brown, M. C., Davis, G. L., & McClendon, S. A. (1999). Mentoring graduate students of color: Myths, models, and modes. *Peabody Journal of Education, 74*(2), 105–118.

Davidson, M. N. & Foster-Johnson, L. 2001. Mentoring in the preparation of ethnically diverse graduate students. *Review of Educational Research,* 71 (4): 549-574.

Daloz, L.A. (1986). *Effective teaching and mentoring.* San Francisco, Jossey-Bass.

Daloz, L.A. (1999). *Mentor: Guiding the journey of adult learners.* San Francisco, Jossey-Bass.

Denzin, N.K. & Lincoln, Y.S. (Eds.) (2005). *The Sage handbook of qualitative research* (3rd ed., pp. 605-639). Thousand Oaks, CA: Sage Publications.

Dohm, F., & Cummings, W. (2002). Research mentoring and women in clinical psychology. *Psychology of Women Quarterly, 26*(2), 163-167

Dohm, F., & Cummings, W. (2003). Research mentoring and men in clinical psychology. *Psychology of Men & Masculinity,4*(2), 149-153

Espinoza-Herold, M., & Gonzalez, V. (2007). The voices of senior scholars on mentoring graduate students and junior scholars. *Hispanic Journal of Behavioral Sciences, 29,* 313-335.

Feixas, G. (1992). A constructivist approach to supervision: Some preliminary thoughts. *International Journal of Personal Construct Psychology, 5*(2), 183–200.

Fischer, C. B., Wertz, F. J., & Goodman, S. J. (2008). Graduate training in responsible conduct of social science research: The role of mentors and departmental climate . In D. Mertens & P. Ginsberg (Eds.) *Sage handbook of social science research ethics.* Thousand Oaks, CA: Sage Publications.

Forehand, R. (2008). The art and science of mentoring in psychology: A necessary practice to ensure our future. *American Psychologist, 63*(8), 744-755.

Gasman, M., Hirschfeld, A., & Vultaggio, J. (2008). "Difficult yet rewarding": The experiences of African American graduate students in education at an Ivy League institution. *Journal of Diversity in Higher Education, 1,* 126-138.

Gergen, K. J. (1999). *An invitation to social construction.* Thousand Oaks, CA: Sage Publishers.

Gilbert, L. A., & Rossman, K. M. (1992). Gender and the mentoring process for women: Implications for professional development. *Professional Psychology: Research and Practice, 23,* 233-238.

Ginott, H. (1972). *Teacher and child.* New York: Free Press

Goodman, L., Liang, B., Helms, J., Latta, R., Sparks, E., & Weintraub, S. (2004). Training counseling psychologists as social justice agents: Feminist and multicultural principles in action. *Counseling Psychologist, 32*(6), 793-837

Green, S., & Bauer, T. (1995). Supervisory mentoring by advisers: Relationships with doctoral student potential, productivity, and commitment. *Personnel Psychology, 48*(3), 537-561.

Green, A. G., & Hawley, G. C. (2009). Early career psychologists: Understanding, engaging, and mentoring tomorrow's leaders. *Professional Psychology: Research and Practice, 40,* 206-212

Hollingsworth, M. A., & Fassinger, R. E. (2002). The role of faculty mentors in the research training of counseling psychology doctoral students. *Journal of Counseling Psychology, 49,* 324-330.

Humble, A. M., Solomon, C. R., Allen, K. R., Blaisure, K. R., Johnson, M. P. (2006). Feminism and mentoring of graduate students. *Family Relations, 55,* 2-15.

Johnson, W. B. (2002). The intentional mentor: Strategies and guidelines for the practice of mentoring. *Professional Psychology: Research and Practice, 33,* 88–96.

Johnson, W. B., & Huwe, J. M. (2002). Toward a typology of mentorship dysfunction in graduate school. *Psychotherapy: Theory/Research/Practice/Training, 39,* 44-45.

Kelly, G. A. (1955). *The psychology of personal constructs* (2 vols.). New York: Norton.

Kelly, S., & Schweitzer, J. (1999). Mentoring within a graduate school setting. *College Student Journal, 33*(1), 130-148.

Kiselica, M., & Robinson, M. (2001). Bringing advocacy counseling to life: The history, issues, and human dramas of social justice work in counseling. *Journal of Counseling & Development, 79,* 387-397

Koocher, G. (2002). Mentor revealed: Masculinization of an early feminist construct. *Professional Psychology: Research and Practice, 33* (5), 509-510.

Lark, J. S., & Croteau, J. M. (1998). Lesbian, gay and bisexual doctoral students' mentoring relationships with faculty in counseling psychology. *Counseling Psychologist, 26,* 754-776.

Leitner, L. M., & Faidley, A. J. (1995). The awful, aweful nature of ROLE relationships. In G. Neimeyer & R. Neimeyer (Eds.), *Advances in personal construct psychology* (Vol. 3, pp. 291-314). Greenwich, CT: JAI.

Love, K., Bahner, A., Jones, L., & Nilsson, J. (2007). An investigation of early research experience and research self-efficacy. *Professional Psychology: Research and Practice, 38*(3), 314-320.

Luna, G., & Cullen, D. (1998). Do graduate students need mentors? *College Student Journal, 32,* 322-331.

Maracek, J., Fine, M., & Kidder, L. (1997). Working between worlds: Qualitative methods and social psychology. *Journal of Social Issues, 53*(4), 631-644.

McNamee, S. (1996). Psychotherapy as social construction. In H. Rosen & K. T. Kuehlwein (Eds.), Constructing reality: Meaning-making perspectives for psychotherapists (pp. 115-137). San Francisco, CA: Jossey-Bass

Neimeyer, R. A. (1995). An invitation to constructivist psychotherapies. In R. A. Neimeyer & M. J. Mahoney (Eds.), *Constructivism in psychotherapy* (pp. 1-8). Washington, DC: American Psychological Association.

Neimeyer, R. A., & Bridges, S. K. (2003). Postmodern approaches to psychotherapy. *Essential psychotherapies: Theory and practice* (2nd ed., (pp. 272-316). New York, NY: Guilford Press.

Raskin, J. D. (2002). Constructivism in psychology: Personal construct psychology, radical constructivism, and social constructionism. In J. D. Raskin & S. K. Bridges (Eds.), *Studies in meaning: Exploring constructivist psychology* (pp. 1-25). New York: Pace University Press.

Raskin, J. D. (2010, this volume). Constructing and deconstructing social justice counseling. In J. D. Raskin, S. K. Bridges, & R. A. Neimeyer (Eds.), *Studies in meaning 4: Constructivist psychotherapy in the real world* (pp. 245-273). New York: Pace University Press.

Russell, G. M., & Horne, S. G. (2009). Finding equilibrium: Mentoring, sexual orientation, and gender identity. *Professional Psychology: Research and Practice, 40,* 194-200.

Schlosser, L., & Gelso, C. (2001). Measuring the working alliance in advisor-advisee relationships in graduate school. *Journal of Counseling Psychology, 48*(2), 157-167

Steele, J. (2008). Preparing counselors to advocate for social justice: A liberation model. *Counselor Education and Supervision, 48*(2), 74-85.

Vidich, A.J. & Lyman, S.M. (2000). Qualitative methods: Their history in sociology and anthropology. In N.K. Denzen & Y.S. Lincoln (eds.), *The Sage handbook of qualitative research* (2nd ed., pp. 37-84). Thousand Oaks, CA: Sage Publications.

Walker, K. L., Hanley, J. H., & Wright, G. (2001). The professional preparation of African American graduate students: A student perspective. *Professional Psychology: Research and Practice, 32* (6), 581–584.

෬ 9 ෭

Gazing at Objectification Theory through a Social Constructionist Lens
Melanie S. Hill

> *The contemporary ravages of the beauty backlash are destroying women physically and depleting us psychologically. If we are to free ourselves from the dead weight that has once again been made out of femaleness, it is not ballots or lobbyists or placards that women will need first; it is a new way to see.*
>
> Wolf, 2002, p. 19

In western industrialized countries it is rare to find a woman who feels good about her body. The dislike many women hold for their bodies has become so widespread that it has often been referred to as a "normative discontent" (Rodin, Silberstein, & Striegel-Moore, 1985). According to recent research, between 50% and 80% of girls and women report being dissatisfied with their appearance (Bearman, Presnell, & Martinez, 2006; Neighbors & Sobal, 2007). This dissatisfaction is not inconsequential. It has been linked to mental health problems for women, such as eating disorders and depression (Grabe, Hyde, & Lindberg, 2007; Johnson & Wardle, 2005). In an effort to improve the psychological well-being of women, a substantial amount of literature has been published attempting to identify the etiology of this discontent, with the ultimate goal of preventing the high rates of depression and eating disorders in women.

In seeking to explain body dissatisfaction, much of the published literature has pointed to the internal psychological processes of women. In particular, the dominant explanation in psychology has been that women's body image disturbances are "caused" by perceptual or cognitive distortions (see Blood, 2005, for a review). For example, much of the research concludes that "perceptual defects" such as unrealistic or irrational expectations and faulty or distorted beliefs prevent high numbers of "normal" women from accurately estimating their body size, which is deemed indicative of body image disturbance. More recent theorizing, however, has begun to focus on the role sociocultural influences play in the development of body dissatisfaction. Feminist theorists, in particular, have argued that the ways in which the female body is viewed and socially constructed shape how women view their own bodies (e.g., Bartky, 1988; Berger, 1972; Bordo, 2003; Orbach, 1988; Kaschak, 1992).

Frederickson and Roberts (1997) proposed a theory that has received a substantial amount of attention. They postulate that living in a culture in which women's bodies are sexually objectified ultimately leads to body dissatisfaction and eating disorders for women (Fredrickson & Roberts, 1997). Since its publication, the constructs put forth in Fredrickson and Robert's objectification theory have dominated the body image literature. In this chapter, I briefly review objectification theory's main tenets, then, through a social constructionist lens, elaborate on some emerging questions and concerns regarding this popular theory and the resulting research. Objectification theory is essentially a synthesis and formalization of many disparate lines of theorizing and research regarding the sexual objectification of women with some roots in social constructionist thinking (e.g., Bartky, Bordo, Foucault). While Fredrickson and Roberts (1997) themselves argue that women's bodies are "constructed through sociocultural practices and discourses" (p. 174), social constructionist theorizing has remained on the periphery. The goal of this chapter is to explore what it would mean to move the tenets of social constructionism to a more central location in the literature on objectification theory.

Social constructionism, as defined by Gergen (1985) and Burr (1995), is rooted in several key assumptions that provide the underpinnings of this chapter. First, social constructionists maintain that one should take a critical stance towards taken-for-granted ways of understanding the world, encouraging people to challenge "the objective basis of conventional knowledge" (Gergen, 1985, p. 267). Second, social constructionists argue that our knowledge of the world is made up of historically and culturally specific social artifacts rather than discovered forces of nature. Third, what people regard as "truth" is not seen as primarily shaped by an objective reality, but instead is seen as the result of social processes such as language and discourse. Fourth, social constructionists contend that how people describe or construct the world prescribes certain avenues of social action and excludes others. It is my hope that by further exploring objectification theory through a social constructionist lens, new and beneficial avenues for social action will emerge.

OBJECTIFICATION THEORY

The core tenet of objectification theory, which reflects the work of many feminist scholars, is that living in a culture in which women's bodies are sexually objectified socializes girls and women to treat themselves as objects (e.g., Bartky, 1990; Berger, 1992; Kaschak, 1992). While the sexualization of women can range from sexual evaluation to sexual violence, the focus of objectification theory is on "objectifying gaze" as it plays out in three arenas: interpersonal and social encounters, visual media that depict interpersonal and social encounters, and visual media that spotlights women's bodies and body parts. According to Fredrickson and Roberts (1997), through such repeated and often ubiquitous experiences of sexual objectification women are "coaxed" or "socialized" to adopt an observer's perspective, ultimately "treating *themselves* as objects to be looked at and evaluated" (p. 177). In other words, sexual objectification leads to self-objectification as women come to value their bodies in observable, appearance-based terms (e.g., "How do I look?") more than in non-observable, competence-based terms (e.g., "How do I feel?" or "What am I physically capable of?"). According to Fredrickson and Roberts, this "self-objectification" and its resulting habitual body surveillance potentially leads to a cadre of negative psychological or subjective experiences for women (e.g, shame, anxiety, decreased peak motivational states, and decreased awareness of internal bodily states), which ultimately may accumulate and contribute to certain psychological disorders (e.g., depression, sexual dysfunction, eating disorders).

In looking at this theory from a social constructionist perspective several questions arise: What is "sexual objectification"? Does it always lead to self-objectification? Can sexual objectification, and for that matter self-objectification, be psychologically beneficial? If self-objectification leads to eating disorders and depression, does that mean the origin of women's dissatisfaction is in their heads? How do the procedures used in conducting research on objectification theory challenge and/or support the objectification of women? Each of these questions is explored in turn, delving into both the perspectives of objectification theory and social constructionism.

QUESTION #1: WHAT IS "SEXUAL OBJECTIFICATION"?

According to objectification theory, many of the psychological consequences and disorders that women experience result from living in a culture where women's bodies are viewed and treated as sexual objects. From a social constructionist perspective, it is thus important to begin by deconstructing the concept of "sexual objectification." For example, who determines what is deemed "objectification"? What makes a certain type of objectification "sexual"? Is the same action (e.g., having someone comment on the pleasing nature of a certain portion of your body) "objectification" regardless of whether the person doing it is a stranger or a lover?

Fredrickson and Roberts (1997) define sexual objectification as "the experience of being treated *as a body* (or collection of body parts) valued predominately for its use to (or consumption by) others" (p. 174, italics in original). In other words, it is the *experience* of objectification that potentially leads to negative psychological consequences for women. Does this mean that it is solely up to the individual experiencing the "objectification" to deem it as such? Clearly, not all women agree on what is sexually objectifying and what is not. Social constructionism can be used to argue that sexual objectification is not only an experience, but also a social construction, a discourse, intimately connected to existing social structures. In other words, whether or not a person experiences a gaze or comment as sexual objectification is shaped by many other factors besides the gaze or comment itself.

Sexual Objectification as a Social Construction

Social constructionists would argue that "sexual objectification" is a socially constructed term and not an objective reality. As such, it may have different meanings for different people in different contexts. For example, having a lover comment on the attractiveness of one's body may carry a different meaning when it is done in the privacy of one's bedroom than when it is done in front of one's coworkers. It also may carry different meaning for someone who has struggled with an eating disorder than for someone for whom this has not been an issue. According to social constructionism, the meaning of language is never fixed (Burr, 1995); language (in this case the gaze or comment) does not refer to some external "reality" but rather carries a multiplicity and varied set of meanings and projections depending on the person, situation, and sociohistorical context.

However, the writing on sexual objectification has generally not taken the potentially varied meanings of the term into account.

Let's return for a moment to the definition of sexual objectification provided by Fredrickson and Roberts (1997):

> the *experience* of being treated as a body (or collection of body parts) valued predominately for its use to (or consumption by) others ... occurs whenever a woman's body, body parts, or sexual functions are separated out from her person, reduced to the status of mere instruments, or regarded as if they were capable of representing her. (p. 174-175, italics added and omitted for emphasis)

The question remains how one determines when this is occurring. Are we free to label something as sexually objectifying as long as it is experienced as such? How does one conclude when a woman's body is separated out from her person? When is it resolved that a woman's body parts are regarded as capable of representing her? Is it objectively clear to anyone who witnesses it or is it based on how the subject (or object) feels?

Research conducted on objectification experiences (my own work included) similarly treats sexual objectification as if it was an objective reality by asking participants to rate how *frequently* "someone has stared at your breasts while talking to you" or "how many times have you been in a situation where someone made evaluative or judging comments on your weight or body shape?" Thus, participants are asked to report the frequency of perceived *behaviors*, not their *experiences* of those behaviors. What each of these perceived behaviors might mean for the participants, or whether or not they even experienced them as "sexually objectifying," is not taken into consideration. Having someone stare at your breasts might be experienced differently when it occurs on a job interview than at a bar, or may evoke different emotions if it occurs when you are 15 versus 50. By not inquiring about the specifics of these experiences, the contexts in which they occur, and the meanings participants ascribe to them, researchers are overlooking a wealth of nuanced information.

While deconstructing the concept of sexual objectification, we begin to see that it refers to something that occurs between people—a relational process, a form of communication that takes place between the objectified and a (real or anticipated) objectifier. Even visual media that spotlights women's bodies is a form of communication between the advertiser/producer and the potential consumer. Viewing objectification in this way encourages people to think of sexual objectification more broadly—not simply as an experience, but as a cultural discourse; a discourse that includes specific experiences, as well as all the multitude of ways people talk about (and depict) women, femininity, sexuality, and self-improvement.

Blood (2005) defines discourses as "groups of statements which cohere around a particular topic or object, providing a way of talking about that topic" (p. 49). She further states that discourses can include objects, events, subjectivity, and experiences. One of the primary discourses regarding sexuality is the romance narrative in which male's sexual desire is ever-present, unrestrained, and uncontrollable while female's sexual desire is virtually non-existent (Kirkman, Rosenthal, & Smith, 1998; Tolman, 2000). Women and girls are, instead, positioned as more or less willing sexual objects. In other words, inherent in the romance narrative is a discourse of sexual objectification—that women are sexual objects to be looked at and evaluated. This discourse is enacted through the male gaze (either in interpersonal encounters or the visual media), but also includes the ways we talk about women's bodies more generally, including seemingly benign comments such as "she looks great; she must have lost weight" or "I wish I had legs like that." By viewing sexual objectification more broadly as a discourse, we shift our gaze from the specific behavior of men and the media and refocus it on the use of language (verbal and non-verbal) more generally—acknowledging how both men *and* women engage in the discourse.

According to objectification theory, sexual objectification experiences influence how women view themselves and their bodies. Reconceptualizing sexual objectification as a discourse allows us a more nuanced perspective as to how it may influence the formation of women's identities. As Burr (1995) asserts: "Identity is constructed out of the discourses culturally available to us, and which we draw upon in our communication with other people" (p. 51). Thus, the cultural discourse of women as sexual objects has the potential to powerfully shape how women see themselves. I will return to this process later in this chapter.

Connection between Discourses and Social Structures

According to social constructionists, in any social and historical context multiple discourses coexist, with some discourses more accessible than others. Further, the discourses that are culturally available at any given time are intimately connected with the existing social structure and power relations, which both "transmit and produce power" (Foucault, 1990, p. 101). Discourses that support and reproduce existing power relations are referred to as "dominant discourses." These discourses appear "natural" and are often regarded as "truth." As such, it can be argued that the romance narrative, more broadly, and the "women are sexual objects" discourse, more specifically, is a dominant discourse (along with other related discourses, e.g., body weight, male sexual desire) in the current historical and social context. It is perceived by many as "natural" and can be used to uphold and sustain existing power inequalities between men and women.

Viewing sexual objectification as a discourse that upholds and reproduces existing power relations between men and women dovetails with what feminists have been articulating for the past several decades. In particular, that the ways in which women's bodies are represented *originate* from women's subordinate position vis-à-vis men in a patriarchal culture and therefore *support* women's continued oppression (e.g., Bartky, 1990; Berger, 1972; Bordo, 1988; Orbach, 1988; Wolf, 2002).

According to Foucault, these discourses are not conspiratorial, intentional, or a matter of top-down coercion; they do not originate from a group of powerful people (in this case, men) thinking them up and then disseminating them. Rather, the existing sociocultural power relations (i.e., inequality between men and women) provide a fertile environment for certain discourses to flourish. However, Foucault adds that once a discourse is culturally available, those that are relatively powerful may be more likely to embrace and engage in it as it ultimately reinforces their power. The following scenario is a good example of how the male gaze functions as a form of communication that ultimately serves to maintain the dominance of men:

> It is a fine spring day, and with an utter lack of self-consciousness, I am bouncing down the street. Suddenly I hear men's voices. Catcalls and whistles fill the air. These noises are clearly sexual in intent and they are meant for me; they come from across the street. I freeze. As Sartre would say, I have been petrified by the gaze of the Other. My face flushes and my motions become stiff and self-conscious. The body which only a moment before I inhabited with such ease now floods my consciousness. I have been made into an object. While it is true that for these men I am nothing but, let us say, a "nice piece of ass," there is more involved in this encounter than their mere fragmented perception of me. They could, after all, have enjoyed me in silence. . . . I could have passed by without having been turned to stone. But I must be *made* to know that I am a 'nice piece of ass': I must be made to see myself as they see me. (Bartky, 1990, p. 27)

In this scenario, and those that many women experience daily, the men do not merely admire the woman passing by but engage in a discourse that is readily available in a culture submerged in gender inequality. Through their gaze and catcalls their "admiration" serves to reinforce their social dominance and power; thus, the existing discourse of women as a 'nice piece of ass,' cannot be disentangled from the social structures that exist.

QUESTION #2: CAN OBJECTIFICATION BE PSYCHOLOGICALLY BENEFICIAL?

While Fredrickson and Roberts (1997) briefly submit that "not all women experience and respond to sexual objectification in the same way," depending on "unique combinations of ethnicity, class, sexuality, age, and other physical and personal attributes" (pp. 174-175), they quickly transition to focusing on what they propose to be a shared set of social and psychological experiences—a vulnerability to be gazed at and evaluated in a sexualized way—and the psychological consequences that result. Indeed, Fredrickson and Roberts (1997) describe their aim as "illuminating the psychological and experiential *consequences* that sexual objectification might have in many women's lives" (p. 177, italics in original). However, the consequences they illuminate are exclusively negative (e.g., increased anxiety and shame, and decreased awareness of internal bodily states and peak motivational states).

Similarly, the majority of the research conducted so far on objectification theory (my own work included) has either (a) disregarded the meaning that individuals attach to their objectification experiences, viewing it as irrelevant; or (b) implicitly assumed that women have a shared experience of cultural objectification—in particular, that it is a negative experience with negative consequences. This limited perspective (often dictated by the use of forced-choice questionnaires) negates the possibility and probability that women experience and construct meaning from being objectified in different ways. The question becomes: can being objectified evoke any other emotions besides negative ones? If so, how? I argue that how women *experience* or make meaning of being gazed at or evaluated varies greatly and thus, the resulting psychological *consequences* may vary as well.

A Range of Emotions

When I teach about objectification theory in my psychology of women course, invariably students raise their hands and comment on positive emotions elicited by objectification experiences (e.g., feeling wanted, desired, sexy). Some of the quantitative and qualitative research I've been doing recently tells a similar story—women report a wide range of emotional reactions (often simultaneously) to being objectified. For example, in response to the single act of experiencing "cat calls" on the street, women reported feeling beautiful, wanted, excited, sexy, dirty, angry, horrified, and embarrassed. Other women, whether because of their race, age, or body shape, bemoaned not being objectified—missing it, wanting it, feeling hurt, sad, and ashamed when it *didn't* happen (Hill, 2010). Indeed there is a discourse evident in the popular media and scholarly articles in which men's evaluative street remarks are presented as flattering at best and innocuous at worst (Gardner, 1980; Kissling & Kramarae, 1991).

As Burr (1995) argues, "our subjective experience is provided by the discourses in which we are culturally embedded" (p. 59). Thus, if one has internalized the dominant discourse that "women are sexual objects" (seeing it as "natural" and reflective of a "truth"), being looked over and told that you are *succeeding* at being a "desirable" object might elicit positive emotions while being "over looked" or deemed not worthy may elicit negative emotions. As Orbach (1988) notes, the words "fat" and "thin" are not merely descriptive, but carry social meaning. Women often feel good about themselves when they are told they look "thin," whereas being told you look "fat" is perceived as negative. Some recent and preliminary research has begun to explore women's experiences of appearance-related compliments. For example, Fea and Brannon (2006) describe a study in which women who viewed their bodies in more appearance based ways reported a less negative mood following appearance related compliments than neutral compliments.

Feelings of Power

Women students in my classes also describe a sense of "power" associated with meeting the cultural ideal of beauty and reaping its implied rewards—for example, having men buy them drinks at bars or getting out of speeding tickets. Thus, women may engage in objectifying themselves in a conscious or unconscious effort to elicit this power. As Foucault argues, power is not something one group possesses and wields over other groups, but something with which all people engage. Burr (1995) describes the power women have access to in relation to the "male sexual drive" discourse as an example of how power is not singular or absolute. While the discourse that men's sex drive originates from a basic biological drive constructs male sexuality as a biological imperative that must be satisfied, Burr argues that it also gives women the power to elicit this desire. Similarly, in the "women are sexual objects to be looked at and evaluated" discourse, men are given the power to evaluate women as commodities while women are given the power to elicit the male's approving gaze (and thus sexual desire) by how they dress or use their bodies.

Consequences

The preceding discussion has focused primarily on women's *experiences* of being treated as a sexual object, not the *consequences* of such treatment. Thus, the question remains whether events experienced as positive result in similar consequences to those as negative. Some preliminary research suggests that even positive objectification experiences may result in negative consequences. Calogero, Herbozo, and Thompson (2009) found that even when compliments about appearance made female participants feel good, the compliments resulted in body dissatisfaction; "indeed, the highest body dissatisfaction scores overall were reported in association with appearance compliments, not appearance criticisms" (p. 128). It should be noted that the majority of the theorizing and research in this area has focused on negative consequences (Moradi & Huang, 2008). Thus, it is possible that objectification experiences could (perhaps simultaneously) lead to both negative and positive consequences (e.g., increased self-esteem) for women, but that we are only finding negative consequences because that is all we are looking for.

QUESTION #3: IS IT ALL IN OUR HEADS?

While acknowledging that the more extreme experiences of cultural sexual objectification (e.g., sexual harassment, sexual assault) may lead directly to negative psychological consequences for women, objectification theory proposes that more ubiquitous experiences affect women indirectly through internalization (i.e., self-objectification). According to objectification theory, women are "taught," "socialized," and "coaxed" to "treat *themselves* as objects to be looked at and evaluated" (Fredrickson & Roberts, 1997, p. 177, italics in original). Thus, it is proposed that it is self-objectification that leads to many of the psychological consequences reported by women.

Essentialism

While objectification theory undoubtedly rejects the perspective that women experience body image dissatisfaction and eating disorders because of a pre-existing set of biological characteristics, the theory ultimately comes from an essentialist perspective. Essentialism argues that people are separate and discrete, possessing their own individual nature that explains how they behave and feel. From an essentialist standpoint, personality and other traits are viewed as stable, definable, and objectively measurable. Essentialism is evident in objectification theory, in particular with the construct of self-objectification. Self-objectification is described by Fredrickson et al. (1998)

as a "trait," a relatively stable individual difference variable. It is measured by asking participants to rate objectively the importance different body attributes have in terms of their "physical self-concept." Such a measure is indicative of a perspective that views self-objectification as an objective reality that can be measured—a stable, fixed and internal entity; something women "have" to varying degrees. As Moradi and Huang (2008) argue, "referring to self-objectification as a trait perpetuates the impression that it is innate, enduring, and resistant to interventions, rather than an experience that is sustained by and sensitive to contextual experiences of sexual objectification" (p. 379).

Social constructionists generally take an anti-essentialist perspective, arguing that people are products of social processes (Burr, 1995; Gergen, 1994). Individuals are not discrete or separate from their contexts and do not have stable, definable, or objectively measurable traits. Social constructionists further argue that there is no objective evidence for something called "self-objectification." Social constructionists are also likely to argue that "traits" such as self-objectification are not really all that stable across time and situations. Do we view our bodies in the same way when we are at a bar packed with good-looking men and women as we do when we are playing bingo with our great-aunt Edna? Do we feel the same way about our bodies when we are running along a secluded path as we do when we are running past a group of construction workers? Indeed, in the infamous "swimsuit study," Fredrickson et al. (1998) found that trying on a swimsuit in front of a full-length mirror was more likely to trigger self-objectification than trying on a sweater (despite no observers actually being present).

This line of reasoning suggests that self-objectification exists *between* not *within* people. Self-objectification does not have meaning without the (real or anticipated) observer; indeed, without the other there would be no observer's perspective to take at all. Further, the extent to which one self-objectifies depends on the unique relationship one has with potential observers. The social constructionist term for this is "joint action" (Shotter, 1993); the way we interact with others, how we talk and behave, is the product of the relationship rather than either person's internal forces. In other words, how I feel about my self and my appearance is different around my sister than it is when I am around my children because of my unique relationship with each of them, not as a result of something within me. As Burr observers, a person's identity is "constantly in flux, constantly changing depending upon whom the person is with, in what circumstances and to what purpose" (p. 40).

Individuals and Society

Objectification theory's argument, namely that the sociocultural context (society) "socializes" girls and women (individuals) to treat themselves as objects, implies that individuals are not only separate from, but products of, the society into which they are born. However, social constructionists maintain that the dichotomy between the individual and society is arbitrary and socially constructed. "In the real world, we never actually see 'society' on the one hand and 'individuals' on the other. It is not like looking at an egg and a hot frying pan and asking what effects each has on the other" (Burr, 1995, p. 104). Rejecting the idea that the explanations for social phenomenon exist either within the individual or the society, social constructionists encourage us to focus on the processes. That is, they emphasize "*how* certain phenomena or forms of knowledge are achieved by people in interaction" (Burr, 1995, p. 8). Thus, the question becomes *how* do discourses and relational processes come to shape one's identity, and in particular, how do women come to identify themselves as observable bodies? While fully delving into the answers to this question is beyond the scope of this chapter, a brief overview of one potential process—disciplinary power—is explored.

Disciplinary Power

From a social constructionist perspective, identity (one's sense of oneself as a person) is constantly being shaped through language and the discourses culturally available at any given time. These discourses are prescriptive in that they have implications for what one can and should do. As such, discourses are instrumental in forming societal "norms" against which people compare, judge, and measure themselves. When individuals internalize a discourse it becomes incorporated into how they see themselves and conceptualize their value as individuals. According to Foucault (1990), people engage with discourses through self-discipline and self-surveillance, comparing themselves to socially accepted norms. Foucault calls this "disciplinary power." It occurs when "people are disciplined and controlled by freely subjecting themselves to the scrutiny of others (especially 'experts') and to their own self-scrutiny" (Burr, 1995, pp. 67-68). In concert with Fredrickson and Roberts' (1997) focus on the gaze, Foucault (1977) observes how such self-surveillance can be triggered by something as subtle as a gaze:

> There is no need for arms, physical violence, material constraints. Just a gaze. An inspecting gaze, a gaze which each individual under its weight will end by interiorizing to the point that he is his [sic] own overseer, each individual thus exercising his surveillance over and against himself. (p. 155)

In applying Foucault's concept of disciplinary power to women, Bordo (2003) argues women are not merely passive victims of "patriarchal desires," but are active agents adopting prescribed discursive or social practices. In comparing themselves to what the dominant discourse prescribes as the "norm," women voluntarily engage in a range of self-regulatory practices such as self-surveillance (or self-objectification) (see Bartky, 1988 for a thorough review of the ways in which women discipline and regulate their bodies).

Such self-surveillance, which many argue promotes a more global disempowerment, can give the individual a sense of control, mastery, and personal triumph (Bartky, 1988). In other words, it is through self-objectification that women engage in power. As Berger (1972) observes, a woman is encouraged "to survey everything she is and everything she does because how she appears to others, and ultimately how she appears to men, is of crucial importance for what is normally thought of as the success of her life" (p. 46). Surveying oneself in this way is further reinforced by a cultural milieu in which meeting or violating the prescribed image for women's bodies often has real social and economic repercussions (see Fredrickson & Roberts, 1997, for a review).

QUESTION #4: DOES RESEARCH CONTRIBUTE TO THE OBJECTIFICATION OF WOMEN?

Most of the research conducted on objectification theory has focused on the construct of trait self-objectification and has used the Self-Objectification Questionnaire (SOQ, Noll & Fredrickson, 1998). The Self-Objectification Questionnaire provides participants a list of 12 body-attributes (six appearance-based, such as physical attractiveness and weight; and six competence-based, such as muscular strength and physical stamina). In completing the questionnaire, participants are asked to rank order the attributes in terms of how important each is to their physical self-concept. In a landmark study exploring the effects of self-objectification on body shame, restrained eating, and math performance (Fredrickson et al., 1998), participants were randomly assigned to try on either a one-piece swimsuit or a V-neck sweater and were asked to complete a series of measures while sitting in front of a full-length mirror. In her review, Blood (2005) critiques the predominant methods used in body dissatisfaction and eating disorder research. She argues that research procedures that ask women to focus their gaze on their body and view it as a series of measurements serve to "intensify and normalize a woman's objectifying gaze of her body" (p. 2), thus reinforcing the idea that the mind and body are separate and distinct. Below, I argue that these concerns are evident in research conducted on objectification theory, as well.

Being Subject to Gaze

Experimental procedures that ask participants to evaluate their body-attributes are asking participants to focus their gaze on their bodies as one would an object, viewing their bodies as a series of parts. Similarly, research that positions women in front of a full-length mirror while trying on a swimsuit or sweater reproduces the anticipated gaze from the perspective of an observer, priming a sense of being on display. What I'm suggesting is that participation in such research could be considered an objectification experience itself because the participants are, in many ways, "being treated *as a body* (or collection of body parts)" (Frederickson & Roberts, 1997, p. 174, italics in original). Given that research has suggested that the degree to which someone self-objectifies varies depending on the context (Hebl, King, & Lin, 2004; Huebner & Fredrickson, 1999; Fredrickson et al, 1998), we need to be careful what conclusions we make about research that perhaps, by the mere measures and methods used, evokes a sense of being observed and/or requires participants to look at their bodies as objects. It is possible that the amount of self-objectification and the associated consequences participants report are sheer artifacts of the research itself.

Dichotomizing Mind and Body

On a larger scale, it has been argued such research reinforces and perpetuates the dominant discourse, one in which a woman's body is viewed as an object separate from the individual or mind that perceives it (Blood, 2005). The argument that women adopt an observer's perspective of themselves implies that the mind (which is taking on the perspective of an observer) is separate from the body (which is being perceived as an object). This dichotomy further shapes, perhaps even limits, the avenues available to women and girls for making sense of their bodies. Again, such research communicates and/or reinforces the belief that women's psychological distress can be understood at the individual level (often by pathologizing the mind of the individual) rather than by examining the available cultural discourses, social structures, and processes through which individuals engage.

QUESTION #5: WHAT ARE THE IMPLICATIONS FOR RESEARCH AND SOCIAL CHANGE?

In conclusion, I think Fredrickson and Roberts were on to something—the ways in which people come to know (or construe) their bodies and themselves is largely influenced by social context (the media people consume, the feedback they receive from others). However, exploring objectification theory through a social constructionist lens brings to the foreground some of the originally proposed tenets of objectification theory and allows us to see ways in which the theory can be enriched. In particular, we are encouraged to explore the multiplicity of potential meanings of sexual objectification, producing varied and sometimes conflicting emotions and consequences. We are persuaded to view sexual objectification experiences more broadly as rooted in discourses that are intimately connected with existing social structures and power inequalities (also social constructions). Both sexual objectification and self-objectification are presented as relational processes rather than objective and discrete entities; processes that are intertwined with power and self-discipline. Such a perspective offers new ways of thinking about research and social change.

In terms of research, it is important to explore what labeling something as "sexual objectification" means for the individual, allowing a space for a multiplicity of meanings—understanding that "subjectivity is both inconsistent and contradictory, rather than unitary and rational" (Blood, 2005, p. 47). As quantitative measures are typically ill-suited for measuring multiplicity, meaning, and contradictions, future research should employ primarily qualitative methods that avoid reinforcing false dichotomies such as "individual/society" and "mind/body." Future research should also avoid procedures that normalize and reproduce an objectifying gaze of the body.

Viewing sexual objectification as a discourse that upholds current power inequalities opens up a new avenue for pursuing social change. Rather than focusing on the individual level (i.e., those who are objectified and those who objectify others), as much of the past literature in this area has done, people are encouraged to focus on available discourses, the social structures that support such discourses, and the ways that each of us engage with these discourses. Doing so opens up the possibility for new ways of conceptualizing action. As Bartky (1988) observes, "We women cannot begin to re-vision our own bodies until we learn to read the cultural messages we inscribe upon them daily" (p. 83), and until we broaden our outlook to see beyond the sense of mastery or power that comes as a result of engaging in dominant discourses. Ultimately, we each have the ability and power to choose to engage with different, perhaps more marginalized, discourses.

REFERENCES

Bartky, S. (1988). Foucault, femininity and the modernization of patriarchal power. In I. Diamond & L. Quinby (Eds.), *Feminism and Foucault: Reflections and resistance* (pp. 61-86). Boston: Northeastern University Press.

Bearman, S. K., Presnell, K., Martinez, E., & Stice, E. (2006). The skinny on body dissatisfaction: A longitudinal study of adolescent girls and boys. *Journal of Youth and Adolescence, 35,* 229-241.

Berger, J. (1972). *Ways of seeing.* London: Viking.

Blood, S. K. (2005) *Body Work: The social construction of women's body image.* New York: Routledge.

Bordo, S. (2003) *Unbearable weight: Feminism, western culture and the body* (10th ed.). Berkeley: University of California Press.

Burr, V. (1995). *An introduction to social constructionism.* New York: Routledge.

Calogero, R., Herbozo, S., & Thompson, K. (2009). Complementary weightism: The potential costs of appearance-related commentary for women's self-objectification. *Psychology of Women, 33,* 120-132.

Fea, C. & Brannon, L. (2006). Self-objectification and compliment type: Effects on negative mood. *Body Image, 3,* 183-188.

Foucault, M. (1977). *Discipline and punish: The birth of the prison.* New York: Random House.

Foucault, M. (1982). The subject and power. In H. Dreyfus & P. Rabinow (Eds.) *Beyond structuralism and hermeneutics* (pp. 208-226). Chicago: University of Chicago Press.

Foucault, M. (1990). *The history of sexuality. Vol.1: An introduction.* New York: Pantheon Books.

Fredrickson, B. L., & Roberts, T. (1997). Objectification theory: Toward understanding women's lived experiences and mental health risks. *Psychology of Women Quarterly, 21,* 173-206.

Fredrickson, B. L., Roberts, T., Noll, S. M., Quinn, D. M., & Twenge, J. M. (1998). The swimsuit becomes you: Sex differences in self-objectification, restrained eating, and math performance. *Journal of Personality and Social Psychology, 75,* 269-284.

Gardner, C. (1980). Passing by: Street remarks, address rights, and the urban female. *Sociological Inquiry, 50,* 328-356.

Gergen, K. J. (1985). The social constructionist movement in modern psychology. *American Psychologist, 40,* 266-275.

Gergen, K. J. (1994). *Realities and Relationships.* Boston: Harvard University Press.

Grabe, S., Hyde, J., & Lindberg, S. (2007). Body objectification and depression in adolescents: The role of gender, shame, and rumination. *Psychology of Women Quarterly, 31,* 164-175.

Hebl, M. R., King, E. B., & Lin, J. (2004). The swimsuit becomes us all: Ethnicity, gender, and vulnerability to self-objectification. *Personality and Social Psychology Bulletin, 30,* 1322-1331.

Hill, M. S. (2010). *Everyday objectification: Exploring its frequency and women's varied emotional responses.* Manuscript in preparation.

Huebner, D. M., & Fredrickson, B. L. (1999). Gender differences in memory perspectives: Evidence for self-objectification in women. *Sex Roles, 41,* 459-467.

Johnson, F., & Wardle, J. (2005). Dietary restraint, body dissatisfaction, and psychological distress: A prospective analysis. *Journal of Abnormal Psychology, 114,* 119-125.

Kaschak, E. (1992). *Engendered lives: A new psychology of women's experience.* New York: Basic Books.

Kirkman, M., Rosenthal, D., & Smith, A. (1998). Adolescent sex and the romantic narrative: Why some young heterosexuals use condoms to prevent pregnancy, but not disease. *Psychology, Health and Medicine, 3,* 355-370.

Kissling, E., & Kramarae, C. (1991). Stranger compliments: The interpretation of street remarks. *Women's Studies in Communication, 14,* 75-93.

Moradi, B., & Huang, Y. (2008). Objectification theory and psychology of women: A decade of advances and future directions. *Psychology of Women Quarterly, 32,* 377-398.

Neighbors, L. A., & Sobal, J. (2007). Prevalence and magnitude of body weight and shape dissatisfaction among university students. *Eating Behaviors, 8,* 429-439.

Noll, S.M., & Fredrickson, B.L. (1998). A mediational model linking self-objectification, body shame, and disordered eating. *Psychology of Women Quarterly, 22,* 623-636.

Orbach, S. (1988). *Fat is a feminist issue: A self-help guide for compulsive eaters* (2nd ed.). New York: Berkley Books.

Rodin, J., Silberstein, L. & Striegel-Moore, R. (1985). Women and weight: A normative discontent. *Nebraska Symposium on Motivation, 32,* 267-307.

Shotter, J. (1993). *Cultural politics of everyday life: Social constructionism, rhetoric and knowing of the third kind.* Toronto: University of Toronto Press.

Tolman, D. (2000). Object lessons: Romance, violation, and female adolescent sexual desire. *Journal of Sex Education & Therapy, 25,* 70-79.

Wolf, N. (2002) *The beauty myth: How images of beauty are used against women.* New York: Harper Perennial.

⋖ 10 ⋗

The Integral Universe, Experiential Personal Construct Psychology, Transpersonal Reverence, and Transpersonal Responsibility[1]

Larry M. Leitner

In this chapter, I want to explore more systematically a little known and understood philosophical principle in constructivist thought: George Kelly's (1955) assumption that the universe is integral and interconnected. I believe this assumption can lead constructivist psychologies in general—and experiential personal construct psychology in particular—into new and interesting areas. In particular, I explore some of the implications of this interconnected universe for the areas I term transpersonal reverence and responsibility. However, before I go there, I need to provide a very brief overview of experiential personal construct psychology to provide a foundation for what is to come.

EXPERIENTIAL PERSONAL CONSTRUCT PSYCHOLOGY

An elaboration of Kelly's (1955) Sociality and Choice Corollaries, experiential personal construct psychology holds

---

[1] This chapter is based upon the Rollo May Award Address, given at the 117th Annual Convention of the American Psychological Association Convention, August 2009, in Toronto, Canada. All clinical material has been falsified to protect client anonymity. Thanks to Alexandra Adame, Jill Thomas, and April Faidley for their helpful comments. See chapter endnote for award acknowledgments.

that meaning is co-created in our dialogical relations to others (Leitner, 1985, 1988). It emphasizes the human need for deep interpersonal connections in order to live a meaningful and fulfilling life. However, deep interpersonal relations, in addition to affirming us, also carry the risk of major psychological injury. Therefore, all of us struggle with the dilemma of relating intimately with an other, with concomitant experiences of richness and meaning plus the potential terror of devastating injury versus retreating from intimate connections and leading a safe yet empty existence. Should we retreat too much from these relationships, we often experience the symptoms associated with psychopathology (literally psyche + pathos – the tragic suffering of the soul) (Leitner, Faidley, & Celentana, 2000). Experiential personal construct psychotherapy engages the client around this central issue.

THE INTEGRAL UNIVERSE

Kelly (1955) rightly is known for his philosophical principle of *constructive alternativism*, the idea that the events of the universe are open to an infinite number of interpretations. However, prior to this famous position, Kelly made it clear that he held certain basic assumptions about the nature of reality. In this chapter, I mention but do not emphasize some of these assumptions that are well worth exploring (e.g., the assumption that the universe is *real* in contrast to how certain scholars continue to portray constructivist thought and the assumption that the universe is a *process unfolding over time*). For our purposes, Kelly was clear that he viewed the universe as *integral*. By integral, Kelly meant that all aspects of the universe are interconnected and related. His belief in the interconnected nature of the universe can be seen in his example that the movement of his hands typing his manuscript in Columbus, Ohio was connected in some way to the price of yak milk in Tibet.

Kelly thus assumed that "every action in the world has

repercussions throughout the world" (Leitner, 2009b, p. 371). Further, as someone who was opposed to mechanistic and reductionistic psychologies, I find it difficult to believe that Kelly would be comfortable defining "action" in strictly behavioral terms. My "actions" then consist of the things I am doing, the things I am thinking, the things I am feeling, and so on. Thus, my feelings about a person I care for, present as I write this chapter, are even now affecting the universe in ways that I cannot comprehend. In other words, the very nature of reality is affected by my thoughts, feelings, and actions. Further, Kelly is very clear that the universe I live in is co-constructed. The reality that I am affecting is the same reality that affirms or disconfirms the meanings I used to affect it. Thus, all of us live in an interconnected matrix in which we are inextricably entwined with one another, as well as with the more-than-human world. As we will see later, this interconnectedness forms the basis of transpersonal constructivist principles within experiential personal construct psychology.

Kelly argued that we cannot see these relationships because we are too bound up in our small time periods and geographic locations. With enough perspective (and enough knowledge), Kelly believed that we could reach the point where we would see this interconnected reality. However, it also is very clear that Kelly only viewed such ultimate knowledge as a *theoretical possibility*. Kelly emphasized that we would reach this point sometime in the infinite future. As a mathematically sophisticated person, Kelly was quite familiar with the technical implications of the term "infinite." It is a future that never arrives because there always is more to come. At any point in time, no matter how far in the future, the "infinite future" is still further away. Thus, at any real time, one never understands all of the interconnections of the universe.

One major implication is that there always will be a certain sense of mystery when we approach the world. The real universe, with all of its interconnectedness, always will be larger than our minds can grasp; than our senses can perceive; than our best mathematical models can describe. Further, given Kelly's assertion that the universe is a process happening over time, its constantly changing nature further insures that we never will know it totally. As a matter of fact, Kelly's philosophy means that our very acts of coming to know the real universe actually change the real universe, meaning that our coming to know always will be (at least) a step behind the reality. More fundamentally, the universe is a process of change over time, just as we are processes of change (Leitner & Thomas, 2003). It is our very process of becoming that makes us most alive (Leitner, 2009a). There is a way, then, that we can speak of the universe as alive, as animate (see Abrams, 1996). One must, therefore, when understanding this, approach the universe with a sense of wonder, reverence, and awe.

Transpersonal Reverence

Overview

The ability to revere an other and be revered by an other is critical to optimal functioning within experiential personal construct psychology (Leitner & Pfenninger, 1994). Adame and Leitner (2009b) state that, when we revere someone, "we stand in awe of another person we have come to know in a deeply intimate way as he or she has come to know us on the same level" (p. 255; see also Leitner, 1988, 1999, 2001; Leitner & Faidley, 1995; Thomas & Schlutsmeyer, 2004). In other words, reverence for an other stems from the intimacy associated with connecting deeply and profoundly with the other. As the other is a part of the universe, implicit in such reverence is a realization that we never can totally know the other—like the universe, the other in some ways always remains a mystery to us (see Romanyshyn, 2002).

Leitner and Faidley (1995) argued that the experience of transpersonal reverence comes out of this stance of interpersonal revering. Leitner and Faidley's position is very similar to Martin Buber's (1957) when he said, "the world is not comprehensible, but it is embraceable: through the embracing of one of its beings" (p. 27). Thomas and Schlutsmeyer (2004) define transpersonal reverence as the "sense of connection with the world and the many others (human and nonhuman) in it" (p. 313). Thomas and Schlutsmeyer's definition leaves open what is meant by the term "world." From my perspective, Rollo May (1983) gave an essentially constructivist definition of world as *"the structure of meaningful relationships in which a person exists and in the design of which he [or she] participates"* (pp. 122-123, emphasis in original). As implied earlier, the integral universe position means that these "meaningful relationships" include relationships with other people, our culture, humanity in general, and the more-than-human world. When we lack such reverence, we (and the entire planet) get into trouble. I now turn to a brief discussion of the problems occurring when reverence is lacking in these areas. However, keep in mind that, in a holistic universe, the division into significant others, cultures, humanity, and more-than-human world is somewhat arbitrary. I only will be using it for illustrative purposes.

Lack of Interpersonal Reverence

Much of what passes for traditional psychopathology can be seen as failures of a person to be revered by significant others and, consequently, being unable to revere others later in life. For example, elsewhere I have described George, who presented for therapy claiming, among other things, that his body was rotting (Leitner, 2007, 2009a). As we explored his life, we saw a childhood that was filled with abuse and neglect. As one example, he was locked in a storage room for days at a time with only water for sustenance. He also was told by his step-father that he could not urinate or defecate on the floor of the room or he would be in "real trouble." He became convinced that the holding in of his feces would make his body rot. I think it is obvious how the lack of reverence George received was critical in his developing his "delusion." (As an aside, I think it is critical to see the ways the delusion both distanced other people from him and was the key to understanding a crucial event in his developmental history.) In this regard, I often am reminded of Norman Cameron's (1963) wise words that it is the birthright of every child to have a schizophrenic parent. What Cameron meant was that we need a parent who honestly, completely, and unshakably believes that we are the best human being to ever grace the planet. Such a fixed, false belief can be seen as a delusion, hence Cameron's point. However, such a belief allows the child to flourish psychologically.

George's problems, though, were not rooted entirely in his past. Because of his injuries, he also could not revere an other in the present. For example, Leitner and Faidley (1995) describe in detail how a component of revering an other is to take in the other's revering of you. How could George truly grasp someone's revering of him when he was rotten on the inside? Given the depth of his preoccupation with his insides rotting, how could George devote time to suspending his concerns and truly understanding an other—a process essential for intimacy? Thus, his psychopathology was related to both not being revered and not being able to revere others.

Lack of Cultural Reverence

As social beings, we naturally form groups and communities. These communities then become validating agents for our life processes (Epting, Pritchard, Leitner, & Dunnett, 1996; Leitner, Begley, & Faidley, 1996). In so doing, they have power over us (Leitner et al., 1996). Because they were, in many ways, created before our birth, there is a way that these cultural confirmations and disconfirmations act as powerful controls over us. However, these cultural institutions also contain a wisdom that has been built up over generations. Therefore, even as we sometimes critique aspects of the culture, we need to be able to revere the culture. In this section, I discuss two interrelated issues: (a) the impact of not being able to reverentially engage with one's culture and (b) the impact of cultures that do not reverentially engage its members.

Let us consider George again. He talked to others about his insides rotting. Others dismissed these idiosyncratic constructions because they were so unusual that others had little way of understanding them. George was unable then to communicate with others who were potential validating agents who might have given him confirmation. Absent any affirmation, George felt more alone, isolated, and alien. As George received continual invalidation, it was very likely that his ways of approaching the world became more tentative, fragile, and chaotic (see Bannister, 1960, 1962, 1963, for empirical confirmation of this point). As such, George's inability to connect deeply with his culture further injured him.

Now let us turn that around. George's inability to connect with his culture also harms the culture. Others do not hear the horrors of his abuse. When multiplied over many seriously damaged persons, we (meaning the culture as a whole) do not see the ways the culture needs to change in order to revere the people in it and reduce the extent to which they are invalidated and damaged. The cultural construction of George as a chemically brain imbalanced schizophrenic allows the culture to avoid wrestling with the implications of what happened to him. As a matter of fact, one could argue that the cultural constructions of George and others as "biologically or genetically defective" and "crazy" allow for the perpetuation of the ills that led to their psychopathology to begin with. *As such, we continue to tolerate intolerable situations.* In addition to racism, sexism, and heterosexism, we, as a culture, tolerate homelessness, inadequate health care, rape, and child abuse (among many other damaging invalidations). This can be seen as the lack of reverence society shows to some of the people in it and, as such, they all fall under our collective responsibility.

Lack of Reverence for Humanity

Leitner and Faidley (1995) showed how, as we develop a capacity for interpersonal reverence, we can turn toward a reverence for all of humanity. As we experience the reverence of confirmation of our very cores in intimate relationships, we can begin to reconstrue our "general tendencies to objectify self and others" (Leitner, 1999, p. 168). As we recognize the interconnected web that holds all of humanity, we come to appreciate how the denigration of any person anywhere on the planet denigrates all of us. As Leitner and Faidley (1995) put it:

> Ethiopians are not starving; Yugoslavians are not at war with one another; inner city Blacks are not out of work; *persons* are starving, *humans* are being exposed to the horrors of living in a kill-or-be-killed world, and *my fellow citizens* are being deprived of the opportunity to grow in more optimal ways. (p. 310, emphasis added)

Sadly, our world is filled with the effects of the lack of reverence for humanity, as any perusal of the daily news cycle can show. People who have not experienced much in the way of reverence from others wind up in positions of political and economic power and use that power in very destructive ways. So we have wars where we tolerate the destruction of human lives because they are the "enemy." We have people exploiting others for economic gain. We accept a world order where 5% of the population of the planet consumes 50% of the planet's resources. Rather than treating other cultures with mutuality and dialogue, we all too often use force or the threat of force to treat others inhumanely.

Let me illustrate this point with a clinical example. Bill presented with classic PTSD symptoms after a tour in Iraq. While deployed, Bill drove an armored vehicle. At the time, the resistance in Iraq utilized a strategy of sending a small child into the road in front of an American convoy. When the lead vehicle for the convoy stopped in order not to run over the child, the rest of the convoy would have to stop, and the resistance would attack. So American drivers were told that, in the future, when a child is in the road in front of them, to not even slow down in order to protect the convoy. Bill drove over one of those children and was haunted by his action, hence his PTSD symptoms.

I would like to make two points here. First, I think Bill's symptoms clearly can be understood as a consequence of our not revering humanity in general. Rather than seeing people who disagree with us as having a legitimate alternative position, we see them as the "enemy" to be destroyed. We do not think of them as fathers and husbands, mothers and wives, or little children. Hence we find ourselves in a conflict where Bill winds up being diagnosed as mentally ill. This leads me to my second point. Who is the mentally ill person here: Bill, who is haunted by what he did, or some other driver who can run over a little child and not be haunted by his action (or the people who ordered Bill and others to engage in such actions)? (Or the culture that puts its young people in the position of needing to make such orders?)

Fortunately (from my perspective), the need to revere humanity and be revered by humanity may be stronger than the powerful effects of such exploitation. It is possible, through the long view of history, to see progress toward revering all others. For example, most Israelis and Palestinians now recognize that a solution to their conflict where both sides can live peacefully and respectfully beside one another is the only solution that will work long term. Even a conservative United States administration decided to devote serious resources to AIDS in Africa. After the tsunami in Indonesia a few years ago, U.S. Marines were dispensing food supplies to stranded Indonesians. The Marines were under orders not to attempt to rescue any of these people due to crowding in the hospitals that were still functioning. However, the Marines, *to a person*, disobeyed these orders and kept bringing injured people back to the port they were working from because they knew, absent evacuation, that these people would die. In this regard, Kelly (1955) was adamant that the long march of history was toward the greater development of the species.

Lack of Reverence for the More-Than-Human World

The integral universe extends beyond just us humans, as Kelly's yak milk metaphor makes clear. Thus, a lack of reverence for the entire planet can be a sign of psychopathology. Abram (1996) has described how the rational, scientific mindset and its associated language casts nature and objects as things to be used for our benefit. As Adame and Leitner (2009b) say, "Instead of dialoguing with the world, revering it, and respecting the balance and order of natural processes, we speak about nature as if we were not a part of the natural order ourselves" (p. 261). We are trained to see the more-than-human world as a *thing* to be manipulated, not something to be reverentially grasped.

Again, the news is filled with the results of not revering the more-than-human world. We are in the midst of the greatest extinction of living organisms since the dinosaurs roamed the earth—an extinction aggravated by our need for exotic chemicals for devices like laptops and cell phones. Global warming threatens the entire planet. One country (China) adds the equivalent of a 20 megawatt coal fired power plant onto the global warming grid each *week*. Polluted streams threaten drinking water around the globe. Many fisheries are on the brink of collapse. After mountains that have stood for millennia are blasted away for natural resources, we discover that the absence of the mountain causes damage to the ecosystem. Deserts appear where once fertile ground was due to mismanagement of the land. The planet groans under the stress of too many billions of people on the earth. (See Adams, 2006, for even further elaboration of these points.)

I want to be clear here. I am suggesting that attitudes of objectification toward the more-than-human world are indicative of psychopathology—a tragic suffering of the human soul. The net result is that we inflict our suffering on the soul of the planet on which we live. To put it in Buber's terms, we have established "I-It" relationships with our fellow persons, humanity in general, and the more-than-human world—and we, our fellow persons, humanity in general, and the entire planet are paying the price for these "I-It" relationships. In contrast, "transpersonal reverence entails a calling toward a purpose in life greater than simply living for the betterment or fulfillment of the self" (Adame & Leitner, 2009b, p. 263). Further, as a part of the interconnected fabric of life on the planet, we all bear some responsibility for what is happening. This point brings me to the issue of transpersonal responsibility.

TRANSPERSONAL RESPONSIBILITY

Overview

Leitner and Pfenninger (1994) described responsibility as one of the essential characteristics of optimal functioning from an experiential personal construct psychology perspective. Leitner and Pfenninger defined responsibility as the willingness to examine one's meaning system in terms of its implications for others. It is possible, given the greater interconnectedness implied by Kelly's integral universe position, to reconceptualize responsibility as our commitment to examine our meaning system in terms of its implications for humanity and the world at large (Adame & Leitner, 2009a). We call this broadened understanding of responsibility *transpersonal responsibility*.

We believe that this commitment flows naturally out of the experience of transpersonal reverence as a part of recognizing the integral nature of our existence with the world. Because, for Kelly (1955) our reality is co-constructed, we are, in some ways, responsible for the role we play with respect to all that is "other" to us. A part of this otherness is the world in which we live. The interconnected universe means that, by definition, transpersonal responsibility flows naturally from the sense of care and commitment to causes and issues greater than us.

Care and Commitment

Because transpersonal responsibility involves an investment in greater things, it should come as no surprise that, from an experiential personal construct psychology perspective, one must commit to some sort of greater action. We must be committed to an ethic of caring for the more-than-human world, as well as for the world of our shared humanity. Now, commitment, like responsibility and reverence, has a specific definition within experiential personal construct psychology. Commitment is the willingness to affirm an other over time (Leitner & Pfenninger, 1994). Although commitment must make itself felt in the realm of our close relationships (Leitner & Faidley, 1995), it also must be associated with the world of humanity in general or the more-than-human world, as Kelly's integral universe makes clear. Therefore, commitment implies being willing to affirm the evolution of something larger than us, more than us. One manifestation of psychopathology is the lack of such an investment and cure often involves such an investment.

For example, Panepinto (2009) has described the ways that women who are recovering from a rape *need* to develop a sense of purpose, usually through political activism. However, Panepinto made clear that the activism had "an element of transpersonal reverence" (p. 244). The purpose of the activism was to "make others less likely to go through the same pain they had experienced" (p. 244). Please note one of the interesting paradoxes about transpersonal responsibility here. The activism was engaged in to make others less likely to be raped (a commitment to a cause greater than the self); however, the activism also winds up being a critical component of the healing process for these women.

Other humanistic and existential writers have made a similar point. May (1967), for example, stated, "When people feel their insignificance as individual persons, they also suffer an undermining of their sense of human responsibility" (p. 31). May (1981) also believed that Eastern philosophies have a better understanding of such commitments:

> In the Western world we experience freedom as individual self-expression. In the East, on the other hand, freedom is experienced as participation. In the latter, one lives more in the context of the community, and one's freedom comes from participating in the group. (p. 78)

He elaborated this point in his discussion of Kierkegaard: "Commitment is an essential element of existence; Kierkegaard said that 'truth exists only as the individual himself [or herself] produces it in action.'" (May, 1983, p. 166)

May (1981) pointed to the importance of committing to something greater than oneself:

> Thus the task is not only to answer 'who am I?' but it goes beyond the problem of identity. For what is this 'I,' this sense of self, except me-in-relation-to-the-universe? It is more fruitful to ask: To what am I called in this world? (p. 128-129)

Similarly, J. W. Walter (2003), in *Martin Buber and the Feminist Ethic*, argued that "the ethics of care is rooted in the fundamental conviction that human life is essentially interdependent" (p. 77). In other words, absent the interdependence of life (or Kelly's integral universe), true care and commitment is impossible. Walter's point, consistent with experiential personal construct psychology, is that an ethic of care arises out of personal connections rather than abstract principles and universalisms.

Existential Guilt

Transpersonal responsibility also connects to a sense of existential guilt. Inevitably, we realize the ways we are not living up to the principles of transpersonal reverence and responsibility. When we do not take responsibility for our unique role in the interconnected universe, when we do not live up to our full potential, we experience existential guilt. Friedman (1992) wrote:

> True guilt does not reside *in* the human person but rather in one's failure to respond to the legitimate claim and address of the world, and the sickness that results from the denial of such guilt is not merely a psychological phenomenon but an event between persons. (p. 114)

In other words, when we do not respond to the suffering of the world, we experience existential guilt. Thus, existential guilt often results from passivity—the resistance to taking on the burden the world gives us.

Fortunately, the experience of existential guilt can stimulate us to act more responsibly in the world. For example, Friedman (1985) concluded that "the acceptance of real guilt is the beginning of responsibility, and responsibility is what enables the person whose relation with the community has been ruptured to reenter into dialogue with the community" (p. 166). Guilt, within constructivism, is the awareness that we are not acting in a manner consistent with our most vital meanings. With awareness, we can re-commit ourselves to the greater good, while, at the same time affirming the deepest and most genuine parts of ourselves that we gift to the universe.

An Act of Faith

As we have seen, Kelly's philosophy of an integral universe means that we are inexorably connected with all things. Through this complex interconnection, we affect the unfolding of the universe and the unfolding universe also affects us. Further, Kelly firmly believed that the long march of the universe was toward a better and more fulfilling world. However, much of this process remains mysterious. Thus, these constructivist principles lead us to the realization that we are trusting in something that cannot be reduced to a scientific proof: "We are talking about *faith*—our belief in things that cannot be proved" (Leitner, 2009b, p. 372).

Now, faith can be a problem for many psychologists. All too often, the concept has been tied up with overly moralistic and literalistic doctrines. However, our view of faith is an audacious one, a daring one. It is a faith we see time and again in the therapy room. For example, all therapists either implicitly or explicitly trust the innate self-healing aspects of the client (Bohart & Tallman, 1999). The workings of this self-healing process are mysterious and cannot be reduced to regression formulas or empirically validated treatment protocols, but involve the interconnection between persons (Leitner, 2009a, 2009b; Leitner & Faidley, 1995). Buber (1957) said:

> In the immediacy of one human standing over against another, the encapsulation must and can be broken through, and a transformed healed relationship must and can be opened to the person who is sick in his relations to otherness—to the world of the other which he cannot remove into his soul. A soul is never sick alone, but always a between-ness also, a situation between it and another existing being. (p. 97)

Therapists, then, often have to take the plunge into the unknown if they are to be of help to the other. We risk the connection and feel the pain of our client's woundedness, trusting that, somehow, in the process of meeting the person in such a place, a healing process can be started. We recognize that our human limitations mean that we fail our clients and can only trust that who we are, as we connect to them, results in more good than bad for them. Further, we recognize that we play a role in all therapeutic failures and that, as a part of the co-constructed reality of the therapy relationship, we cannot say that a failed therapy was due to a "bad" client.

Essentially, then, Kelly was being consistent here. He was using the same principles that he used to understand persons to understand the entire universe. Leitner (2009b) said:

> Just as people are continuous processes of evolution within PCP... the universe is a consistent process of evolution. Just as touching the process of the other's being reveals the wonder and mystery of the other... experiencing the process of the more than human reveals the wonder and mystery of the universe. (p. 372)

Truly, Kelly was asking for a courageous leap of faith. He wanted us to have the courage to act with boldness for the greater good (Kelly, 1980). One of the paradoxical aspects of Kelly's challenge is that we never can know whether any action ultimately leads to greater goodness. For example, "if I rescued a child from a potentially fatal accident and that child grew up to be the next Hitler, would I have done something good or something bad" (Leitner, 2009b, p. 371)? Having the courage to act in the face of such uncertainty is an important aspect of faith.

An Act of Humility

One aspect of faith that needs to be discussed more specifically I am calling *humility*. While I am acting for the greater good, I must be cognizant that my actions are only a part of the evolving cosmos. Others, who may be acting for a very different good, also are a part of the mysterious evolving universe. I must simultaneously, then, have the courage to stand for my beliefs and the humility to realize that others who go in a different direction also will be used by the interconnected fabric of the world for its greater evolution. Where faith comes back in is the belief that, over the course of time, the cosmos will continually evolve toward greater wholeness, cohesiveness, goodness. In other words, with time, our contrasting notions of goodness wind up being synthesized, utilized, or discarded as the course of cosmic development becomes clearer.

If I can combine this courage and humility, I can wind up, through my connections with others, evolving to the place where I recognize my connection with the cosmos. As such, I have close relationships that nourish me and that I nourish, infusing my life with richness and meaning. I become aware that I have played a part, perhaps a small but an essential part nonetheless, in the evolution of the universe, knowing there will come a time, "perhaps in the infinite future, when we all can grasp the interconnected wondrous mystery that infuses all things, human and non-human, animate and inanimate, in the universe" (Leitner, 2009b, p. 372).[*]

REFERENCES

Abram, D. (1996). *The spell of the sensuous: Perception and language in a more-than-human world.* New York: Vintage.

Adame, A. L., & Leitner, L. M. (2009a). *Dialogical constructivism.* Unpublished manuscript.

Adame, A. L., & Leitner, L. M. (2009b). Reverence and recovery: Experiential personal construct psychotherapy and transpersonal reverence. *Journal of Constructivist Psychology, 22,* 253-267.

Adams, W. (2006). The ivory-billed woodpecker, ecopsychology, and the crisis of extinction: On annihilating and nurturing other beings, relationships, and ourselves. *The Humanistic Psychologist, 34,* 111-133.

Bannister, D. (1960). Conceptual structure in thought disordered schizophrenics. *Journal of Mental Science, 106,* 1230-1249.

Bannister, D. (1962). The nature and measurement of schizophrenic thought disorder. *Journal of Mental Science, 108,* 825-842.

Bannister, D. (1963). The genesis of schizophrenic thought disorder: A serial invalidation hypothesis. *British Journal of Psychiatry, 109,* 680.

Bohart, A. C., & Tallman, K. (1999). *How clients make therapy work: The process of active self-healing.* Washington, DC: American Psychological Association.

Buber, M. (1957). *Pointing the way: Collected essays.* New York: Harper & Brothers.

Cameron, N. (1963). *Personality development and psychopathology: A dynamic approach.* Boston: Houghton Mifflin.

Epting, F. R., Pritchard, S., Leitner, L. M., & Dunnett, N. G. M. (1996). The case for personal and social constructivism. In D. Kalekin-Fishman & B. Walker (Eds.), *The construction of group realities: Culture, society, and personal construct theory* (pp. 309-322). Melbourne, FL: Krieger.

Friedman, M. (1985). *The healing dialogue in psychotherapy.* New York: Jason Aronson.

Friedman, M. (1992). *Religion and psychology: A dialogical approach.* St. Paul, MN: Paragon House.

Kelly, G. A. (1955). *The psychology of personal constructs* (2 vols.). New York: Norton.

Kelly, G. A. (1980). A psychology of the optimal man. In A. W. Landfield & L. M. Leitner (Eds.), *Personal construct psychology: Psychotherapy and personality* (pp. 18-35). New York: John Wiley.

Leitner, L. M. (1985). The terrors of cognition: On the experiential validity of personal construct theory. In D. Bannister (Ed.), *Issues and Approaches in Personal Construct Theory* (pp. 83-103). London: Academic.

Leitner, L. M. (1988). Terror, risk, and reverence: Experiential personal construct psychotherapy. *International Journal of Personal Construct Psychology, 1,* 261-272.

Leitner, L. M. (1999). Terror, numbness, panic, and awe: Experiential personal constructivism and panic. *The Psychotherapy Patient, 11* (1/2), 157-170.

Leitner, L. M. (2001). The role of awe in experiential personal construct psychology. *The Psychotherapy Patient, 11* (3/4), 149-162.

Leitner, L. M. (2007). Theory, technique, and person: Technical integration in experiential constructivist therapy. *Journal of Psychotherapy Integration, 17,* 33-49.

Leitner, L. M. (2009a). Doing(?) experiential personal construct psychotherapy. In L. M. Leitner & J. C. Thomas (Eds.), *Personal constructivism: Theory and applications* (pp. 193-214). New York: Pace University Press.

Leitner, L. M. (2009b). Theory, therapy, and life: Experiential personal construct psychology and the "desert places" of a therapist. In R. J. Butler (Ed.), *Reflections in personal construct theory* (pp. 361-374). Chichester, UK: Wiley-Blackwell.

Leitner, L. M., Begley, E. A., & Faidley, A. J. (1996). Sociality, commonality, individuality, and mutuality: A personal construct approach to non-dominant groups. In D. Kalekin-Fishman & B. Walker (Eds.), *The construction of group realities: Culture, society, and personal construct theory* (pp. 323-340). Melbourne, FL: Krieger.

Leitner, L. M., & Faidley, A. J. (1995). The awful, aweful nature of ROLE relationships. In G. J. Neimeyer & R. A. Neimeyer (Eds.), *Advances in personal construct psychology*. (Vol. 3, pp. 291-314). Greenwich, CT: JAI.

Leitner, L. M., Faidley, A. J., & Celentana, M. A. (2000). Diagnosing human meaning making: An experiential constructivist approach. In R. A. Neimeyer & J. D. Raskin (Eds.), *Construction of Disorders: Meaning-making frameworks for psychotherapy* (pp. 175-203). Washington, DC: American Psychological Association.

Leitner, L. M., & Pfenninger, D. T. (1994). Sociality and optimal functioning. *Journal of Constructivist Psychology, 7*, 119-135.

Leitner, L. M., & Thomas, J. C. (2003). Experiential personal construct psychotherapy. In F. Fransella (Ed.), *International handbook of personal construct psychology* (pp. 257-264). London: John Wiley.

May, R. (1967). *Psychology and the human dilemma*. Princeton, NJ: Van Nostrand.

May, R. (1981). *Freedom and destiny*. New York: W.W. Norton.

May, R. (1983). *The discovery of being: Writings in existential psychotherapy*. New York: W. W. Norton.

Panepinto, A. R. (2009). A constructivist conceptualization of meaning reconstruction after a rape. In L. M. Leitner & J. C. Thomas (Eds.), *Personal constructivism: Theory and applications* (pp. 229-252). New York: Pace University Press.

Romanyshyn, R. D. (2002). *Ways of the heart: Essays toward an imaginal psychology*. Pittsburgh: Trivium.

Thomas, J. C., & Schlutsmeyer, M. W. (2004). A place for the aesthetic in experiential personal construct psychology. *Journal of Constructivist Psychology, 17*, 313-335.

Walter, J. W. (2003). *Martin Buber and feminist ethics: The priority of the personal*. Syracuse, NY: Syracuse University Press.

---

[*] As an awards speech, the talk began with the following acknowledgment: First, I would like to thank Division 32 for this award. I cannot describe how honored I feel. As most of you know, experiential personal construct

psychology is fundamentally a relational approach to human existence. As such, it should come as no surprise that I am here accepting this award because of the relationships I have had in my life. So, I would like to thank some people, without whom my life would have seen an entirely different course. First, my parents, Marion and Marguerite Leitner: so much of who I am comes from you. I wish you were alive and could be here today. I am so pleased that my three daughters, Laura, Shannon, and Joy are here today. Two professors, colleagues, and friends, Franz Epting and Al Landfield, have played an instrumental role in my career. Colleagues at Miami University, particularly Ray White, Steve Hinkle, Pat Capretta, and Roger Knudson helped a young faculty member find his voice. Throughout my career, I have been blessed with some of the brightest and best graduate students a professor could have. Many of them have challenged me and pushed me to grow in ways I could not have imagined prior to meeting them. I am so grateful that they chose to work with me and with experiential personal construct psychology. Colleagues from Division 32, particularly Art Bohart, Dave Elkins, Connie Fischer, Del Jenkins, Art Lyons, Maureen O'Hara, and Will Wadlington, have been trusted friends and intellectual peers. Constructivist scholars such as Peter Cummins, Sally Robbins, Alan Thomson, Gavin Dunnett, Jim Mancuso, Beverly Walker, Linda Viney, Spencer McWilliams, Gerald and Kate Forster, Bob and Greg Neimeyer, Seth Krieger, Sara Bridges, and Jon Raskin also have played key roles in my development. Life would not be what it is without the presence and support of good friends. In that regard, I would like to acknowledge John and Sue McIlvried, Cindy and Basel Noblet, Tom and Nancy Heilman, Steve and Barb Tegarden, Cyndi and Doug Alte, David Surber, and Jack Barta, among many others. I also want to humbly acknowledge the many human beings who have entrusted me with their lives—my clients. They were and still are the true test of experiential personal construct psychology. I am grateful for the ways they allowed me into their areas of darkest suffering. It was a privilege to be of whatever help I could be. To the extent that I (and the theory) failed them, I take responsibility and am sorry. Finally, I want to acknowledge April Faidley, my wife, my best friend, my greatest collaborator, and my toughest critic. You have transformed my life both professionally and personally. In many ways, I believe that you should be up here—not me.

∞ 11 ∞

Constructing and Deconstructing Social Justice Counseling[1]

Jonathan D. Raskin

Marriage and family therapist Scott Johnson (2001) recounts a meeting of the Association of Marriage and Family Therapy. During the meeting, one speaker asked attendees, "What is being done to heal this country?" Another asked, "What, 'as a profession' could be done . . . to end the discord between native peoples and those of European descent in northern America?" (p. 3). The implication, according to Johnson (2001), was that "it was manifestly the mission of the clinical profession of family therapy to solve national and international problems of conflict and bigotry" (p. 3). Such sentiments are not unique to marriage and family therapists. Counseling psychologists and their peers in related disciplines are increasingly emphasizing social justice, the idea that their usual focus on clients' inner lives should be supplemented with more direct measures to reform the often oppressive social systems in which clients live (Aldarondo, 2007; Goodman et al., 2004; Lee & Walz, 1998; Toporek, Gerstein, Fouad, Roysircar, & Israel, 2006). For example, Goodman et al. (2004) note that "in recent years, an increasing number of counseling psychologists have echoed

---

[1] Portions of this chapter were presented at the 116th Annual Convention of the American Psychological Association, August 2008, in Boston. Thanks to Sara K. Bridges, Jay S. Efran, Melanie S. Hill, and Robert A. Neimeyer for their feedback.

calls from critical, community, and liberation psychologists that we engage more systematically in social justice work" (p. 793). Similarly, Constantine, Hage, Kindaichi, and Bryant (2007) speak of "counselors' and counseling psychologists' ability to commit to and actualize an agenda of social justice" (p. 24).

As these quotes illustrate, a social justice orientation has taken root amongst counselor educators (Aldarondo, 2007; Toporek et al., 2006). Backers of such an orientation contend that psychologists and counselors have all too often been derelict in their professional duties by failing to fulfill the role of social justice agent. To rectify this, they endeavor to inculcate a social justice orientation in the counseling professions. Their clarion call advocates strongly and compellingly for social justice concerns to be integrated into all aspects of clinical training, research, and practice because "counselors and counseling psychologists are situated in an optimal position to help society's inhabitants understand the undue effects of social injustices for the well-being of the larger society" (Constantine et al., 2007, p. 28).

The idea of social justice, generally speaking, is something everybody finds appealing and agreeable. Further, criticizing social justice perspectives runs the risk of getting one accused of favoring injustice. For these reasons, few have critically scrutinized the philosophical and practical issues arising from the move toward a social justice orientation in counseling and related professions. This chapter employs ideas from constructivism and social constructionism in examining social justice in psychology and counseling. After establishing social justice counseling as a distinct theoretical orientation, a constructivist critique of this orientation is developed. Social justice counseling is criticized as: (a) espousing naïve realism; (b) being theoretically unelaborated; (c) imposing values; (d) being hubristic; and (e) going beyond psychology and counseling's range of convenience. Social justice counselors are urged to articulate a detailed theoretical approach that restricts its focus of convenience to counseling and demonstrates its utility compared to existing counseling approaches.

SOCIAL JUSTICE COUNSELING AS A THEORETICAL ORIENTATION

Although I use the term throughout this chapter, social justice counselors do not generally use the phrase "social justice counseling." Consider the titles of two seminal volumes: *Handbook of Social Justice in Counseling Psychology* (Toporek et al., 2006) and *Advancing Social Justice through Clinical Practice* (Aldarondo, 2007). In both instances, social justice is separated from counseling, something *in* it or accomplished *through* it. This seemingly trite observation is important because how people talk reflects an underlying worldview that shapes lived realities (Gergen, 1994; Glasersfeld, 1984; Maturana & Poerksen, 2004; Maturana & Varela, 1992). Both titles suggest that there is *social justice* and there is *counseling*—and that they are independent of one another, with the latter being a mechanism for accomplishing the former. This semantic difference is noteworthy because seeing social justice and counseling as distinct from one another encourages *reification*, or what George Kelly (1968/1969, p. 294) called "hardening of the categories." When reification occurs, social justice takes on an atheoretical connotation; it becomes a universal "thing" that all counselors are assumed to agree on and be able to work toward in clinical practice. However, saying social justice should be the goal of all counseling is a bit like saying all counseling should uncover unconscious conflicts, or eradicate irrational thinking, or neutralize chemical imbalances. These goals only make sense from within the respective traditions from which they emerged. Just like psychoanalysis, cognitive therapy, or the medical model of mental illness, social justice constitutes a particular theoretical orientation.

Therefore, when I use the term "social justice counseling," I refer to an approach that conceptualizes human experience as shaped primarily by often oppressive social forces and sees the redistribution of societal resources in more equitable ways as the central goal of counseling practice. This contrasts with other counseling traditions that espouse different goals—for example psychoanalytic counseling (which stresses working through unconscious conflicts as the goal of counseling), humanistic counseling (which sees reaching one's full human potential as the goal of counseling), or cognitive counseling (which sees clear and logical thinking as the goal of counseling). Like any theoretical orientation, social justice counseling has its own truth claims, practice implications, and ethical imperatives. In other words, truths about counseling are always *truths within traditions* (Gergen, 1994, 1999, 2001). Thus, in keeping with constructivism's philosophy of "as if" (Vaihinger, 1952), counselors may adopt a social justice counseling perspective whenever they consider that it might be clinically helpful. Identifying social justice counseling as a theoretical viewpoint (rather than a profession-wide imperative) clears a space for counselors not only to use it, but also to critique it without feeling as if they are being unjust, immoral, or disloyal to the bedrock goals of their profession. All criticisms that follow are offered from this "as if" standpoint, with the idea that readers should try my arguments on for size and take from them whatever they feel is useful. My goal is not to offer assessments that are universally true or final in some kind of essential way. Rather, my critique is meant to invite social justice counselors to consider how their approach might develop were they to entertain my point of view.

Criticism #1: Social Justice Counseling Too Often Espouses Naïve Realism

Deconstructing Consciousness-Raising

From a constructivist perspective, social justice counseling too often tends toward naïve realism, the notion that our theories carve nature at its joints. For example, social justice counselors regularly encourage the use of *consciousness-raising* (Goodman et al., 2004; Morrow, Hawxhurst, Montes de Vegas, Abousleman, & Castañeda, 2006; Toporek & Williams, 2006). In that practice, the "personal is rendered political" by "helping clients understand the extent to which individual and private difficulties are rooted in larger historical, social, and political forces" (Goodman et al., 2004, p. 804). The assumption is that when people have their consciousness raised, they escape a state of *false consciousness* (Prilleltensky & Fox, 1997). Despite acknowledging multicultural concerns about imposing hegemonic beliefs on others, social justice counselors continue to encourage consciousness-raising because "political education and political literacy are part of the answer" (Prilleltensky, Dokecki, Frieden, & Ota Wang, 2007, p. 24). In this conception, counseling involves "assisting clients to become more knowledgeable of the economic/sociopolitical/psychological implications that result from being oppressed" (Crethar, Torres Rivera, & Nash, 2008, p. 273).

While the motivations behind such sentiments are noble, consciousness-raising is worrisome from a constructivist standpoint because it rather paternalistically presumes—as even social justice counselors sometimes acknowledge (Toporek & Williams, 2006)—that the consciousness raiser has a better grasp on the actual state of affairs than the person whose consciousness is to be raised:

> The basic assumption underlying this view is that there is a real, material state of affairs (e.g., that employers pay their employees less than the full value of the work they do, and are thereby able to extract a profit: the real state of affairs is that the workers are exploited), but that people do not recognize (and therefore revolt against) this reality because it is obscured by widely accepted ideas and beliefs. (Burr, 1995, p. 79)

From Consciousness-Raising to Consciousness-Raising-Within-a-Tradition

In a constructivist vein, consciousness-raising must be reconsidered. Instead of seeing it as something that brings people into direct contact with an extra-linguistic reality, consciousness-raising is always *consciousness-raising-within-a-tradition*. This shift encourages social justice counselors to continue their work, but with a subtle and important difference. Rather than seeing themselves as dispensers of a higher truth, they are asked to settle for seeing themselves as advocates of a particular framework for living. They invite clients to try on their preferred discourse, with the idea that perhaps it might open new avenues of understanding. At the same time, they remain cognizant—in a manner similar to Foucault (1980; Rabinow, 1984)—that every discourse (their own included) sometimes oppresses and at other times liberates.

This contrasts with the naïve realist perspective social justice counselors often adopt, wherein they mistake their theoretical framework for reality itself. When operating from this naïve realist viewpoint, social justice counselors insist that, despite erroneous claims to the contrary, the fundamental cause of client problems is—without exception—societal oppression. All effective psychotherapy, therefore, must concern itself with rectifying this. For example, Morrow et al. (2006) assert that "counselors and psychotherapists earn their living trying to heal the wounds inflicted by an unjust society" (p. 241). Similarly, Roy (2007) states, "it is in the interrelationship of material facts and internalized oppression that the work of 'therapy' lies" (p. 67). More ominously, Waldegrave (2005) warns that when therapists fail to see that client problems are, at their very essential core, problems of oppression, they "silence the voice of poor people as they unintentionally help make them happy in poverty" (p. 272). Conceptualizations that do not recognize oppression as the root cause of client problems are seen as *illusory* and *wrong*.

This suggests that social justice counseling does not merely offer one among many conceptualizations a counselor or psychologist might entertain, but instead provides a window onto truth itself. All other alternatives are foreclosed.

Some of the certitude that all counseling is about alleviating oppression seems to be an understandable reaction against often equally naïve realist constructions holding that all client problems are due to discrete mental disorders or individual dilemmas. However, just as it is troublesome to insist that all client problems are products of faulty brain chemistry, genetic anomalies, psychological complexes, or other individual deficits, it is equally limiting to insist that all client problems are due to economic disparities and/or societal oppression. When counselors enter the consulting room already firmly settled on the reality of their clients' difficulties, clients who don't share the view being imposed on them are justified in not returning for future sessions. The old stereotype of the psychoanalyst who remains adamant that all presenting problems really must be about patients' relationships with their mothers (regardless of the problem at hand) seems apropos. A social justice perspective is one potentially generative tradition for conceptualizing and working with clients, but not the only one.

Criticism #2: Social Justice Counseling Remains Theoretically Unelaborated

Constructivism holds that people always come at things from a particular vantage point. Rather than having direct, unmediated access to the world as it is, people must rely on constructed frameworks to organize and make sense of experience (Gergen, 1994, 1999; Glasersfeld, 1984, 1995; Kelly, 1955/1991a, 1955/1991b; Mahoney, 1988; Maturana & Poerksen, 2004; Maturana & Varela, 1992; Poerksen, 2004). Consequently, our theories matter because when unelaborated they frequently let us down. If social justice counseling constitutes a theory developed for the purpose of aiding clinical practice, then it requires a model of the person and the social—one that leads to specific strategies to be used in conducting counseling. While some approaches associated with social justice—critical psychology and radical psychiatry, to name two examples (Parker, 1999; Prilleltensky & Fox, 1997; Roy, 2007)—do try to attend to this, those encouraging counseling psychologists to make social justice the central focus of their discipline have yet to articulate much in the way of theory (Goodman et al., 2004; Speight & Vera, 2004; Toporek et al., 2006). The seminal article by Goodman et al. (2004) on social justice in counseling psychology is a good example of this shortcoming. They outline six principles that they claim are central to social justice counseling: *ongoing self-examination, sharing power, giving voice, facilitating consciousness-raising, building on strengths,* and *leaving clients tools to work toward social change.* These principles are a perfectly reasonable starting point, but they are never elaborated into a full-blown psychological theory whose implications provide a rationale for conducting counseling in a particular manner. Thompson and Shermis, in a response to Goodman et al. (2004), seem aware of this problem, noting that Goodman et al. (2004) offer "no explicit philosophical position. The authors' convictions, with which we agree, appear to be intuitively based, but the fact that their intuitions are sound does not exempt them from articulating a more coherent philosophical base" (Thompson & Shermis, 2004, p. 869). They continue:

> A paradox arises: They ask their counseling psychology students to make judgments, but they do not provide a coherent philosophical basis for them to do so. So from what base do these judgments derive? From egalitarianism? From democratic theory? From socialism? We do not know. Their arguments would be more persuasive, more coherent, and easier to defend had they provided a more explicit philosophy. (p. 870)

Two principles of Goodman et al. (2004) (ongoing self-examination and building on strengths) are so general that they apply to just about any counseling theory. After all, how many counseling theories actively discourage self-examination or building on strengths? The other four principles are a bit more distinctive, but because no broader theoretical frame is offered, they remain vague both conceptually and in their practice implications. Consider sharing power, for example. We are told that social justice counselors aim to "facilitate shared power between clinicians or researchers and the individuals with whom they work" (p. 800). We are also told that sharing power "enhances the growth of each collaborator" (p. 802). Yet Goodman et al. (2004) never address, from a theoretical angle, exactly what power is and how it operates. Nor do they explain how sharing it allows "the voices of marginalized and oppressed groups to emerge" (p. 802).

Goodman et al. (2004) do try to give an example of sharing power, but it does little to clarify matters. It describes a community-organizing project for helping low-income women with depression. Participants are empowered by giving them "an opportunity to reflect on their own lives and situations and then make desired changes," as well as a chance "to comment on their experience of each meeting . . . so that participants can hear and give feedback that can be put to use immediately to shape the program itself" (p. 814). While this strategy seems intuitively sensible, Goodman et al. (2004) do not explain what makes it an exemplar of social justice. Doesn't all effective counseling, even in very structured formats, involve soliciting input from clients and using that input to guide future work? If so, then don't counselors of all stripes regularly share power? Why doing so should be considered an act of social justice remains theoretically ambiguous, especially because it seems like the ordinary practice one expects.

The basic definition of social justice counseling offered by Goodman et al. (2004) further illustrates a lack of theoretical clarity: "We conceptualize the social justice work of counseling psychologists as scholarship and professional action designed to change societal values, structures, policies, and practices, such that disadvantaged or marginalized groups gain increased access to these tools of self-determination" (p. 795). This sounds great. But when we move from the general to the specific, questions arise: Which societal values, structures, policies, and practices should be changed? What should they be changed to? By what means should they be changed? What constitutes a disadvantaged or marginalized group? Do counselors' determinations of who is disadvantaged or marginalized take precedence over the determinations of others, including members of the presumed marginalized group? On what theoretical grounds should social justice counselors answer these questions?

When counselors and counseling psychologists call on one another to advance social justice in this overly general way, the implications are so vague that nobody has sufficient grounds to object. Whatever the case might be, who would answer "No" when asked "Are you for social justice?" This is nowhere more evident than when Fouad et al. (2006) base their social justice counseling approach on the Webster's Dictionary definition of social justice: "the distribution of advantages and disadvantages within a society" (Fouad et al., 2006, p. 1). This definition doesn't say what makes a particular distribution of advantages and disadvantages just or unjust. Should advantages and disadvantages be distributed based on merit, on inheritance, on everyone sharing equally, or on some other scheme? The implications of the dictionary definition Fouad et al. (2006) offer are too broad to guide clinical work. What is needed is a psychosocial theory from which precise and operational definitions of social justice and its counseling implications derive.

CRITICISM #3: SOCIAL JUSTICE COUNSELING RIGHTEOUSLY IMPOSES VALUES

Feeling one has a certain hold on truth invites righteous imposition of one's values (Butt, 2000; Gergen, 1994; Raskin, 2001; Stojnov, 1996). When one is sure one's account catches truth in a bottle, then stamping out false alternatives is heroic, not tyrannical. In this respect, social justice counselors who insist that they know best because they have truth on their side fall into the same imperious trap as their purportedly oppressive adversaries.

As a general example, consider the repressed memory debate, which has been raging on and off for many years. Some counselors believe that repressed memories of past abuse are extremely common and that counselors must educate their clients about the issue so that clients recognize the truth of what happened to them and how it has impacted their current life problems. Others argue that repressed memories are rare or non-existent and that overzealous counselors talk vulnerable and suggestible clients into falsely believing they were abused. Depending on which of these positions a counselor believes, the implications for socially just professional conduct vary. In many respects, these contradictory positions are less damaging unto themselves than the certitude with which their adherents often push them. When psychoanalytic practitioners of the past vehemently insisted that sexual abuse was rare and, when reported, almost always the product of projected fantasies, they clearly harmed many of their patients. At the same time, many current therapists may do just as much harm when they interpret every utterance and behavior their clients put forth as evidence of abuse and as the one and only explanation of what really happened. Righteous certainty may make one feel like an agent of justice, when precisely the opposite may be the case.

Now consider an example more specific to social justice counseling. Some social justice advocates have recommended placing ethical sanctions on psychologists who fail to utilize the "transformative potential of psychology in working for the liberation of oppressed peoples" (Speight & Vera, 2004, p. 114). Along these lines, Brown (1997) criticizes the American Psychological Association for not demanding that its members combat oppression. "To be an ethical APA member," she laments, "one need not actively fight racism, sexism, heterosexism or other forms of oppression in the profession and the world" (p. 59). But what does it mean to fight these things in practice? What and how much must one do? Are there specific positions a counselor must adopt in order to be socially just? Must he or she support affirmative action? Argue that homosexuality is biologically innate? Oppose prescription privileges for psychologists? Endorse the use of treatment manuals in psychotherapy? If we are not careful, we will quickly descend into the "McCarthyism and persecution" (Brown, 1997, p. 57) that the APA ethics code sought to avoid by distinguishing between the psychologist's professional conduct and personal beliefs, a distinction which Brown (1997) feels "has lost its value" because "the academic and social climate has become more open" (p. 57). Yes, the climate is more open—if you believe all the same things Brown does. If not, then you are unethical and oppressive.

Similarly, Brown (1997, p. 59) argues that "the researcher who collects information with all the appropriate consent mechanisms in place, and then interprets the findings so as to lead to the ridicule of a vulnerable group" is behaving unethically; said person is not "simply exercising his or her opinion about the meanings of the research" (p. 59), but is actively oppressing people in a malevolent way that must be stopped. But who gets to decide what is malevolent and oppressive, or what constitutes a vulnerable group? Given that Democrats currently control the U.S. presidency and both houses of Congress, might Brown's statement plausibly be interpreted as meaning that Amodio, Jost, Master, and Yee's (2007) recent research offering neurocognitive explanations for why conservatives are more rigid than liberals is unethical because it demeans conservatives? Brown's view encourages the censorship of any and all research agendas whose implications can reasonably be deemed objectionable. Such righteous certitude leaves little room for honest disagreement. Thus, even if we find ourselves personally in concurrence with some of Brown's specific political positions, we may simultaneously oppose her supposition that alternative perspectives are quintessentially unethical and must be silenced.

What would happen if we started ethically regulating counselors who failed to push a social justice agenda rooted in the particular political ideology that social justice counseling typically espouses? Would we sanction the counselor who believes that intervening in a client's life outside the consulting room is clinically contraindicated (as many psychoanalytic counselors do)? If so, then a counselor might be labeled unethical if he does not specifically advocate that his client confront her professor (or actively intervene himself) when he feels the professor has treated the client in a sexist manner. Would we discipline the counselor who thinks her economically disadvantaged client's money problems are due to irresponsible spending habits rather than oppressive social conditions? After all, from a social justice perspective, this counselor may be "unintentionally . . . adjust[ing] people to poverty" (Waldegrave, 2005, p. 268) and, therefore, practicing unethically. Counselors disagreeing on what constitutes effective, or even justifiable, counseling is nothing new. However, righteous certitude can egg on counseling professionals to frame all their theoretical and political preferences as moral imperatives. Feeling one has truth and God on one's side can be hazardous. Warns Gergen:

> [W]hen we venture out to identify the "something beyond the convention of representation"—the realm of the "really there"—we implicitly arrogate ourselves to the status of minor gods. In our transcending the clouded vision of mere mortals, we position ourselves to declare certain forms of discourse (and their attendant traditions) ignorant, misguided, primitive, backward and expendable. (Gergen, 2001, p. 425)

CRITICISM #4: SOCIAL JUSTICE COUNSELING BRIMS WITH HUBRIS

"I'm for Social Justice! (Anyone Who Disagrees with me is Not!)"

The discursive strategy of casting ourselves as social justice agents makes us right and all those who think otherwise wrong. As such, it is a way of asserting power and privilege, of hubristically holding oneself up as a moral exemplar. Thus, when counseling psychology professors tell their students and clients that they espouse a social justice agenda they make it discursively much more difficult to disagree with them. I recall a conservative Republican graduate student who took umbrage at the social justice scholarship that argues that individualism and capitalism are the root causes of client difficulties (A. G. Johnson, 2001). This student offered a spirited defense of these "isms" and argued that counselors who repudiate them do more harm than good, even when doing so in the name of social justice. Fellow students and faculty members were incensed. They condemned this student's perspective as not only socially regressive, but also unprofessional. Though he held his ground for a while, in the end this student stopped speaking up in class. His voice had been silenced. If privilege involves "something of value that is denied to others simply because of the groups they belong to" (A. G. Johnson, 2001, p. 23), then this student lost the privilege of speaking out because he belonged to a dissenting group, in this case conservative Republicans. Surprisingly, none of the students or faculty opposing him found it troublesome that his voice was effectively dismissed as a result of their extensive moral condemnation. Should they not have been concerned with making sure dissenting voices are heard, respected, and even seriously considered—especially in light of their identifying so fervently with a social justice agenda that favors dialogue, power sharing, and attention to issues of privilege?

What I am arguing is that "the luxury of obliviousness" (A. G. Johnson, 2001, p. 24) that commonly accompanies privilege applies in many instances, not just those where gender, race, and sexuality are at issue. Surely social justice counselors deserve kudos for offering their colleagues a theoretical orientation that addresses issues of discrimination and oppression in challenging and generative new ways. At the same time, it seems important to note that in different contexts different groups are privileged and that the privileged group in counseling psychology these days may be social justice counselors themselves. This is especially so when, holding the majority of positions that warrant voice in professional circles, they work to make their brand of social justice the categorical imperative for the field. We may wish to acknowledge that invoking social justice is a way of warranting voice for our own preferred agenda while undermining the discursive power of those with whom we disagree.

The Counseling Professions are Not a Hive Mind

What too many of us forget is that being counselors and psychologists doesn't guarantee that all of us share the same ideas about justice. Yet it often seems that counselors and psychologists advocate for social justice based on the assumption that such a consensus exists simply because of our shared professional pedigree. But why would counselors and psychologists—simply by being counselors and psychologists— necessarily share the same conceptions of justice? The realm of counseling and psychology is one context in which we dwell, but it is by no means the only one. Each of us comes from particular families with their own unique constructions of the social world. Further, each of us comes from a dazzling panoply of religious, political, ethnic, and racial backgrounds that have constituted—perhaps to a much greater extent than psychology has—our particular constructions of social justice. Psychology is merely one of multiple contexts within which each of us exists.

To assume that all psychologists and counselors share the same set of values and attitudes simply because they are psychologists and counselors seems implausible. It overlooks the immense complexity, messiness, and struggle involved in constructing accounts of social justice, and in so doing does a disservice to the very concept of social justice.

Perhaps an example might help demonstrate the idea that counseling and related psychologists are not of one mind on important and timely social justice issues. Consider the recent controversy about whether it was ethical for psychologists to serve at those U.S. military installations where the principles of the Geneva Conventions were not being upheld (Carey, 2008a, 2008b). Psychologists who believed that it was unethical for their peers to work in settings where torture, as defined by the Geneva Conventions, was taking place made one argument. Those who felt that psychologists should be present in such settings because their presence supplied a voice of reason provided another argument. A third, if less often heard, argument some psychologists offered was that they must be present at such installations to use their psychological knowledge for gaining information from suspected terrorists and preventing terror attacks. All three arguments are rooted in conflicting definitions of social justice and psychologists have endorsed all three. Though the membership of the American Psychological Association ultimately did vote that psychologists cannot ethically be present in settings where torture might occur (American Psychological Association, 2008), there remains a great deal of dissension surrounding this issue (Carey, 2008a; Ephron, 2008). Debates about prescription privileges, empirically supported treatments, psychotherapy manuals, nature versus nurture, and a myriad of other historical conflicts among members of the profession also can be used to make the point that psychologists do not necessarily share ideas about what is just simply because they are psychologists. What is deemed "just" emerges from the theoretical frameworks we employ—and psychologists and counselors subscribe to many different, often contradictory, frameworks.

Psychologists Aren't Any More Just than Anyone Else

Psychologists and counselors might also bear in mind that they do not have any better access to what social justice is than anybody else. Consider again the issue of whether psychologists should have been present at military installations not abiding by the Geneva Conventions. Some contended that the presence of psychologists in such places served as an ethical corrective; namely, psychologists both prevented and cleaned up negative occurrences (Carey, 2008a). This argument seems to be that psychologists could do nothing but positively impact the climate at military installations where questionable interrogation techniques were practiced. That is, in a Kohlbergian sort of way (Kohlberg & Hersh, 1977), psychologists presumably have a more developed sense of social justice, thus their presence made torture less likely. Unfortunately, those making this argument minimized (a) the many regrettable examples of psychologists behaving unethically, and (b) extensive social psychology research suggesting that the power of the situation usually overwhelms the power of the person (Benjamin & Simpson, 2009; Burger, 2009; Darley & Latane, 1968; Latane & Darley, 1968; Milgram, 1963)—even if that person is a psychologist.

In an era in which many psychologists demand that interventions be empirically validated before being implemented, it is interesting that no controlled experimental studies have been offered to support the implicit assumption that psychologists are ethically more sophisticated than others and therefore less prone to the social pressures that would otherwise undermine their social justice barometers. What makes psychologists think that they are better attuned to what social justice is than, say, historians or computer scientists or linguists? Indeed, anecdotal evidence suggests that psychologists are not immune to behaving unjustly. It was, in the end, a pair of psychologists who helped to convince the C.I.A. that only harsh interrogations could yield confessions from terror suspects (Shane & Mazzetti, 2009). My point is that too much of the social justice literature in psychology seems premised on the idea that psychologists are trained arbiters of social justice issues. This risks minimizing the enormous complexity of negotiating and implementing ever-changing constructions of social justice. It encourages psychologists to see themselves as enlightened in the ways of justice purely because they are psychologists. Radical constructivist Humberto Maturana cautioned:

> My view is that we should never believe that we are in any way special as far as morality or anything else is concerned. . . . Those who think they are immune will be the first, I believe, to become torturers in certain situations. They are not aware of their own seducibility. (Poerksen, 2004, p. 68)

More narrowly, psychoanalyst Lawrence Friedman (1976) wryly observed: "Describing therapy in terms of the therapist's virtues rather than his skills invites a grandiosity of the humbler-than-thou variety" (p. 261). Too many political and religious viewpoints have been sullied by such self-important thinking and its tendency to exclude or dismiss all contradictory viewpoints. Good intentions notwithstanding, this is a domain in which psychologists are urged to proceed with caution.

There is No Politics Unique to Counseling and Psychology

So why do social justice counselors assume that their peers share their ideas about social justice solely because they work in the same profession? One tentative hypothesis is that, while psychologists and counselors disagree about many issues within their field, they nevertheless share a vocation that attracts people who tend to occupy the same quadrants of the political spectrum. To put it more bluntly, most psychologists and counselors are political liberals. Thus, when we sit down together to discuss issues beyond the immediate scope of our profession, we often find ourselves in agreement. This easily fosters the illusion that, when we speak to one another about social justice, the solutions we reach are bona fide universal truths rather than socially constructed accounts. All the same, it is important to remember that *there is nothing in the science or practice of psychology that demands loyalty to a particular political ideology.* To assume otherwise is to reach beyond our profession's purview. This issue of purview, or range of convenience, is the topic we turn to next.

CRITICISM #5: SOCIAL JUSTICE COUNSELING OVEREXTENDS ITS RANGE OF CONVENIENCE

Counseling and Psychotherapy's Range of Convenience

The constructs we develop have both foci and ranges of convenience, defined as follows:

> A construct has its focus of convenience—a set of objects with which it works especially well. Over a somewhat larger range it may work only reasonably well; that is, its range of convenience. But beyond that it fades into uselessness and we can say the outer array of objects simply lies beyond that range of convenience. (Kelly, 1970/2003, p. 11)

While we are always free to extend a construct's range of convenience beyond the focus for which it works best, sometimes we go too far and the construct stops being functional. George Kelly warned about people in one profession setting out to wise up those in another. For example, problems often result

> when a physician bursts into the field of psychiatry after several years of preoccupation with medicine, or when a physicist, suspecting that the social scientists are not keeping up with him,

> decides to take a year off and bring "scientific enlightenment" into the collapsing world of interpersonal relations. Yet it may be some time after the man changes his letterhead before he begins to grasp constructs whose focus of convenience is in the area in which he has come to work. (Kelly, 1955/1991a, p. 128)

The same sort of difficulty occurs when counselors, fearing the world is going to hell, decide that only their special brand of wisdom can salvage matters. Yet their forays into social engineering beg the question: if we stretch counseling's range of convenience that far, at what point does it break down or morph into something else entirely? Of course, this implies that we have already precisely defined what we mean in the first place when we speak of *counseling* or *psychotherapy* (terms used interchangeably here). However, I'm not sure we have, a sentiment reflected in George F. J. Lehner's (1952) famous observation: "I am afraid that in spite of our efforts we have left therapy as an undefined technique which is applied to unspecified problems with nonpredictable outcome. For this technique we recommend rigorous training" (p. 547).

Much of the problem in defining psychotherapy can be tied to differences in theoretical orientation. However, I contend that, despite these differences, therapy's basic contours can nonetheless be sketched. It typically involves a client and a counselor (sometimes more than one of each, as in couples and family counseling) sitting down together for a prescribed period of time to help the client resolve conflicted meanings through (a) naming the difficulty at hand, and (b) working to achieve defined tasks (Friedman, 1976). The client usually identifies the problems therapy should address, though sometimes others (e.g., relatives, friends, and judges) do, too. Typically the client and counselor talk regularly (e.g., once a week) about the client's difficulties and, through the course of these conversations and other (often structured) activities that serve as symbolic communications (Frank, 1979/2006), the client develops new ways to consider and resolve them. The theoretical approach of the counselor makes a big difference because, depending on the orientation employed, the client's problems may be explained as due to unconscious conflicts, environmental circumstances, faulty thinking, a failure to self-actualize, chemical imbalances, or something else entirely. The counselor is usually financially compensated for the services provided, though not always directly by the client. Training in strategies for initiating client change is required of counselors, though the specifics of this training vary depending on the theoretical approach of those providing it. Regardless of theoretical bent, the counselor is typically educated in some version of a scientist-practitioner model, whereby good practice is informed by research in an effort to use "the primacy of communication as the medium of healing" (Frank, 1979/2006, p. 60).

While this definition of psychotherapy is far from perfect or comprehensive, it paints a general picture that most of us recognize and can subscribe to. That is, even if every element of counseling is not thoroughly agreed upon, we typically share a basic conception of what it is. Thinking about this in personal construct terms, in good measure we define something by contrasting it with its perceived opposite, or what it isn't (Kelly, 1955/1991a, 1955/1991b). Another way to say this is that people draw distinctions and then live according to them (Maturana & Varela, 1992; Poerksen, 2004). I distinguish counseling as a certain kind of activity that precludes other activities. To wit, counseling is not teaching a class or dribbling a basketball or eating in a restaurant or chatting with a friend or writing a paper or dancing at a party. People make such distinctions not because they are written in stone, but because they help make life more understandable and manageable. I am suggesting that maintaining a distinction between social activism and counseling remains important if each is to retain coherence as a discrete activity.

An Example: Conflating Social Activism and Counseling

Consider a chapter about social justice by counseling psychologist Lawrence Gerstein, in which he outlines his work as an activist in the movement to free Tibet from Chinese rule (Gerstein & Kirkpatrick, 2006). After providing a detailed history of the conflict, Gerstein discusses his work as part of the International Tibet Independence Movement (ITIM). Although his devotion to a cause he obviously cares deeply about is admirable, his activities are at best only tangentially related to counseling. He describes organizing marches and provides advice on preparing and exhibiting protest signs, noting that (a) sign size, text color, and contrast are critical to visual effectiveness, and (b) when protestors displaying signs become preoccupied with socializing, they hold their signs too close together for passing motorists to read (Gerstein & Kirkpatrick, 2006, p. 460). This advice, while helpful to the aspiring protestor, does not require counseling psychology expertise. However, the implication is that it does, an implication also made when Gerstein notes that at biweekly ITIM meetings, he must

> facilitate the discussions, promote creative problem solving, strive to strengthen cohesion in the group, empower participants' involvement, attempt to balance the needs of the participants with the objectives of the organization, honor the cultural differences between the participants and make every effort to provide the participants with a rewarding experience. (Gerstein & Kirkpatrick, 2006, p. 457)

While these activities seem more related to counseling than sign preparation, they are in no way distinctive to counseling. Indeed, they involve the very same skills required of any leader managing an organization and its staff. Effective leadership is not specifically tied to being a counseling psychologist or even knowing anything about counseling as a profession—which is why the team leader at Target, the manager of the New York

Yankees, and President Obama may all excel in their roles despite little or no exposure to the counseling profession. Yes, the good "people skills" that sometime (though not always!) accompany being a counseling psychologist may prove beneficial when leading others (again, not always—some leaders are successful despite extensive interpersonal deficits). However, to imply that leadership success is contingent upon being trained as a counseling psychologist is unconvincing, as Gerstein himself seems to understand when he admits that "not all counseling psychologists have the skills to effectively lead such a diverse group of individuals" (Gerstein & Kirkpatrick, 2006, p. 457). Both activism and counseling are valuable and may sometimes complement one another, but they are not the same thing. Counseling trainees enter their graduate programs with the promise that they will be taught how to become professional counselors, not how to paint protest signs, organize rallies, or free Tibet. In other words, social activism and counseling are best not construed as one and the same.

Put another way, *lots of activities that help people—social activism included—simply have little or nothing to do with counseling.* Many of these activities fall outside counseling's range of convenience. The same goes for other endeavors we might find worthwhile, such as building a house for Habitat for Humanity, donating food to the local homeless shelter, or providing old cell phones to victims of domestic violence. Useful activities all, but none are counseling. When counseling is defined as *any* activity a counseling psychologist takes up or *anything* having to do with interacting with, coordinating, or helping others, we have so overextended its range of convenience that it becomes devoid of meaning. Not only that, we have parochially implied (intentionally or not) that only those with counseling training can be effective leaders and save the world.

A CHALLENGE TO SOCIAL JUSTICE COUNSELING

I began this chapter by quoting Scott Johnson's experience at a conference where social justice was invoked as counseling's professional purpose. Johnson's response was that such tendencies were grandiose, Messianic even. He advocated for a much more limited focus for counseling:

> In the end, the theories that we nurture must be judged not for ending famine or injustice, war or pollution or imperialism, though they may—and should—speak to such vital questions. But what must matter in the end—at least for us as a discipline—is how well our ideas improve human relationships. (S. Johnson, 2001, p. 10)

I contend that we would do well to heed Johnson's call. This does not mean social justice must be banished from counseling and psychology, but it does mean that it should be clearly demarcated as a theoretical approach so that clients know what they are buying. Requesting that counselors declare their intentions up front is not something we should restrict to social justice counselors. Given how many different perspectives on counseling and psychotherapy there are, asking counselors to be frank about their orientations so that clients can make informed decisions about what they're getting themselves into makes a great deal of sense. Perhaps we should do less labeling of clients and more labeling of counselors.

But it is not enough for social justice counselors to be open about their theoretical proclivities. They must develop more substantive models of counseling and psychotherapy, justifying particular kinds of counseling interventions. Without a clear model of the person and the social, there is no rationale for social justice counselors to practice in prescribed ways. Of course, once distinct models are offered, social justice counselors must also attend to whether their approach helps people. Calling something social justice counseling does not automatically mean that it yields social justice. Not only must social justice counselors decide what social justice is by rooting it in particular theoretical conceptualizations, they must also address whether the resulting counseling practices deliver what they purport to accomplish. Outcomes are important and should be measured. This need not necessarily be done according to the demands of the empirically supported treatment crowd (whose preference for narrowly experimental methodologies unfairly favor more concrete and structured approaches to the detriment of less traditional alternatives). Methodological diversity in examining therapy effectiveness is important, but some demonstration that social justice counseling is generative, helpful, and worthy of continued use and development is nevertheless required. Do clients of social justice counseling report greater satisfaction and more positive outcomes compared to those who undergo psychoanalytic, cognitive-behavioral, and humanistic counseling? If so, show us!

Conclusion: We All Work for Justice in Our Own Way

I am not advancing the argument, made famous by constructivism-influencing philosopher F. A. Hayek (1976), that there is no such thing as social justice. Social justice is something: it is a social construction, one that guides our collective sense of right and wrong. The notion of social justice helps us know what causes to work for and what actions we wish to take on behalf of others. Thus, it provides the motivation and framework for potentially doing much good in the world, especially when the concept is not reified or used to ignore and dismiss those espousing contrary perspectives. Social justice counseling, as an emerging theoretical orientation that draws on social justice scholarship and community activism, should maintain a narrower range of convenience than social justice proper. It should take the time to develop a more thorough theoretical rationale, one that preserves a focus on the pragmatics of counseling and psychotherapy. To that end, I encourage psychologists and counselors to reexamine whether invoking social justice as something their entire discipline unquestioningly agrees upon (and, by implication, works toward as a profession) is necessarily wise or called for. Each of us works for social justice in our own way. To suggest that there is a singular "psychology" or "counseling" way to do social justice is to dismiss the many ongoing and often contradictory dialogues occurring within these professions. It also mistakes a theoretical orientation for a discipline-wide directive.

Social constructionism holds that reality springs from relationships and there are as many realities as there are relationships for constructing them (Gergen, 1994). Social justice is a noble goal in the abstract, but one that is complicated and messy in the specific. Social constructionists do not attempt to find a final truth that trumps all others. Rather, they believe that we must simply "keep the conversation going" as respectfully and cooperatively as possible (Lax, 1992; Rorty, 1979). One sure way to foreclose conversation is to label one's own perspective as socially just and, implicitly or explicitly, derogate other perspectives as unjust. From my socially constructed viewpoint, remaining humble and open to dialogue with those coming from alternative perspectives is critical to the goal of "keeping the conversation going."

References

Aldarondo, E. (Ed.). (2007). *Advancing social justice through clinical practice.* Mahwah, NJ: Lawrence Erlbaum.

American Psychological Association. (2008, September 17). *APA members approve petition resolution on detainee settings.* Retrieved from http://www.apa.org/releases/petition0908.html

Amodio, D. M., Jost, J. T., Master, S. L., & Yee, C. M. (2007). Neurocognitive correlates of liberalism and conservatism. *Psychophysiology, 45*(1), 11-19.

Benjamin, L. T., Jr., & Simpson, J. A. (2009). The power of the situation: The impact of Milgram's obedience studies on personality and social psychology. *American Psychologist, 64,* 12-19.

Brown, L. S. (1997). Ethics in psychology: *Cui bono?* In I. Prilleltensky & D. Fox (Eds.), *Critical psychology: An introduction* (pp. 51-67). London: Sage.

Burger, J. M. (2009). Replicating Milgram: Would people still obey today? *American Psychologist, 64*, 1-11.

Burr, V. (1995). *An introduction to social constructionism.* London: Routledge.

Butt, T. (2000). Pragmatism, constructivism, and ethics. *Journal of Constructivist Psychology, 13*, 85-101.

Carey, B. (2008a, August 15). Psychologists clash on aiding interrogations. *The New York Times.* Retrieved from http://www.nytimes.com

Carey, B. (2008b, September 17). Psychologists vote to end interrogation consultations. *The New York Times.* Retrieved from http://www.nytimes.com

Constantine, M. G., Hage, S. M., Kindaichi, M. M., & Bryant, R. M. (2007). Social justice and multicultural issues: Implications for the practice and training of counselors and counseling psychologists. *Journal of Counseling and Development, 85*, 24-29.

Crethar, H. C., Torres Rivera, E., & Nash, S. (2008). In search of common threads: Linking multicultural, feminist, and social justice counseling paradigms. *Journal of Counseling and Development, 86*, 269-278.

Darley, J. M., & Latane, B. (1968). Bystander intervention in emergencies: Diffusion of responsibility. *Journal of Personality and Social Psychology, 8*(4), 377-383.

Ephron, D. (2008, October 27). The biscuit breaker. *Newsweek,* 49-50.

Foucault, M. (1980). *Power/knowledge: Selected interviews and other writings, 1972-1977* (C. Gordon, Ed.; C. Gordon, L. Marshall, J. Mepham, & K. Soper, Trans.). New York: Pantheon Books.

Frank, J. D. (2006). What is psychotherapy? In S. Bloch (Ed.), *An introduction to the psychotherapies* (4th ed., pp. 59-76). Oxford: Oxford University Press. (Original work published 1979)

Friedman, L. (1976). Defining psychotherapy. *Contemporary Psychoanalysis, 12*, 258-269.

Gergen, K. J. (1994). *Realities and relationships.* Cambridge, MA: Harvard University Press.

Gergen, K. J. (1999). *An invitation to social construction.* London: Sage.

Gergen, K. J. (2001). Construction in contention: Toward consequential resolutions. *Theory & Psychology, 11*, 419-432.

Gerstein, L. H., & Kirkpatrick, D. (2006). Counseling psychology and non-violent activism: Independence for Tibet! In R. L. Toporek, L. H. Gerstein, N. A. Fouad, G. Roysircar, & T. Israel (Eds.), *Handbook for social justice in counseling psychology: Leadership, vision, and action* (pp. 442-471). Thousand Oaks, CA: Sage.

Glasersfeld, E. von. (1984). An introduction to radical constructivism. In P. Watzlawick (Ed.), *The invented reality: How do we know what we believe we know? Contributions to constructivism* (pp. 17-40). New York: Norton.

Glasersfeld, E. von. (1995). *Radical constructivism: A way of knowing and learning.* London: The Falmer Press.

Goodman, L. A., Liang, B., Helms, J. E., Latta, R. E., Sparks, E., & Weintraub, S. R. (2004). Training counseling psychologists as social justice agents: Feminist and multicultural principles in action. *The Counseling Psychologist, 32,* 793-837.

Hayek, F. A. (1976). *Law, legislation, and liberty: A new statement of the liberal principles of justice and political economy. Vol. 2. The mirage of social justice.* Chicago: The University of Chicago Press.

Johnson, A. G. (2001). *Privilege, power, and difference.* Boston: McGraw-Hill.

Johnson, S. (2001). Family therapy saves the planet: Messianic tendencies in the family systems literature. *Journal of Marital and Family Therapy, 27*(1), 3-11.

Kelly, G. A. (1991a). *The psychology of personal constructs: Vol. 1. A theory of personality.* London: Routledge. (Original work published 1955)

Kelly, G. A. (1991b). *The psychology of personal constructs: Vol. 2. Clinical diagnosis and psychotherapy.* London: Routledge. (Original work published 1955)

Kelly, G. A. (1969). The role of classification in personality theory. In B. Maher (Ed.), *Clinical psychology and personality: The selected papers of George Kelly* (pp. 289-300). New York: John Wiley. (Original work published 1968)

Kelly, G. A. (2003). A brief introduction to personal construct theory. In F. Fransella (Ed.), *International handbook of personal construct psychology* (pp. 3-20). Chichester, UK: John Wiley. (Original work published 1970)

Kohlberg, L., & Hersh, R. H. (1977). Moral development: A review of the theory. *Theory into Practice, 16*(2), 53-59.

Latane, B., & Darley, J. M. (1968). Group inhibition of bystander intervention in emergencies. *Journal of Personality and Social Psychology, 10*(3), 215-221.

Lax, W. D. (1992). Postmodern thinking in a clinical practice. In S. McNamee & K. J. Gergen (Eds.), *Therapy as social construction* (pp. 69-85). London: Sage.

Lee, C. C., & Walz, G. R. (Eds.). (1998). *Social action: A mandate for counselors.* Alexandria, VA & Greensboro, NC: American Counseling Association & ERIC Counseling and Student Services Clearinghouse.

Lehner, G. F. J. (1952). Defining psychotherapy. *American Psychologist, 7,* 547.

Mahoney, M. J. (1988). Constructive metatheory: I. Basic features and historical foundations. *International Journal of Personal Construct Psychology, 1,* 1-35.

Maturana, H. R., & Poerksen, B. (2004). *From being to doing: The origins of the biology of cognition* (W. K. Koek & A. R. Koek, Trans.). Heidelberg, Germany: Carl-Auer.

Maturana, H. R., & Varela, F. J. (1992). *The tree of knowledge: The biological roots of human understanding* (Rev. Ed.; R. Paolucci, Trans.). Boston: Shambhala.

Milgram, S. (1963). Behavioral study of obedience. *Journal of Abnormal and Social Psychology, 67*(4), 371-378.

Morrow, S. L., Hawxhurst, D. M., Montes de Vegas, A. Y., Abousleman, T. M., & Castañeda, C. L. (2006). Toward a radical feminist multicultural therapy: Renewing a commitment to activism. In R. L. Toporek, L. H. Gerstein, N. Fouad, G. Roysircar, & T. Israel (Eds.), *Handbook for social justice in counseling psychology: Leadership, vision, and action* (pp. 231-247). Thousand Oaks, CA: Sage.

Parker, I. (1999). Critical psychology: Critical links. *Radical Psychology, 1,* 3-18. Retrieved from http://www.radicalpsychology.org/vol1-1/Parker.html.

Poerksen, B. (2004). *The certainty of uncertainty: Dialogues introducing constructivism* (A. R. Koeck & W. K. Koeck, Trans.). Exeter, UK: Imprint Academic.

Prilleltensky, I., Dokecki, P., Frieden, G., & Ota Wang, V. (2007). Counseling for wellness and justice: Foundations and ethical dilmmas. In E. Aldarondo (Ed.), *Advancing social justice through clinical practice* (pp. 19-42). Mahwah, NJ: Lawrence Erlbaum.

Prilleltensky, I., & Fox, D. (1997). Introducing critical psychology: Values, assumptions, and the status quo. In I. Prilleltensky & D. Fox (Eds.), *Critical psychology: An introduction* (pp. 3-20). London: Sage.

Rabinow, P. (Ed.). (1984). *The Foucault reader.* New York: Pantheon.

Raskin, J. D. (2001). On relativism in constructivist psychology. *Journal of Constructivist Psychology, 14,* 285-313.

Rorty, R. (1979). *Philosophy and the mirror of nature.* Princeton, NJ: Princeton University Press.

Roy, B. (2007). Radical psychiatry: An approach to personal and political change. In E. Aldarondo (Ed.), *Advancing social justice through clinical practice* (pp. 65-90). Mahwah, NJ: Lawrence Erlbaum.

Shane, S., & Mazzetti, M. (2009, April 21). In adopting harsh tactics, no inquiry into their past use. *The New York Times.* Retrieved from http://www.nytimes.com

Speight, S. L., & Vera, E. M. (2004). A social justice agenda: Ready or not? *The Counseling Psychologist, 32,* 109-118.

Stojnov, D. (1996). Kelly's theory of ethics: Hidden, mislaid, or misleading? *Journal of Constructivist Psychology, 9,* 185-199.

Thompson, C. E., & Shermis, S. S. (2004). Tapping the talents within: A reaction to Goodman, Liang, Helms, Latta, Sparks, and Weintraub. *The Counseling Psychologist, 32,* 866-878.

Toporek, R. L., Gerstein, L. H., Fouad, N., Roysircar, G., & Israel, T. (Eds.). (2006). *Handbook for social justice in counseling psychology: Leadership, vision, and action.* Thousand Oaks, CA: Sage.

Toporek, R. L., & Williams, R. A. (2006). Ethics and professional issues related to the practice of social justice in counseling psychology. In R. L. Toporek, L. H. Gerstein, N. Fouad, G. Roysircar, & T. Israel (Eds.), *Handbook for social justice in counseling psychology: Leadership, vision, and action* (pp. 17-34). Thousand Oaks, CA: Sage.

Vaihinger, H. (1952). *The philosophy of "as if"* (C. K. Ogden, Trans.). London: Routledge.

Waldegrave, C. (2005). "Just therapy" with families on low incomes. *Child Welfare, 84,* 265-276.

PART IV

THEORY REVISITED

❧ 12 ☙

The Hierarchy of Epistemological Beliefs: All Ways of Knowing Are Not Created Equal

Tabitha R. Holmes

Over the last several decades, psychologists have grown increasingly interested in understanding how individuals think about the nature of knowledge and themselves as knowers. Research in this area has primarily focused upon the relationship between personal epistemologies and how individuals learn in settings of formal education. Against this backdrop, different epistemological perspectives have been presented as part of a hierarchical, developmental sequence anchored by dualistic, objective epistemologies at one end, and contextual, constructed ways of knowing at the opposite end. Embedded in such a trajectory is the implicit (and often explicit) assumption that not all epistemological beliefs are created equally; some are viewed as cognitively complex and superior, while others are positioned as primitive and less than ideal. Such a view discounts how different ways of knowing may be adaptive and functional across different ecological contexts. Similarly, it ignores the possibility that many individuals have objectives that differ from those promoted and rewarded by institutions of higher education. With this in mind, the purpose of this chapter is to address the biases and limitations inherent in current models of epistemological development. Using several theoretical models that explain the dynamic interweaving of psychological and social processes, epistemic perspectives will be examined as systems of meaning-making that reflect the values, goals, and practices of diverse social groups.

EPISTEMOLOGICAL ELITISM

Epistemology, the study of knowledge or justified belief, began as the purview and product of philosophers who were interested in the structure, source, and limits of knowledge (Steup, 2008). Over the last 50 years, however, this area of scholarship has grown far-reaching tentacles that extend across disciplinary boundaries. Researchers from all backgrounds, favoring all types of theoretical orientations, have described, deconstructed, and debated how knowledge is created and disseminated across cultures (e.g., the East vs. the West; Harding, 1996), disciplines (e.g., the "hard" sciences vs. the humanities; Muis, Bendixen, & Haerel, 2006), and historic periods (e.g., Period of Enlightenment; Moodie, 2003). Most of this work has emphasized the merits and pitfalls of different intellectual traditions, be it rational-empirical modes of knowing or constructivist approaches, with particular attention given to the epistemological consequences of cultural hegemony, imperialism, and colonialism.

In the literature that examines epistemological differences, the "West" is often portrayed as an epistemic bully, advancing rational-empiricism and heralding the merits of scientific evidence and methodology while repressing and ridiculing alternative ways of knowing (Moodie, 2003). In a critique of intellectual traditions and ways of knowing, for example, Moodie points out that "Western society continues to arrogate to itself the right to judge what is 'superstitious' or 'mumbo-jumbo' and what is 'scientific,' what is invalid and what is valid in the total field of human knowledge" (p. 15). Smith (1999) makes a similar point by suggesting that "The globalization of knowledge and Western culture constantly reaffirms the West's view of itself as the center of legitimate knowledge, the arbiter of what counts as knowledge and the source of 'civilized' knowledge" (p. 63). As these quotes illustrate, scholarship in this area often has an overt political tenor that links Western ways of knowing to dehumanizing practices, sciences, and technologies that have failed around the world (e.g., Harding, 1996).

Psychologists and educators have generally taken a different approach to understanding theories of knowledge by focusing upon personal epistemology, "how the individual develops conceptions of knowledge and knowing and utilizes them in developing an understanding of the world" (Hofer, 2002, p. 4). This work examines the variability in people's beliefs about how knowledge is defined, acquired, and evaluated, thereby shifting the conversation to the epistemological diversity found *within* communities, cultures, and contexts. Clearly, all Western knowers are not shackled by positivist, mechanistic beliefs about knowledge; rather, there are a range of epistemological perspectives found side-by-side within most cultures. Such plurality raises questions about epistemological elitism at the local level of analysis—how certain beliefs about knowledge are valued more than others within classrooms, organizations, and cultural institutions. This requires a better understanding of *how* and *why* individuals develop diverse ways of knowing.

THE EPISTEMOLOGICAL STAIRCASE: FROM SIMPLE TO COMPLEX WAYS OF KNOWING

Perry (1970) launched an interest in personal epistemology with his landmark study that explored how students' beliefs about knowledge evolve as a function of formal education. Interviewing a group of mostly male undergraduates attending Harvard University, he questioned participants on their intellectual and ethical experiences, exploring the systematic changes that occurred between students' freshman and senior years of college. Perry went on to develop a nine-part developmental scheme that describes the positions from which individuals think about knowledge claims as they relate to the self and larger world. Positions can be grouped into four main categories that reflect qualitative differences in epistemic cognition: Dualism, Multiplicity, Contextual Relativism, and Commitment (Moore, 2002).

In the first category, Perry suggested that most students enter college with a *dualistic* way of thinking that is characterized by a reverence for expert authorities, who are viewed as the gatekeepers of knowledge. For these individuals, knowledge exists independent of the self and is understood as absolute and certain, "right" or "wrong." Accordingly, dualistic knowers have no tolerance for ambiguity, "gray areas," or alternate points of view. Eventually, as students begin to see that experts offer contradictory, unknown, or uncertain answers, they move from a dichotomous orientation to one of *multiplicity,* a perspective characterized by pluralistic awareness of the subjectivity and diversity found in knowledge claims. Importantly, these individuals acknowledge that truth and knowledge can be temporarily unknown and ambiguous, a dramatic departure from a dualistic orientation; however, they also believe that true knowledge can be excavated through the use of proper tools and procedures. Over time, some individuals become less confident that certain answers exist, a positioning that prompts reliance on individualized knowing. These students acknowledge that others can have different perspectives and opinions, each equally valid and legitimate. Accordingly, evaluation of knowledge is viewed as neither necessary nor useful.

As students continue their education in Western institutions, Perry suggested that many experience a "revolutionary restructuring" in epistemological perspective as knowledge begins to be viewed as contextual, contingent, and relative. Viewed as one of the most dramatic and important changes that occur in the epistemological trajectory, some students embrace *contextual relativism,* an epistemic approach characterized by the awareness that knowledge cannot be extricated from the context in which it exists, nor can it be understood without acknowledging that individuals are active creators of meaning. Finally, the emphasis shifts from the intellectual realm to the ethical realm (Moore, 2002) as some students enter a phase of *commitment* in which they are aware of the need to make conscious decisions about ideas, values, and life decisions, often in the face of contradictory and competing knowledge claims. These commitments help individuals craft and define their identities in a relativistic world.

Using Perry's work as a launching pad, many researchers have continued to explore the nature, progression, and content of epistemological beliefs (see Hofer & Pintrich, 1997, for a detailed review). Belenky, Clinchy, Goldberger, and Tarule (1986), for example, responded to the privileged male sample in Perry's original work by interviewing a group of women from diverse economic and educational backgrounds (all in the United States) about their epistemic beliefs. They identified five distinct epistemological perspectives: (1) *silenced knowing*, in which women think of themselves as incapable of learning from others, "deaf and dumb" in their approach to new information and experiences; (2) *received knowing*, characterized by the listening, absorbing, and adopting of the words and ideas offered by experts; (3) *subjective knowing*, marked by an appreciation for subjective experiences, intuition, and individualized ways of arriving at truth; (4) *procedural knowing*, in which people believe that there are systematic, effortful ways that a person can arrive at truth by utilizing established methods and procedures; and (5) *constructed knowing*, characterized by the belief that knowledge and truth are contextually situated constructions of humankind (Belenky et al., 1986; Belenky, Bond, & Weinstock, 1997; Bond, Belenky, & Weinstock, 2000).

A similar progression is seen in the Epistemological Reflection Model developed by Baxter Magolda (1992), which begins with Absolute Knowing and ends with Contextual

Knowing, a stage in which "self-authorship" becomes critical as people shift from dependence on an external authority to recognition of an internal authority. The Reflective Judgment Model (King & Kitchener, 1994) also offers a description of how individuals develop more complex reasoning skills and judgments over time that reflect different epistemic assumptions. This model begins with *Prereflective Reasoning*, which is characterized by an individual's reliance on authority-based, absolute approaches to knowledge. This is followed by *Quasi-Reflective Reasoning* in which judgments and reasoning are viewed as idiosyncratic, and *Reflective Reasoning*, an approach characterized by evidence-based knowing that acknowledges the fluid and contextual nature of knowledge.

BLINDERS AND BIASES IN THE STUDY OF EPISTEMOLOGIES

Although models of epistemological development differ in nomenclature and focus, common patterns are apparent across theoretical frameworks and research methodologies, underscoring Hofer's (2002) observation that "Regardless of the number of stages, positions, or perspectives, the sequence [of epistemological development] invariably suggests movement from a dualistic, objective view of knowledge to a more subjective, relativistic stance, and ultimately to a contextual constructivist perspective of knowing" (p. 7). Importantly, this observation suggests that developmental models converge in the assumption that individuals' beliefs about knowledge progress from simple to complex. Thus, embedded in the epistemological discourse is the presumption that certain types of knowers are more competent and mature than their "simpler" counterparts. This is despite the fact that some researchers have tried to avoid describing ways of knowing on a developmental continuum. In describing the Women's Ways of Knowing Model (WWK), for example, Goldberger (1996) notes:

> Although in WWK we resisted calling our five perspectives developmental stages, we did imply that the fifth perspective, Constructed Knowing, was somehow superior in that it encompassed multiple approaches to knowing and avoided overvaluation of any one way of knowing. This is a debatable point. (p. 362)

Regardless of intent, the literature on epistemological perspectives has categorized epistemic beliefs in ways that are largely judgmental and pejorative.

Working under the assumption that some ways of knowing are superior to others is particularly problematic given the homogeneous samples on which the developmental models were constructed. Most models were developed and refined based on individuals immersed in a system of formal education within the United States. This obviously limits the degree to which they reflect the many varied ways in which knowledge may be experienced and evaluated in groups with diverse social, educational, and cultural practices. In response to this lack of generalizability, researchers have begun to acknowledge that cultural-level processes may play a role in how knowledge and knowing are perceived (e.g., Khine, 2008); however, most of this work has emphasized specific beliefs (e.g., the degree to which knowledge is certain or uncertain, innate or based on ability) rather than the systems of beliefs that are integrated and coordinated in developmental models (Hofer, 2008). In addition, this research has largely been cross-cultural in nature, an approach that focuses on the transporting and testing of current models with an eye on establishing universal, pan-human constructs and processes (Georgas, Berry, van de Vijver, Kagitcibasi, & Poortinga, 2006). Such a research agenda tends to privilege one worldview over others, defining diverse systems of meaning-making in terms of deficits and deficiencies.

Lack of attention to cultural context in the research on personal epistemology is surprising given definitions of what constitutes a sophisticated approach to knowledge. Contextual approaches to knowledge are identified as the most complex, yet research in this area has not paid homage to the constructed knowers' dictum that "truth is a matter of the context in which it is embedded" (Belenky et al., 1986, p. 138); ways of knowing have generally not been described as the product of a particular time and place. This is not to suggest that discussions of context are completely absent from the discourse on epistemological development. A large body of research has recently focused on the ways in which diverse educational settings promote and privilege certain ways of knowing depending on the domain of knowledge in question (e.g., see Muis et. al., 2006, for a review). It is important to note, however, that most of this work explores "context" in terms of academic environments. Accordingly, context is typically parsed apart and analyzed based on differences between academic disciplines, college majors, or pedagogical practices, all within institutions of formal education. Such a narrow definition ignores informal mechanisms of learning and socialization that occur across a broad array of social settings.

In addition to offering a myopic view of context, research on epistemological development has failed to consider the values implicit in the epistemological hierarchy. It should come as no surprise that procedural, evidence-based epistemologies are seen as more mature than intuitive or authority-based ways of knowing given the very context that has cultivated the research agenda. Most research on epistemological development has been conducted within the halls of academia by researchers immersed in a social system that embraces and reveres "justified knowledge" grounded in reason (Olson & Bruner, 1996). Given that communities have different ecological demands that require diverse roles, skills, and competencies (Wang, Ceci, Williams, & Kopko, 2004), not all individuals aspire to the same endpoint. Thus, reasoned reflection and analysis are not likely to be meaningful, useful, or adaptive across all social and cultural contexts. Such a possibility requires a fresh look at the notion of epistemological development, beginning with use of the word "development" and all its accompanying baggage.

By positioning different epistemological perspectives on a *developmental* continuum, different ways of knowing are automatically compared, judged and rank-ordered. A more useful strategy calls for the examination of different patterns of construing knowledge and knowing in light of cultural practices, products, and institutions. This requires acknowledging that epistemic changes do not only occur within an individual; rather, they are mutually constituted through social interactions. Thus, personal epistemologies cannot be understood by symbolically sequestering the individual from the social and cultural context. To do so is tantamount to relying on only one of your senses to understand a piece of chocolate cake.

With this in mind, the rest of the chapter illustrates how personal epistemologies are likely negotiated between individuals and the social world. To explore this position, several different types of social processes are examined through the lens of theories identified with cross cultural and cultural psychology, sub-disciplines at the forefront of examining social interactions at the micro and macro levels. For the purpose of this chapter, culture is broadly defined as "patterns of representations, actions, and artifacts that are distributed or spread through social interaction" (Markus, Uchida, Omoregie, Townsend, & Kitayama, 2006, p. 11). Thus, both within and between nation examples are used to illustrate the importance of going "outside of the head" to understand individual functioning. This allows epistemic development to be conceptualized beyond a stage-like progression from simple to complex.

KNOWING IN LIGHT OF CULTURAL VALUES

One approach to understanding the relationship between social and psychological processes is to focus upon the dominant norms, values, and beliefs that characterize certain cultural communities. This strategy is generally used by cross-cultural researchers who view culture as an overarching "recipe" for thought and action that organizes how people function in the world (e.g., Triandis, 1982; Hofstede, 1980; Hofstede & Hofstede, 2005). The ingredients of this recipe, or *dimensions* as they are typically called, are dominant values that inform cultural institutions and practices. These collective values serve as a point of comparison, providing insight into cultural differences in patterns of behavioral, emotional, and cognitive tendencies. Interestingly, many of the value dimensions that have been identified in the literature have direct implications for how individuals construe knowledge and knowing. In his seminal work on employee work habits, for example, Hofstede (1980) identified several dimensions that differ as a function of national culture (i.e., country is viewed as a proxy for culture), two of which are particularly salient to epistemological beliefs—individualism/collectivism and acceptance of power differentials.

Since Hofstede (1980) introduced individualism and collectivism to the psychological community, these constructs have served as a powerful tool for understanding cultural differences. In general, individualism is defined as personal independence, while collectivism centers upon an individual's obligation and duty to others in his or her ingroup (Oyserman, Coon, & Kemmelmeier, 2002). Triandis (1996) described these dimensions as "cultural syndromes" that influence how individuals in different cultural communities define, think about, and behave toward the self and others, a set of characteristics that has implications for processes of knowledge acquisition. Nisbett (2003), for example, described how there are dramatic differences between how Asians and North Americans address conflict and negotiation. He wrote:

> Debate is almost as uncommon in modern Asia as in ancient China. In fact, the whole rhetoric of argumentation that is second nature to Westerners is largely absent in Asia. North Americans begin to express opinions and justify them as early as the show-and-tell sessions of nursery school ("This is my robot; he's fun to play

with because..."). In contrast, there is not much argumentation or trafficking of opinions in Asian life. (p. 73)

In models of epistemological development, the art of crafting and defending arguments and opinions with evidence is viewed as a sophisticated, advanced approach to knowledge production (Belenky et. al., 1997; King & Kitchener, 1994). This clearly is a flawed appraisal in the context of cultures that do not value such rhetoric. For people with a collectivist orientation, asserting an opinion and touting supporting evidence is an uncomfortable assertion of self that works against the communal goal of harmony and group consensus. Thus, engaging in debate and playing "devil's advocate" is not a route to knowledge endorsed by all people.

This was a finding that emerged in the work of Belenky and colleagues (1997), who focused specifically upon women's ways of knowing. Unlike Perry's original work which looked at the epistemological development of men, they found that women whose epistemic beliefs center upon procedures fall into two different categories of knowers, separate and connected. As described by Clinchy (2002), separate knowers believe that knowledge is the product of debate and challenge, with an emphasis on validity, justification, and objective detachment (i.e., a "scientific" approach). Conversely, connected knowers believe that knowing requires meaning-making, adopting the perspective of others, and immersion in that which is unknown. These differences in personal theories of knowledge are not simply a matter of preference; rather, they reflect differences in people's opportunities, experiences, and values. Women and men in the United States have traditionally occupied different cultural niches, replete with different norms, expectations, and activities. These, in turn, contribute to different ways of knowing (Harding, 1996).

A second value dimension that has implications for a person's epistemological beliefs involves how cultures address and think about power differentials. Hofstede (1980) suggested that cultures socialize different ways of thinking about authority figures and inequality such that members of some communities are more comfortable and accepting of power disequilibrium than others. This informs norms and common practices across social settings and institutions, most notably in schools. In countries that endorse a large power differential, for example, teachers are revered for their unquestionable wisdom; students are forbidden to contradict their instructors, who command respect and allegiance (Hofstede & Hofstede, 2005). Conversely, in countries where small power differentials have been identified, students are often treated as valued, equal members of the educational community and encouraged to contribute to intellectual dialogues. Contradiction, challenge, and engagement with instructors are viewed as part of the learning process.

This suggests that beliefs about power differentials have possible implications for how epistemological perspectives may be cultivated within social settings. In China, a culture that has historically scored very high on the Power Distance Index (indicating high degrees of acceptance for inequality; Hofstede, 1994), the education system can be traced to a Confucian model of learning that embraces respectful knowing, a form of education that encourages obedience of authority figures whom society has identified as knowledge exemplars (Tweed & Lehman, 2002). Thus, in many Chinese communities truth and knowledge are not seen as the product of an individual's active engagement in questioning, reasoning, and evaluating, as found in Western, "Socratic" institutions. Instead, knowledge is believed to be that which is reproduced from pre-existing sources. Thus, some "dimensions of constitution" (Markus & Hamedani, 2007) may influence how individuals interact in the social world with direct implications for personal approaches to knowledge.

KNOWING IN SOCIOHISTORICAL CONTEXT

At the heart of a sociohistorical approach to development is the notion that individuals cannot be understood as separate entities removed from their social context. Culture does not simply influence or inform development; rather, people and culture are inextricably connected. Individuals contribute to, modify, and perpetuate cultural ideas and objects at the same time that cultural ideas and objects contribute to, modify, and perpetuate how individuals think, feel, and behave (Rogoff, 2003). As Markus and Hamedani (2007) suggest, "[people] are active agents who are socioculturally shaped shapers of themselves and their worlds. The arrows between social and psychological formation are bidirectional; the constitution is mutual" (p. 5). They further point to the importance of understanding socially situated meanings, practices, and products, both in situ and as they evolve.

Applying this approach to the study of epistemological development, it is important to consider that ways of knowing are most likely established through engagement in social practices within social institutions using socially constituted products. Surely the child learning to count on an abacus under the direction of a sibling will think of knowledge differently than the child independently doing algebra on a computer. Moreover, subjective and conventional meanings of constructs also play important roles, as they are shared and shaped within communities. For example, the socially constructed meaning of "experts" and "opinions," "intuition" and "reason" are likely to differ across social contexts. Such differences may then inform (and be informed) by cultural practices such as how to engage with teachers or how to solve problems, practices that bear on how knowledge and knowing are construed.

In working under the assumption that epistemological development is both a public and private endeavor, "cultures of class" become particularly salient for understanding epistemological development. This is evident in the United States, where individuals in the middle and working classes are often systematically exposed to different material, symbolic, and social experiences. Working-class individuals, for example, are typically immersed in work settings that provide few opportunities for autonomy and self-direction, while middle- and upper-class individuals are privileged with more control and choice (Markus, Uchida, Omoregie, Townsend, & Kitayama, 2006). Accordingly, if a factory worker or store clerk has a circumscribed set of duties that are clearly defined and monitored, there is little room for independent expression and creativity. This, in turn, may have implications for ways of knowing.

As an example of such implications, consider the finding that many workers with low-level jobs do not construe well-being as related to independent expression of thought and self (Markus et al., 2006). Furthermore, individuals with low-level jobs are more likely to value obedience and conformity as life skills that are necessary for survival (Kohn, 1963, 1977). Thus, working-class work environments may restrict opportunities for valuing and practicing subjective epistemologies, instead encouraging authority-based ways of knowing. As Belenky et al. (1986) posit, subjective ways of knowing typically develop when personal voice is exercised in a supportive and flexible environment. In working-class environments, exposure to such an environment may be the exception rather than the rule.

In addition to providing distinct social settings and systems of meaning, work environments also provide differential access to artifacts and material objects. Professors have the opportunity to participate in shared governance and brainstorming sessions; however, they also have almost unlimited access to reading material, computers, and technological tools that have the potential to directly influence epistemic thought. As sociohistorical theorists point out, cultural artifacts influence cognition, while also providing continuity between successive generations (Rogoff, 2003). Cultural artifacts and tools, however, are not equally distributed throughout cultural communities. As these examples illustrate, beliefs about knowledge are intertwined with local meanings, practices, and products.

KNOWING IN AN ECOLOGICAL CONTEXT

If work settings have the potential to influence directly people's epistemic beliefs, they also have the potential to influence indirectly the epistemic beliefs of people's children. In Bronfenbrenner's (1979) ecological model, "environment" is divided into a set of four nested, bidirectional contexts that involve varying degrees of distal and proximal influences. Of particular interest for this discussion is the relationship between the microsystem and exosystem. The *microsystem* represents face-to-face interactions between a child and others in the immediate environment (e.g., parent-child interactions) while the *exosystem* refers to distal processes that indirectly affect a child's social world (e.g., a parent's pay raise). As an example of this relationship, research suggests that the experiences that parents have in the workplace indirectly influence developing children at home through parent-child interactions (e.g., Bronfenbrenner, 1986; Mason, Cauce, Gonzales, Hiraga, & Grove, 1994). As argued previously, parents in low-wage, working-class jobs may regularly experience lack of autonomy, which promotes authority-based epistemologies. In turn, these parents may create contexts at home, complete with endorsed values and practices, which socialize children to adopt specific ways of thinking about knowledge and the self as a knower.

In support of this possibility, research suggests that low-income parents are less likely than middle-income parents to engage their children in "academic lessons" within the family and less likely to negotiate meaning with their children through dialogue (Rogoff, 2003). In practice, this means that children from middle-income families, when compared with their peers who live in working-class homes, tend to be asked more questions, asked more frequently about their opinions, and asked to provide evidence for their positions and ideas. Although this work does not explicitly address epistemological development, there are important implications. Children who grow up in homes where they participate in the construction of knowledge will most likely believe that knowledge is procedural and contextual. Conversely, parents who dispense knowledge from expert to novice will socialize their children to embrace knowledge as absolute, immutable, and generated by those in positions of authority. As Rogoff (2003) suggests, development is based on how individuals *participate* in shared socio-cultural activities.

Although research has not specifically looked at the relationship between parents' work environment and epistemological transmission, research does support the idea that there is a relationship between parents' epistemologies and the contexts that they create and maintain within families. For example, Bond, Belenky, Weinstock, and Cook (1996) found that mothers' views on knowledge, their own minds, and the minds of their children influence the types of settings that children are placed in and the types of activities that evolve in these settings. Mothers with different epistemologies have also been shown to place different cognitive demands on their children and to interact with them in fundamentally different ways (e.g., Bond et. al, 1996; Holmes, Bond, & Byrne, 2008). These differences presumably influence children's cognitive styles, including how they view themselves in the knowledge process. Again, epistemological development is likely to occur in the midst of social interaction.

KNOWING IN AN ECOCULTURAL CONTEXT

One way to understand how and why parents create contexts that socialize different ways of knowing is to draw from the ecocultural approach to development (Berry, 1976).

This theoretical orientation focuses on two contexts, the sociopolitical and ecological, both of which "constrain, pressure, and nurture cultural forms, which in turn shape behavior" (Segall, Dasen, Berry, & Poortinga, 1999, p. 26). Embedded in these contexts are discrete environmental conditions, such as the climate, types of food production, and economic resources that require cultural adaptation. As an application of this theory, some research suggests that parenting strategies are adaptations to perceived environmental demands. Parents in low-income families, for example, often have dualistic, authority-based parenting beliefs and parenting strategies (that socialize authority-based epistemologies) because this is the best way to keep their children safe (e.g., Lamborn, Mounts, Steinberg, & Dornbusch, 1991). In other words, within high-crime, dangerous neighborhoods, it may be adaptive for children to learn that they need to follow directions from adults without asking for evidence and the reasoning behind decisions; a dualistic way of knowing may be critical to survival.

Adding to the theoretical discussion, Super and Harkness (1986, 1997) describe a developmental niche model that pertains specifically to the socialization and enculturation of children. This model contains three subsystems, each posited to influence how a particular child develops in a particular time and place. These include: *the settings* (i.e., where and with whom the child physically spends time); *the customs* (i.e., child-rearing practices), and *the psychology* of the caretaker (i.e., beliefs about raising children). Theoretically, these three components work in concert, each influencing the other. Importantly, this model contributes to the idea that parents' systems of meanings—their beliefs and constructions of parenting goals, expectations, and values—are related to what they find adaptive in specific environments. These meanings, in turn, are related to the customs and settings that define a child's world. As Kohn (1963, 1977) argues, parents look to what is adaptive in their own jobs to define what is adaptive for their children. This, in turn, informs how parents socialize their children to be successful members of society. Although this work does not explicitly examine individuals' beliefs about knowledge, it does suggest that individuals have culture-specific ways of defining competence (i.e., successful adaptation). By extension, to be competent, one needs to understand local knowledge and ways of knowing. The type of knowledge that is valued is linked to how individuals think about knowledge acquisition, characteristics, and standards of evaluation (Zambrano & Greenfield, 2004).

A large body of cross-cultural literature compares the indigenous views of cognition and intelligence endorsed by people living in Western Africa (e.g., Ruzgis & Grigorenko, 1994). Competence for many of these populations includes "responsible intelligence" that manifests itself in social responsibility. As Nsamenang and Lamb (1995) point out, "Socialization is not organized to train children for academic pursuits or to become individuals outside the ancestral culture. Rather, it is organized to teach social competence and shared responsibility within the family system and the ethnic community" (p. 137). Accordingly, individuals in these communities most likely have little need for a view of knowledge as the product of logic, analysis, and debate; rather, there is a greater need for practical "hands-on" knowledge that is experienced rather than deduced.

Such an emphasis on experiential knowledge is typical of communities that do not emphasize school based knowledge systems. One example of this can be seen in what Goldberger (1996) defines as "body knowledge." This knowledge is visceral rather than cerebral, subjective rather than objective. It has been shown to be endorsed and useful in ghetto communities that value intuition (Ogbu, 1981), Inuit communities that endorse "seeing as believing" (Tulviste, 1991), and in some Mayan groups where one attains knowledge through ongoing practice and habitual engagement (Zambrano & Greenfield, 2004). Clearly, there is an inextricable relationship between local meanings of competency, cultural practices, and ways of knowing.

These examples can be compared with views of competence often applied in the psychology classroom. Most psychology research methods textbooks begin by briefly discussing different ways of knowing; these include descriptions of authority, use of reason, experience, intuition, tenacity and common sense (e.g., Goodwin, 2008). After describing the flaws in these epistemologies, "scientific knowing" is revealed as the prize-winning route to knowledge. Students who embrace and master the scientific method are deemed competent and rewarded with a good grade; students who demonstrate other ways of knowing tend to struggle in the course. While this is an obvious simplification of what actually occurs in the classroom, this scenario illustrates how certain contexts define which epistemologies are sanctioned "end points" and which are inferior. A subjective epistemology will not serve students well in a research course. Similarly, procedural-based epistemologies will not be useful to individuals in communities whose developmental goals are not wedded to institutions of formal education. Thus, again, it is obvious that different ways of knowing serve different purposes and meet certain culture-specific ecological demands.

FUTURE DIRECTIONS

This chapter has critiqued theories of personal epistemology that include developmental trajectories advancing from simple to complex ways of knowing. To challenge the idea that ways of knowing change in a predictable, stage-like progression, I have argued that epistemological development must be conceptualized as a social enterprise guided by norms and goals rather than as a personal plight measured in degrees of sophistication. Such a perspective is aligned with work in the tradition of cultural psychologists such as Rogoff (2003), who suggests that "people develop as participants in cultural communities. Their development can only be understood in light of the cultural practices and circumstances of their communities—which also change" (pp. 3-4). With this in mind, the remaining chapter will consider new directions for advancing our understanding of how and why individuals develop certain beliefs about knowledge and the implications of endorsing such epistemologies within certain contexts.

A Focus on Process and Pragmatism

Research on epistemological development has largely focused upon describing different ways of knowing and the behaviors that are associated with such epistemologies (e.g., study skills, intellectual competencies, parenting behaviors). Importantly, this work has not delved into the processes and mechanisms that lead to certain epistemic cognitions. One way to address this gap in the literature may be for researchers to apply some of the principles espoused in the pragmatist school of thought to the study of personal epistemology. Such an approach will address many of the issues raised in this chapter, most notably the need to conceptualize epistemic beliefs as the adaptive product of social interaction.

At its most basic level, pragmatism advances the idea that knowledge claims should be evaluated based on the practical consequences and effectiveness of certain ideas and beliefs (Stone, 2006). John Dewey championed this approach by discussing the "instrumental character of thought" that is couched in everyday problem-solving (as cited in Barone, Maddux, & Snyder, 1997, p. 16). He went on to posit that thinking and behavior are transactional, situated in a particular culture, social time, and social space. Thus, people's ideas and beliefs are "a vehicle of both the orientation of an individual body to its environment and coordination of the actions of individuals in shared undertakings" (Miettinen, 2006, p. 394).

Using pragmatism as a lens to interpret differences in epistemological perspectives can contribute to the literature in several ways. First, pragmatism moves the discussion away from judgment and hierarchy to purpose and function; it reorients the conversation to the consequences, or pros and cons, of having a particular epistemic belief. Against this backdrop, epistemologies are not more or less complex or sophisticated; rather, they are more or less useful and efficacious within a particular context. As Bruner (1990) suggests, an idea or belief should be evaluated according to how it is used in daily life and the degree to which it is effective. Building on this idea, epistemology research would benefit from a better understanding of when and why certain ways of knowing are adaptive. When, for example, does it make sense for someone to endorse an authority-based, dualistic way of knowing? Why are medical students more likely than psychology students to be classified as dualists (Lonka & Lindblom-Ylanne, 1996)? When might it be harmful to approach something with a constructed epistemology? Answers to such questions will provide a good beginning to our understanding of how certain ways of knowing may be beneficial in one context, problematic in another.

Second, as Miettinen (2006) suggests, pragmatism can be viewed as a type of activity theory in which thinking is transformed through participation in shared activities with shared artifacts and cultural symbols. As such, future research should attend to the bidirectional relationship between beliefs and practices and the materials (e.g., objects, vocabulary) that inform both. Rogoff (2003), for example, described the tendency of middle-class American parents to prime their children to understand that knowing emerges from question-posing and answering. Children of these parents learn that it is common for adults to ask questions even when they already know the answers (a type of social interaction that is ubiquitous in settings of formal education). Conversely, children in some communities are taught that such known-answer questions are often a form of trickery, insult, or an aggressive challenge; an adult or person of authority would never waste time on a question for which the answer is already known. These children are taught that knowledge is not mutually constructed; rather it is dispensed from experts. Although epistemological development was not the topic of inquiry in Rogoff's (2003) research, this work illustrates that beliefs about knowledge can be cultivated through social interaction and social artifacts (e.g., multiple-choice questions). Studies designed specifically to look at these types of experiences will add to our understanding of how epistemologies are socialized, a topic rarely considered in the literature on epistemic beliefs.

In sum, pragmatism may serve as a useful tool for understanding epistemological development. Accordingly, researchers need to evaluate epistemologies as a measure of the fit between an individual's personal epistemology and the communities' epistemic norms, goals, and expectations. Moreover, it requires that we view *individuals* as pragmatists who adopt ideas and beliefs based on the degree to which they work meaningfully in their lives.

When Epistemological Elitism Makes Sense

This chapter advocates for a better understanding of how different epistemologies make sense in different communities with different goals and values. Although the general tenor has been to acknowledge the relativistic nature of epistemic cognition, further discussion needs to occur regarding when some epistemologies may, in fact, be "superior." As an example, recent work has examined the indigenous knowledge beliefs of people in Africa regarding the transmission and treatment of AIDS (e.g., Liddell, Barrett, & Bydawell, 2006). Clearly, if a community's goal is to prevent HIV transmission, a collective epistemology that rejects knowledge based on scientific evidence may be harmful. Thus, the point of this chapter is not to suggest that all epistemologies should be created equally in all settings at all times. Rather, the point is to start a conversation about how and why certain epistemologies evolve and how they may be useful or detrimental to individuals who participate in different ecologies.

Such a conversation must begin by utilizing the litmus test offered by pragmatism; the evaluation of epistemologies should occur against the backdrop of the *usefulness* of certain beliefs toward achieving culturally-endorsed goals. In systems of formal education in the United States, for example, it is important, if not necessary, to cultivate a belief that knowledge is the product of what individuals perceive, analyze, and evaluate through systematic procedures and practices. Thus, in Western classrooms instructors tend to favor procedural or evidence-based ways of knowing that reward overt questioning and doubting, the expression of personal hypotheses, and self-directed learning (Tweed & Lehman, 2002). This epistemological perspective is illustrated in the types of assignments and tasks that are used as a basis for evaluation (e.g., participation in class) and reward. Although this leaves students with incompatible ways of knowing at a systematic disadvantage, it is no different than any other expectation espoused in the classroom, be it the requirement of correct grammar or organizational skills. Essentially, mastery of a particular epistemology may be viewed as a skill that differentiates successful from unsuccessful students.

This raises interesting questions about domain specificity. Although an evidence-based epistemology is favored in many classrooms in the United States, it is not favored in all classrooms. Accordingly, one important question involves how certain educational contexts socialize individuals to endorse different epistemological perspectives and how students navigate such differences across academic contexts. Students in math, for example, tend to illustrate dualistic, authority-based epistemologies as they view knowledge as the purview and product of experts. As an illustration of this, Lampert (1990) describes common beliefs in mathematics as involving the idea that math is associated with certainty and right and wrong answers, the following of discrete rules, and evaluation of correct and incorrect answers by teachers. Similarly, Schoenfeld (1992) suggests that many students believe that math problems have only one correct answer and that there is only one route to a mathematical solution. This raises the possibility that disciplines lend themselves to different epistemologically salient "lessons" about knowledge and the self as a knower through distinctive instructional environments that shape and/or reinforce students' epistemological perspectives (Paulsen & Wells, 1998). This seems likely given the different goals, interests, and philosophical underpinnings that exist between disciplines.

With this in mind, research needs to examine the degree to which individuals can learn to adapt different epistemologies to different settings depending on the changing ecological demands, goals, and expectations. Can, for example, a Chinese student utilize a Socratic, procedural way of knowing in the United States and a Confucian, authority-based epistemology in China, switching epistemologies as easily as one might switch languages? Can an academic wedded to a constructivist perspective endorse a received way of knowing when interacting with a medical doctor, mechanic, or accountant? And, if so, is the hallmark of a "superior" epistemology one that can adapt to diverse ecological demands in a fluid, responsive manner? This issue should be studied in light of the diverse epistemological contexts that exist side by side.

Beyond the Theoretical: Possible Consequences of Epistemological Elitism

Although it is important to acknowledge that some epistemologies are justifiably privileged and viewed as superior in some contexts, it is also important to acknowledge that when only one way of knowing is valued, to the exclusion of all others, there are consequences. As an initial point, assuming that some epistemologies are more worthwhile than others can result in the pursuit and construction of knowledge that is not relevant for all people. By extension, knowledge that *is* relevant may be deemed invalid and dismissed or ignored by those in positions of power. Using the field of psychology as an example, Sinha (1997) describes how, despite the fact that there are scholars in psychology from around the world, most non-Western academic contributions are not acknowledged as scientific. Thus, psychologists endorsing a positivist paradigm of knowing have historically served as the gatekeepers of knowledge about human behavior, dictating the questions, methods, and conclusions that are appropriate. This has resulted in a body of knowledge that may not represent the constructs, problems, and solutions of all groups of individuals. As Azuma states, "when a psychologist looks at non-Western culture through Western glasses, he may fail to notice important aspects of the non-Western culture since the schema for recognizing them are not provided by his science" (as cited in Sinha, 1997, p. 135).

Making a similar argument, Harding (1996) notes that "all knowledge claims are socially situated; historically local; shaped by culturally distinctive locations in nature, interests, discursive, resources, and ways of organizing the production of knowledge" (p. 446). She goes on to cite the dominant biomedical system of knowledge as an example. Before women, with their diverse ways of knowing, were invited to sit at the metaphorical research table, knowledge on women's bodies and health was confined to the questions, methods, and concerns of male scientists. This resulted in systematic ignorance and knowledge claims that did not necessarily reflect that which was meaningful to women. A similar point was made by indigenous scholars who suggest that many researchers use an imposed etic (Berry, 1969; 1999) to generate knowledge about "others." In such an approach, research is conducted by an "outsider" with little knowledge of the questions, concerns and meaning systems of those being studied (Smith, 1999). This results in a body of knowledge that may be meaningless to the very people it is designed to understand, empower, or assist.

As the above examples illustrate, one of the consequences of privileging some epistemologies over others involves the possibility of posing limitations on the kind of knowledge that is constructed, accessible, and available for understanding the world. In the field of psychology, for example, qualitative research has a history of being undervalued, scorned, and viewed as a flawed source of knowledge. This bias has driven journal content (i.e., dissemination), which directly influences the cycle of research (e.g., what questions are cultivated from published material) and, ultimately, what we claim to know about human behavior. Importantly, qualitative and quantitative inquires reflect more than different epistemic perspectives; rather, they are driven by different questions. Qualitative research is generally concerned with how people interpret and make sense of their own world, while quantitative inquiries are focused on questions of causation (Creswell, 2009). Thus, when some epistemological pathways are valued and rewarded more than others, certain types of knowledge are marginalized in a way that can narrow and restrict our knowledge base.

A second consequence of valuing some epistemologies more than others occurs when individuals with differing social positions have incompatible epistemological beliefs. In many cases, different epistemologies are relatively inconsequential. A friend who describes her intuition as the basis for a decision, for example, may be easily dismissed by someone who values the use of procedures to evaluate the pros and cons of a choice. Similarly, partners approaching conflict from different epistemic vantage points may feel misunderstood and annoyed when their ways of knowing clash, yet they can walk away from the argument. In many other instances, however, epistemological "mismatches" have important implications, particularly when individuals with culturally elevated positions do not acknowledge and value diverse ways of knowing. This is particularly true if we acknowledge that "how one knows and what one is allowed to know differ according to cultural assignments (by gender, race, and class) and social power differentials" (Goldberger, 1996, p. 363).

The therapeutic relationship is one place where epistemological mismatches may pose unique challenges. Therapists and counselors, by virtue of their position, guide interactions during therapy sessions—they decide on the questions to ask their clients, the methods that will best elicit information, and the conclusions that are drawn, all decisions that are informed by personal beliefs about knowledge. When a therapist and client are operating from different epistemic vantage points, problems may arise. How might a therapist with a procedural or constructed way of knowing, for example, interact with a client who uses body knowing (Goldberger, 1996) that is based on visceral feelings rather than thoughts and interpretations? How do therapists and clients interact when questions such as "How do you feel?" and "What do you think?" have different epistemic meanings? How might a therapist with a dualistic epistemology respond to someone with a spiritual epistemology (for which Western developmental research has no label or understanding) given Smith's (1999) assertion that "the arguments of different indigenous peoples based on spiritual relationships to the universe, to the landscape and to stones, rocks, insects and other things, have been difficult arguments for Western systems of knowledge to deal with or accept" (p. 74).

The above questions are particularly important given past research that has begun to identify a relationship between counselors' epistemological perspectives and how they work with clients. As an example of this work, McAuliffe and Lovell (2006) compared how counselor trainees with different epistemological orientations conducted helping interviews. Using a thematic qualitative analysis, findings revealed that dualists and relativists differed in several areas of counselor functioning, including how therapeutic evidence was used, how ambiguity was approached and addressed, and the degree to which counselors were reflective.

Epistemological preferences also appear to influence the work of seasoned psychotherapists. In a study conducted by Neimeyer, Lee, Gizen, Aksoy-Toska, and Phillip (2008), therapists who endorsed a rationalist epistemology tended to differ from those preferring a constructivist epistemology on therapeutic qualities, styles of interaction, and the techniques used when conducting psychotherapy. Therapists with constructivist ways of knowing, for example, tended to be more flexible and tolerant of ambiguity than those with a rationalist perspective.

If the epistemological preferences of some therapists have direct, practical implications for how they interact with clients, it stands to reason that the epistemological preferences of clients will also have implications for how clients interact with their therapists, and, by extension, what they take away from therapy. As an example, imagine that a client with a dualistic, authority-based epistemology enters therapy with a counselor who endorses a constructivist epistemology. Such a counselor would most likely view therapy as a collaborative endeavor, while minimizing, if not abdicating, his or her position as an expert (Sutherland, 2007). Such an approach may be quite problematic and unproductive for someone who views knowledge as external to the self, created and dispensed by those in positions of authority. Instead, he or she may be looking for advice, a diagnosis, or a prescription for happiness that the therapist with a constructed epistemology will not provide. Such epistemic mismatches may contribute to ineffective therapy and therapeutic relationships (Lyddon, 1991). This is particularly true given that clients' epistemological perspectives may be related to how they view their therapists (e.g., as experts or co-collaborators), how questions are perceived (e.g., as necessary or a waste of time), or how they view their own role in therapy (e.g., as active or passive), among other things.

In sum, there has been a paucity of research devoted to discussing the implications for individuals and groups of privileging some personal epistemologies over others. Our understanding of this issue may benefit from work that considers the implications of having the knowledge gatekeepers—be it journal editors, teachers, therapists, or politicians—make their epistemic assumptions transparent and available to others. At a basic level, this might help clarify epistemic misunderstandings that occur on a regular basis. Chinese students operating under a Confucian style of knowing, for example, tend to endorse a received epistemology in which information from instructors is memorized and, at least initially, perceived as truth. Such students are often uncomfortable questioning professors and participating in an active exchange of ideas. In response to this, Western instructors often articulate negative perceptions of Chinese students, viewing them as uninterested in ideas, deep thinking, and original contributions (Barker, Child, Gallois, Jones, & Callan, 1991; Biggs, 1996). Such misperceptions could be avoided if personal epistemologies were better understood and recognized as an important lens for understanding people. As discussed previously, epistemological beliefs are not simply ideas about knowledge; rather, they encompass a person's ideas about reality, authority, and the self as a knower, all issues that are important in determining how people interact. Sensitivity and appreciation for diversity in beliefs about knowledge can contribute to better understanding between different knowers, along with the construction of better, more useful bodies of knowledge.

Conclusion

In closing, this chapter begins to explore the various ways in which models of epistemological development have assumed that some notions of knowledge production, acquisition, and evaluation are more advanced and superior to other epistemic possibilities. Such a perspective has contributed to a narrow view of human cognition that assumes universal values and universal developmental goals. Moreover, research in this area has generally ignored the ways in which social processes are related to epistemic processes. In response, this chapter has argued that epistemological development should be studied as a social process that occurs in the midst of social institutions, social products, and social meanings.

Interestingly, it is not only researchers who have strong opinions about epistemological beliefs about knowledge. In mainstream American culture many people have strong ideas about how knowledge and knowing should be defined and evaluated. This was evidenced during the Bush Administration when a barrage of criticism was leveled at Michael Chertoff, the Director of Homeland Security, when he pointed to his "gut feeling" as evidence that a terrorist attack was imminent. Chertoff's subjective epistemology was the brunt of many a late night comedy routine and demonstrated how implicitly and explicitly individuals respond to others' ways of knowing when they are discordant. Such "knowledge discrepancies" happen on a regular basis. Every day, teachers must respond to students with differing ways of knowing, be it the student who copiously takes notes word for word, hanging on the expertise of his professor, or the student who relies on anecdote and personal experiences to back up her points. Doctors must interact with patients who simply "know" something is wrong. Qualitative researchers must respond to those who sneer at inductive methodologies. Thus, understanding how knowledge evaluation is practiced and endorsed by different communities is more than an intellectual exercise: it has real-world implications for individuals who interact in a diverse, pluralistic world.

References

Barker, M., Child, C., Gallois, C. Jones, E., & Callan, V. J. (1991). Difficulties of overseas students in social and academic situations. *Australian Journal of Psychology, 43,* 79-84.

Barone, D. F., Maddux, J. E., & Snyder, C. R. (1997). *Social cognitive psychology: History and current domains.* New York, Springer.

Baxter Magolda, M. B. (1999). *Creating contexts for learning: Constructive-developmental pedagogy.* Nashville, TN: Vanderbilt University Press.

Baxter Magolda, M. B. (1992). *Knowing and reasoning in college: Gender-related patterns in students' intellectual development.* San Fransisco: Jossey Bass.

Belenky, M. F., Bond, L. A., & Weinstock, J. S. (1997). *A tradition that has no name: Nurturing the development of people, families and communities.* New York: Basic Books.

Belenky, M. F., Clinchy, B. M., Goldberger, N. R., & Tarule, J. M. (1986). *Women's ways of knowing: The development of self, voice and mind.* New York: Basic Books.

Berry, J. W. (1969). On cross-cultural comparability. *International Journal of Psychology,* 4(2), 119-128.

Berry, J. W. (1976). *Human ecology and cognitive style: Comparative studies in cultural and psychological adaptation.* New York: Sage/Halsted.

Berry, J. W. (1999). Emics and etics: A symbiotic conception. *Culture and Psychology,* 5, 165-171.

Biggs, J. B. (1996). Western misperceptions of the Confucian-heritage learning culture, In D. A. Watkins & J. B. Biggs (Eds.), *The Chinese learner: Cultural, psychological, and contextual influences* (pp. 45-67). Hong Kong: Comparative Education Research Centre.

Bond, L. A., Belenky, M. F., & Weinstock, J. S. (2000). The Listening Partners Program: An initiative toward feminist community psychology in action. *American Journal of Community Psychology,* 28, 697-730.

Bond, L. A., Belenky, M. F., Weinstock, J. S., & Cook, T. (1996). Imagining and engaging one's children: Lessons from poor, rural New England mothers. In S. Harkness & C. M. Super (Eds.), *Parents' cultural belief systems: Their origins and consequences* (pp. 467-495). New York: Guilford Press.

Bronfenbrenner, U. (1979). *The ecology of human development: Experiments by nature and design.* Cambridge, MA: Harvard University.

Bronfenbrenner, U. (1986). Ecology of the family as a context for human development: Research perspectives. *Developmental Psychology,* 22(6), 723-742.

Bruner, J. (1990). *Acts of meaning.* Cambridge, MA: Harvard University Press.

Clinchy, B. M. (2002). Revisiting women's ways of knowing. In B. H. Hofer & P. R. Pintrich (Eds.), *Personal epistemology: The psychology of beliefs about knowledge and knowing* (pp. 63-87). Mahwah, NJ: Lawrence Erlbaum.

Creswell, J. W. (2009). *Research Design: Qualitative, Quantitative, and Mixed MethodsApproaches* Los Angeles, CA: Sage.

Georgas, J., Berry, J.W., Vijver, F.J.R. van de, Kagitcibasi, C., & Poortinga, Y.H. (Eds.). (2006). *Families across cultures.A 30-nation psychological study.* Cambridge: Cambridge University Press.

Goldberger, N. (1996). Cultural imperatives and diversity in ways of knowing. In N. Goldberger, J. Tarule, B. Clinchy, & M. Belenky (Eds.), *Knowledge, difference, and power* (pp. 335-371). New York: Basic Books.

Goodwin, J. (2008). *Research in psychology: Methods and design* (5th ed.). Hoboken, NJ: John Wiley and Sons.

Harding, S. (1996). Gendered ways of knowing and the "epistemological crisis" of the West. In N. Goldberger, J. Tarule, B. Clinchy, & M. Belenky (Eds.), *Knowledge, difference, and power,* (pp. 431-454). New York: Basic Books.

Hofer, B. (2002). Personal epistemology as a psychological and educational construct: An introduction. In B. H. Hofer & P. R. Pintrich (Eds.), *Personal epistemology: The psychology of beliefs about knowledge and knowing* (pp. 3-14). Mahwah, NJ: Lawrence Erlbaum.

Hofer, B. (2008). Personal epistemology and culture. In M. S. Khine (Ed.), *Knowing, knowledge and beliefs: Epistemological studies across diverse cultures,* (pp. 3-22). Dordrecht, The Netherlands: Springer.

Hofer, B. K., & Pintrich, P. R. (1997). The development of epistemological theories: Beliefs about knowledge and knowing and their relation to learning. *Review of Educational Research, 67*(1), 88-140.

Hofstede, G. (1980). *Culture's consequences: International differences in work related values.* Thousand Oaks, CA: Sage Publications.

Hofstede, G. (1994). Uncommon sense about organizations: Cases, studies, and field observations. Thousand Oaks, CA: Sage Publications.

Hofstede, G., & Hofstede, G. J. (2005). *Cultures and Organizations: Software of the Mind,* Revised and expanded 2nd edition. New York: McGraw-Hill.

Holmes, T. R., Bond, L.A., & Byrne, C. (2008). Mothers' beliefs about conflict and mother-adolescent conflict. *Journal of Social and Personal psychology, 25*(4), 561-586.

Lamborn, S. D., Mounts, N. S., Steinberg, L., & Dornbusch, S. M. (1991). Patterns of competence and adjustment among adolescents from authoritative, authoritarian, indulgent, and neglectful families. *Child Development, 62*(5), 1049-1065.

Lampert, M. (1990). When the problem is not the question and the solution is not the answer: Mathematical knowing and teaching. *American Educational Research Journal, 27,* 29-63.

Liddell, C., Barrett, L., & Bydawell, M. (2006). Indigenous beliefs and attitudes to AIDS precautions in a rural South African community: An empirical study. *Annals of Behavioral Medicine, 32*(3), 218-225.

Lonka, K., & Lindblom-Ylanne, S. (1996). Epistemologies, conceptions of learning, and study practices in medicine and psychology. *Higher Education, 31*, 5-24.

Lyddon, W. J. (1991). Epitsemic style: Implications for cognitive psychotherapy. *Psychotherapy, 28*(4), 588-597.

Khine, M. S. (2008). (Ed.). *Knowing, knowledge and beliefs: Epistemological studies across diverse cultures.* New York: Springer.

King, P. M., & Kitchener, K. S. (1994). *Developing reflective judgment: Understanding and promoting intellectual growth and critical thinking in adolescents and adults.* San Francisco: Jossey-Bass.

Kohn, M. L. (1963). Social class and parent-child relationships: An interpretation. *American Journal of Sociology, 68*, 471-480.

Kohn, M. L. (1977). *Class and conformity: A study in values* (2nd ed.). Chicago: University of Chicago Press.

Markus, H. R., & Hamedani, M. G. (2007). Sociocultural psychology: The dynamic interdependence among self systems and social systems. In S. Kitayama & D. Cohen (Eds.), *Handbook of cultural psychology* (pp. 3-39). New York: Guilford.

Markus, H. R., Uchida, Y., Omoregie, H., Townsend, S. S. M., & Kitayama, S. (2006). Going for the gold: Models of agency in Japanese and American contexts. *Psychological Science, 17*, 103-112.

Mason C., Cauce, A. M., Gonzales, N., Hiraga, Y., & Grove, K. (1994). An ecological model of externalizing behaviors in African-American families: No family is an island. *Journal of Research on Adolescence, 4*(4), 639-655.

McAuliffe, G., & Lovell, C. (2006). The influence of counselor epistemology on the helping interview: A qualitative study. *Journal of Counseling and Development, 84*, 308-317.

Miettinen, R. (2006). Epistemology as transformative material activity: John Dewey's pragmatism and cultural-historical activity theory. *Journal of the Theory of Social Behavior, 36*(4), 389-408.

Moodie, T. (2003). Alternate ways of knowing—doing justice to non-Western intellectual traditions in a postmodern era. *Journal of Education, 31*, 7-26.

Moore, W. S. (2002). Understanding learning in a postmodern world: Reconsidering the Perry scheme of ethical and intellectual development. In B. K. Hofer & P. R. Pintrich (Eds.), *Personal epistemology: The psychology of beliefs about knowledge and knowing,* (pp. 17-36). Mahwah, NJ: Lawrence Erlbaum.

Muis, K. R., Bendixen, L. D., & Haerel, F. C. (2006). Domain-generality and domain-specificity in personal epistemology research: Philosophical and empirical questions in the development of a theoretical model. *Educational Psychology, 18*, 3-54.

Neimeyer, G. J., Lee, J., Aksoy-Toska, G., & Phillip, D. (2008). Epistemological commitments among seasoned psychotherapists: Some practical implications of being a constructivist. In J. D. Raskin & S. K. Bridges (Eds.). *Studies in meaning 3: Constructivist psychotherapy in the real world* (pp. 31-54). New York: Pace University Press.

Nsamenang, B. A., & Lamb, M. E. (1995). The force of beliefs: How the parental values of the NSO of Northwest Cameroon shape children's progress toward adult models. *Journal of Applied Developmental Psychology, 16,* 613-627.

Nisbett, R. E. (2003). *The geography of thought: How Asian and Westerners think differently ... and why.* New York, NY: Free Press.

Ogbu, J. U. (1981). Origins of human competence: A cultural-ecological perspective. *Child Development, 52,* 413-429.

Olson, D. R., & Bruner, J. S. (1996). Folk psychology and folk pedagogy. In D. R. Olson & N. Torrance (Eds.), *Handbook of education and human development: New models of learning, teaching and schooling* (pp. 9-27). Oxford: Blackwell.

Oyserman, D., Coon, H. M., & Kemmelmeier, M. (2002). Rethinking individualism and collectivism: Evaluation of theoretical assumptions and meta-analyses. *Psychological Bulletin, 128,* 3-72

Paulsen, M. B., & Wells, C. T., (1998). Domain differences in the epistemological beliefs of college students. *Research in Higher Education, 39,* 365-384.

Perry, W. (1970). *Forms of intellectual and ethical development in the college years: A scheme.* New York: Holt, Rinehart, and Winston.

Rogoff, B. (2003). *The cultural nature of human development.* New York: Oxford.

Ruzgis, P., & Grigorenko, E. (1994). Cultural meaning systems, intelligence, and personality. In R. Sternberg & P. Ruzgis (Eds.). *Personality and intelligence* (pp. 248-270). Cambridge: Cambridge University Press.

Schoenfeld, A. H. (1992). Learning to think mathematically: Problem solving, metacognition, and sense making in mathematics. In D. A. Grouws (Ed.), *Handbook of research on mathematics teaching and learning* (pp. 334-370). New York: Macmillan.

Segall, M. H., Dasen, P. R., Berry, J. W., & Poortinga, Y. H. (1999). *Human behavior in global perspective: An introduction to cross-cultural psychology* (2nd rev. ed.). Needham Heights, MA: Allyn & Bacon.

Sinha, D. (1997). Indigenizing psychology. In J. W. Berry, Y. H. Poortinga, & J. Pandey (Eds.), *Handbook of cross-cultural psychology: Vol. 1. Theory and method* (2nd ed., pp. 129-169). Needham Heights, MA: Allyn & Bacon.

Smith, L. T. (1999). Decolonizing methodologies: Research and indigenous peoples. New York: St. Martin's Press, LLC.

Steup, M. (2008). Epistemology. *The Stanford Encyclopedia of Philosophy.* Retrieved April 15, 2009 from http://plato.stanford.edu/archives/win2008/entries/epistemology/

Stone, R. (2006). Does pragmatism lead to pluralism? Exploring the disagreement between Jerome Bruner and William James regarding pragmatism's goal. *Theory and Psychology 16*(4), 553-564.

Super, C., & Harkness, S. (1986). The developmental niche: a conceptualization at the interface of child and culture. *International Journal of Behavioral Development, 9,* 545–570.

Super, C. M., & Harkness, S. (1997). The cultural structuring of child development. In J. W. Berry, P. R. Dasen, & T. S. Saraswathi (Eds.), *Handbook of cross-cultural psychology: Vol. 2. Basic processes and human development* (2nd ed., pp. 1-39). Needham Heights, MA: Allyn & Bacon.

Sutherland, O. (2007). Therapist positioning and power in discursive therapies: A comparative analysis. *Contemporary Family Therapy, 29,* 193-209.

Triandis, H. C. (1982). Culture's consequences. *Human Organization, 41*(1), 86-90.

Triandis, H. C. (1996). The psychological measurement of cultural syndromes. American Psychologist, 51, 407-415.

Tulviste, P. (1991). *The cultural-developmental development of verbal thinking.* Commack, NY: Nova Science Publishers.

Tweed, R. G., & Lehman, D. R. (2002). Learning considered within a cultural context: Confucian and Socratic approaches. *American Psychologist, 57,* 89-99.

Wang, Q., Ceci, S. J., Williams, W. M., & Kopko, K. A. (2004). Culturally situated cognitive competence: A functional framework. In R. J. Sternberg & E. Grigorenko (Eds.), *Culture and competence* (pp. 225-249). Washington, DC: American Psychological Association.

Zambrano, I., & Greenfield, P. (2004). Ethnoepistemologies at home and at school. In R. J. Sternberg & E. L. Grigorenko (Eds.), *Culture and competence* (pp. 251-272). Washington, DC: American Psychological Association.

⋄ 13 ⋄

Psychotherapist-as-Philosopher-of-Science[1]

Dušan Stojnov

Even a superficial glance at personal construct theory shows the salience and importance of the model of person used throughout Kelly's work (Kelly, 1955/1991). As a matter of fact, the *person-as-scientist* is one of the most fundamental constructs in PCP. Presumably, it was the consequence of Kelly's resistance to the prevailing worldviews dominant in the psychology of his time. To use Bannister's (1966b) humorous metaphors, Kelly was reluctant to portray human beings as psychoanalysis and behaviorism had done—as rather nervous clerks refereeing sexual assaults on Victorian women by sexually frustrated apes (1966a); or as ping-pong balls with a memory, respectively.

The alternative Kelly presented as a "model of man" clearly contradicted the mainstream psychology of his time. It was constructive and elegant in its simplicity: people are neither to be seen as machines determined by implacable causes nor as animals driven by uncontrollable instincts. On the contrary, each person—young or old, educated or uneducated, left- or right-wing or whatever—should be construed as a *scientist*:

---

[1] This article is a result of the project "Education for knowledge-based society" No 149001 (2006-2010), financially supported by the Ministry for Science and Environmental Protection, Republic of Serbia.

> The long view of man leads us to turn our attention toward those factors appearing to account for his progress rather than those betraying his impulses. To a large degree—though not entirely—the blueprint of human progress has been given the label of "science". Let us then, instead of occupying ourselves with man-the-biological-organism or man-the-lucky-guy, have a look at man-the-scientist. (Kelly, 1955, p. 4/1991, Vol. 1, p. 4)

In saying that all persons can be construed as scientists, Kelly did not mean that "all men and women wear white coats, have PhDs or are interminably dull in their discourses" (Bannister, 2003, p. 34). Instead, he meant that all people have theories—sublime or ridiculous, confused or clear, discursive or intuitive —but some sort of theory about what kind of person somebody is; what sort of behavior someone should manifest in order to achieve something or who is going to win the elections. Even if people are not "proper" scientists and their construct systems are not dignified by being called theories, for Kelly they still *are* theories in that they are based on hypothetical thinking. Call them a "bunch of hunches" or a "set of assumptions" or predictions, expectations, anticipations or something else—they would be hypothetical because they are based on our opinion about the world we populate and about ourselves and others in that world. If they are hypothetical in their nature, no harm is done if they are called "hypotheses." But in order to become proper theories (something like "deep convictions," "core beliefs" of an elaborated system guiding someone's life), they need to be tested in light of their outcomes. Instead of being tested through rigorous experimental procedure in a laboratory populated with "real" scientists, they are tested through human behavior in the world, a wider laboratory populated with other persons-as-scientists. Be it a laboratory experiment of a "real" scientist or a behavioral experiment of the average human, it will cast some light on the hypothesis being tested—either in the form of validation or invalidation. Whatever the outcome is, persons-as-scientists are capable of modifying, changing or reformulating their hypotheses, or framing them as their deepest convictions. And following the same process over and over enables acquisition of that precious control that helps humans cope with the inexorable vicissitudes of life. The process of formulating and subsequently testing hypotheses gives humans the possibility of making some choices in their daily conduct. Thus Kelly stated that "it is ... their human character that makes scientists what they are" (1970, p. 8) and further that "the aspirations of the scientists are essentially aspirations of all men" (1970, p. 23) offering a deeply human account of scientific behavior—as well as the possibility of understanding human behavior in terms of scientific enterprise.

The ability to formulate hypotheses and to choose between them also makes human beings *persons*—individual embodied agents having *intentions* and the possibility of choosing among several anticipated ways of realizing these intentions. It gives them an opportunity to be far more in control of their contingent lives than their evolutionary ancestors—reactive beings driven by necessities of natural laws and instinctual drive.

> What I think this view of man as the paradigm of the scientist—and vice versa—does mean is that the ultimate explanation of human behavior lies in examining man's understandings, the questions he asks, and strategies he employs, rather than in analyzing the logical pattern and impact of the events with which he collides. (Kelly, 1969, p. 16)

Personal Science: The Good and the Bad of It

So far, it may appear that this chapter is advocating for Kelly's model of the person in the sublime light of a civil, controlled and "committed scientist successfully carving out truth from nature" (Gergen, 1998, p. 116). However, it actually has more to do with the elaboration of the opposite pole of person-as-scientist: an unsuccessful, fruitless, and clumsy acolyte in a white coat disguise—a *bad* scientist doing *bad* science. As such, this work can be construed as a continuation of those occasional works committed to further exploration of Kelly's metaphorical model of the person. For example, Neimeyer (1987, p. 5) foreshadows the present argument by considering that

> if we assume that the client—like more formally accredited members of the scientific establishment—is actively interpreting, hypothesizing, and theorizing on the basis of her experience, then even "disturbed" behavior can be seen as an experiment... designed to test important implications of the client's personal theory. Stated differently, symptoms have significance... they represent urgent but often muddled questions about what can be expected of oneself and other people. For example, the sharp escalation of client demands on a therapist's time through an endless series of "crisis" calls, walk-ins and prolonged therapy hours may represent a behavioral test of a deeply held prediction: "even my therapist will reject me in the end." This enacted hypothesis may turn out to be part of a larger self-theory that stresses one's essential unlovability. By attempting to grasp the anticipatory meaning of a client's behavior, we as therapists are better able to help clients recognize when their predictions border on self-fulfilling prophecies.

Despite the promise of this approach, considering the dimension of "normal vs. pathological" from the perspective of good versus bad science is clearly eclipsed by the prevailing medical discourse that Leitner and Phillips (2003) call the "ontologically evident" approach to pathology, such as the *DSM-IV* (American Psychiatric Association, 1994). Instead, it was developed in the hope that it might provide more dignifying treatment for persons with psychological disorders, perhaps offering more adequate and emancipatory management of their problems than the mainstream approach to pathology of psychiatry and clinical psychology. In order to heal clients, *DSM-IV* assumes they must be diagnosed and labeled with categories of mental disorder. Although well intentioned, this process often puts people with psychological problems in the unpleasant situation—albeit in the cause of treatment, and perhaps temporarily—of stigmatization of their condition.

Given its importance, it is surprising that little has been written addressing the person-as-scientist metaphor. There are some exceptions to this—like Fransella's paper, "What Sort of Scientist is the Person-as-Scientist" (Fransella, 1983). In this article Kelly was placed in the company of influential and avant-garde scientists such as Albert Einstein and David Bohm, thus implying that the construction of science and scientist is far from monolithic. But the early attempts to analyze Kelly's affiliation to philosophy of science come from Rychlak (1968; 1988)—suggesting a "Kantian outlook" and a "dialectic" nature of PCP, as well as from Bannister and Fransella's overview of personal construct theory, claiming that it is "a psychological theory which admits that values are implicit in all psychological theories and takes as its own central concern the liberation of the person" (1986, p. 112). Another important contribution comes from Mancini and Semerari (1988) placing Kelly shoulder to shoulder with Popper and his constructivist view of knowledge. Probably the most comprehensive examination of personal construct psychology in relation to philosophy of science was undertaken by Warren in his cogent research on the philosophical dimensions on PCP (1998) and its affiliation to Galilean modes of thought.

Other provocative reconstructive assaults questioning certain foundations of Kelly's theory were undertaken in several papers initiated by Walker and others, where the viability of such basic notions as (in)validation, disorder and the science metaphor were reconsidered (Walker, 2002; Walker et al., 2002; Walker & Winter, 2005). Explaining *nonvalidation,* one of the core outcomes of their research, Walker and Winter (2005) claim that it can be considered as a protective strategy intended to avoid construct revision, which otherwise may lead to threat or the conglomeration of negative emotions. The consequence of nonvalidation is that people remain stuck, immobile or unable to move forward—simply stated: unable to reconstrue. Thus, the "nonvalidation project" throughout Walker's research convincingly shows that that there is definitely more than meets the eye in the validation-invalidation circle and that one has to be cautious to avoid an overly one-sided and mechanistic interpretation of the experience cycle.

Although pointing in the important direction of articulating the non-optimal functioning of the person-as-scientist, Walker's elaboration seems to be highlighting new strands for exploration rather than being conclusive. Replacing one existing word with a negation prefix (*in*-validation) with another negative expression (*non*-validation) simply does not do the trick. If we want to understand why people opt for non-validation, we have to understand their choice much more deeply. Choosing between validation and nonvalidation may be an option for a person only if by choosing nonvalidation they anticipate the greater possibility for extension and definition of their system. But Kelly explicitly warns that intelligible choices can be pursued successfully only if alternatives are formulated in positive way, and not as negations:

> Psychologically we cannot choose between a "something" and a "nothing"; we have to choose between two "somethings". To tell a person simply to "stop worrying" is not to offer him a real alternative to his present course of action. Instead, one has to tell him to "start" something which will alleviate his confusion. (Kelly, 1955, p. 895/1991, vol. 2, p. 236)

A similar point was made by Gregory Bateson (1972) when he said that "animals cannot *not* do" (p. 146). In order to get a desired reaction from the animal you have to communicate to it what it has to do and not what *not* to do. Furthermore, the vast majority of actors, following the "Method"—Stanislavski's (2004) famous theory of acting—know that their instructions have to be formulated in positive way. For example, if a director instructs an actor "not to pay attention to someone," the options for ways to not "pay attention" are wide open. But if the same actor is instructed to "look at other people in the room, sing, look at the papers or play with their mobile phone," then this instruction provides much clearer direction compared with the negative formulation "not to pay attention."

When people do not validate their construing, they do not choose "to be immobile, unable to move forward, and unable to reconstrue" (Walker et al., 2002, p. 103) and *not* to do. Their choice is probably aimed at *doing* something which is not easily noticed by outsiders. Whatever it is, by definition it is an alternative through which people anticipate the greater possibility for extension and definition of their system. This definitely cannot be articulated as "*non*-engagement in," or "*non*-completion of" the validation cycle as Walker et al. (2002) suggest. It is engagement in an alternative which represents a better choice and which has to be patiently explored in the joint negotiating efforts of client (person-as-scientist) and therapist (person-as-philosopher-of-science). Although Walker's work is highly relevant, we will not be able to understand the subtle nuances of human *ad interim* logic if we continue to formulate human endeavors through negative expressions.

Nevertheless, Walker seems to be right in her caveat that we have to beware of simplified constructions of science and scientist because the

> scientist metaphor has implications beyond the advocacy of explanation as a desirable way to live. It suggests a particular form of that process. It proposes a staged sequence of events that corresponds to the ideal or stereotype of science. This sequence entails formulating a theory, developing hypotheses based on that theory, constructing an experiment to test out the theory, carrying that out, analyzing the results, and revising the theory in the light of those results. Those of you who know even a little about science will realize that possibly most science does not follow this kind of sequence. However, this is the ideal of scientific process that is so inaccurately taught in many different contexts, especially in psychology. (Walker, 2002, p. 52-53)

In his effort to answer the critiques of Mischel and Reid, Tschudi (1983) has elaborated the idea of "bad science": He emphasized a difference between the "incipient and accomplished scientist" (p, 119) and pointed out the fact that incipient scientists can be trained to avoid exercising bad science. As a viable alternative to universities and laboratories—a context in which accomplished scientists are trained—Kelly has offered somehow a different context for training incipient scientists: *Psychotherapy as a form of experimentation*, thus making an offer too generous to be ignored by his successors. In the rest of this chapter the idea of psychological disorder will be explored in light of the opposite pole of science proper: doing science in a wrong way. Simply stated, a continuous invalidation does not have to be seen only as "a pursuit of nonvalidation"—it may also be construed as pursuit of validation gone wrong—or (methodologically) done in an erroneous way. Persons-as-scientists do not always *choose* their mistakes out of hostility; they also make them accidentally out of negligence, thinking that they are doing the right thing—as many incipient scientists do. In order to prevent this, a potential expansion of Kelly's scientific discourse is offered by the addition of a new metaphor of *psychotherapist-as-philosopher-of-science* to the existing metaphor of person-as-scientist. This suggests that psychotherapy may be looked at as a process of methodological counseling taking place between person-as-scientist (client) and psychotherapist-as-philosopher-of-science (counselor), an elaboration not that far from Kelly's original position. In order to understand both the metaphor of person-as-*scientist* and psychotherapist-as-philosopher-of-*science*, one needs to explore the meaning of the word *science* a little more. And there is no better way of doing this than taking a look at its opposite.

SCIENCE AS OPPOSED TO WHAT?

Because every construct is dichotomous, the same logic applies to person-as-scientist—an emergent pole of a bipolar construct. Or—because Kelly himself has not equipped us with a clear-cut name for the opposite pole of scientist (except for his man-the-biological-organism and man-the-lucky-guy metaphors)—one can wonder what the relevant contrast may be. Kelly was hinting at an opposite pole more than once in his two volumes, contrasting proper science with "stereotyped thinking"; "biased expectations"; "throwing loaded dice"; or simply "cooking the books."

If people function as scientists, they are trying to formulate hypotheses in a propositional manner and to test them in their behavioral experiments:

> When a scientist formulates a hypothesis as a propositional construct he says, in effect "Here is a proposition. Let us act as if it were true. Then we can see if what we expect to happen will actually happen. If it does happen, we will try a related experiment. If it does not happen, our whole world will not collapse as a result; we need then only modify this one proposition. Other truths are not necessarily affected by the outcome of this one experiment." This is the kind of thinking which permits the true scientist to face the outcome of his experimentation with equanimity, while the person whose thinking is stereotyped is frightened at the prospect that some of his constructs will be invalidated. When the scientist performs an experiment, only his hypothesis is at stake. When the stereotyped thinker faces his research data, a whole way of life is at stake. (Kelly, 1955, p. 598/1991, vol. 2, p. 30)

Yet, people do not always appear to choose a "scientific" way of approaching life. Sometimes they do not want to discover more; they do not wish to find what lies over the hill in the next valley; they seem not to be ready to check where their hypotheses lead to and they act as if they do not want an answer to questions they have posed:

> Questions are restless bed fellows. When they are behaviorally activated they disturb all sleep nestled in foregone conclusions and elicit dreams of unprecedented replies. Ask the most foolish question you can imagine and, sure enough, someone will offer an answer. Even a stunned silence in the midst of an animated conversation is an outcome not to be ignored. And before the questioner's ears have told him what is happening in the room he will begin to sense his own internal response to the venture. One so often remembers his foolish question longer than he does his sensible ones, and he wonders over and over why on earth he asked them. Behavior is like that; it puts itself into perspective by exploring its own outlandish possibilities. (Kelly, 1969a, p. 22)

The reluctance to keep a languid attitude during the restless venture of the question-asking project may be accounted for by Kelly's opinion that people have not mastered their endeavors sufficiently, which in the perspective of centuries makes them "incipient scientists" (1955, p. 12). Perhaps this happens for all sorts of reasons. Some people may be unwilling to find out more because they may be afraid of their lack of ability to control an anticipated far-reaching surplus of knowledge. They might have been frightened by certain outcomes lying outside their "I can cope with it" list. But there is no reason to fear: fear is *the* reason. In PCP, fear is not understood as in traditional psychological discourse as the product of certain physiological arousal states of the body stirring up emotions preparing people to do something out of their despair. On the contrary, it rests in the realm of their constructive enterprise—the awareness that their anticipations are doing the job poorly and therefore have to be replaced.

Stated otherwise, some people may be thoroughly threatened by the awareness that life will not pay healthy dividends to their particular way of looking at things. So there is only one ray of hope left—and it is to somehow help Mother Nature treat them right to whisper to her softly what it is that they expect from their lives or perhaps to shout it out loud, if she is becoming a little deaf with age. Or simply try to extort some validation from her—Mother Nature, a stubborn old lady, offering only merciless alternatives which do not fit nicely with the "wishing well" approach to life. It is in this very moment that scientists stop performing proper science and become *hostile*, showing a continued tendency to extort validational evidence for certain social predictions which have already proven to be a failure:

> The hostile client is unwilling to sit at the feet of nature and learn. He does not perform experiments; he tries only to stage demonstrations. He does not try to discover what is right; he seeks only to prove that he was right at the first place. When the therapist asks him to experiment, he approaches the exercise with the attitude that he will use the experience to show the therapist just what happens. It is not hard to imagine what the outcome of such a venture might be. (Kelly, 1955, p. 1135/1991, vol. 2, p. 403)

When people stop performing proper experiments, they also cease to deal with probabilities. When scientists do not try to discover what is right and try instead to stage demonstrations, they begin to deal with *necessities*. And these necessities are based on the anticipations with which they would like to pigeonhole Mother Nature. Instead of trying to predict what life will bring them and how to make the best of it, they act as if they are expecting life to be Santa Claus and conform to their expectation list. Suffice it to say that this change forms Kelly's demarcation line between proper and bad science. If someone is not ready to face whatever life has to offer, that person is not a scientist.

If people cannot face what life has to offer in response to their behavioral experiments, it is likely to lead them towards hostility. Unfortunately, this is not the end of the path because they can move further along and become really stuck. This is simply because in Kelly's opinion only one step beyond hostility is *psychological disorder* or "any personal construction which is used repeatedly in spite of consistent invalidation" (Kelly, 1955, p. 831/1991, vol. 2, p. 193). In such a case, it seems that such people, in the desperate attempt to gain the control over their lives and circumstances—even at the price of extortion—somehow have lost the ability to control their conduct in the light of the validational outcome of their behavioral experiments. Furthermore, there is a substantial difference between the definitions of "hostility" and "disorder," in that there is a lack of the "social" in the latter, signifying perhaps some sort of relational void. This means a lack of any effort to construe the conduct or construing of others, even to the point of giving up extortion of validation in social realm, but still repeating the same experiments based on the same anticipations and followed by the same invalidation *ad nauseam* and without any reconstructive attempts to change anything. It may also be construed as an example of minimization of freedom, mainly the freedom of choice, because Kelly's definition of pathology shows that "the number of degrees of freedom" in human conduct is drastically decreased in the case of pathology. A good theory, if nothing else, provides a base broad enough for the achievement of freedom, perhaps the most important project facing the human race. Theories are important because they help us gain control and freedom and enable us to enter the most complex realm of collective relations in which we become *persons*—in Kelly's view the highest achievement of the human enterprise of social becoming:

> Theories are the thinking of men who seek freedom amid swirling events. The theories comprise prior assumptions about certain realms of these events. To the extent that the events may, from these prior assumptions, be construed, predicted, and their relative courses charted, men may exercise control, and gain freedom for themselves in the process. (Kelly, 1955, p. 22/1991, vol. 1, p. 16)

Without a good theory, life becomes complicated. Without a personal construct system that is doing a good job in predicting, the questions to Mother Nature are vague and answers appear fuzzy. Constructs based on vague questions and fuzzy answers become poor guidelines for actions—they become the guidelines for becoming stuck instead. The ghost of anxiety creeps in. With high anxiety and without proper control and freedom of choice people make lousy theories. They become poor scientists. Their science begins to suffer. They become an easy prey for pathology.

Tschudi (1983) has prudently verbalized a caveat that there are pronounced differences between the prediction of an *accomplished* scientist and some preverbal behavioral experiments of the person-as-incipient-scientist, suggesting that a person in psychological trouble may be construed as similar to scientists who mess up their experiments and need training in order to conduct them properly. It is important to keep in mind that development is a two-fold process leading both to growth and deterioration. Thus, "normal" development can be accounted for in terms of assimilating viable principles of science as opposed to "pathology" which can be viewed as a product described as deterioration and collapse of the ability to exercise proper science. Not very remote from this point is Kelly's basic concern in personal construct theory—"the psychological reconstruction of life" (1955, p. 23), an endeavor aimed to help incipient scientists do a better job of doing science.

FROM SCIENTIST TO PHILOSOPHER OF SCIENCE

Unfortunately, a lot of scientific research has been done to date without substantial concern for the meta-perspective of science. Many "hard scientists" pursued their academic careers and never asked themselves how we know what we (scientifically) know: What is science? What is the structure of science? How is it different from other forms of epistemological and spiritual inquiry? What are the foundations of building science? What is a scientific revolution? What is the "truth" and what criteria do we use in order to reach it? Is there any progress in scientific knowledge? Which are the possibilities and boundaries of science in explaining and understanding reality? What is the goal and purpose of science?

These questions may equally disturb every lay epistemologist and thoroughly educated critic or reviewer of scientific texts, even the scientists themselves. Although there is a chorus of critical science giving voice to different opinions today, the majority of scientists in all branches of science are less interested in these issues than one might assume. Simply stated, the majority of scientists work, but they do not care about the assumptions of their work. They create theories, but they avoid considering what a theory is. They question certain objects, but do not ask themselves about the nature of "reality" and the possibilities of knowing it. They are doing the scientific work, but the end purpose of their work they do not see, because the question of meaning is above the boundaries of their work. To put it succinctly: scientists often show poor reflexivity and do not ask themselves what science is because they are convinced that they already know—and therefore leave this question to others.

Concerning this description a far reaching conclusion can be drawn: Psychological theory and method are clearly almost entirely non-empirical, yet no satisfactory account of this fact has been available. Such a statement may appear quite unflattering to the majority of proponents of mainstream psychology, but one does not have to look long at psychology to discover that huge portions of it are practiced *a priori*. A simple scratch on the surface shows that all of the methodology of psychological research is *a priori*. Theories or models of experimental design and of statistical analysis and of measurement and of operationalization are *a priori*. Influential general theories are *a priori* in that they are not falsifiable. There is no observation that would tell us that in fact behavior is not a way of discharging instinctual energy, or that behavior is not the inevitable outcome of a learning history and present circumstances. The way psychologists have presented themselves to the scientific community is that their enterprise is thoroughly empirical. So strong is this attitude that decades of protests by dissenting insiders and psychologically equipped outsiders have succeeded in publishing nonempirical studies only in the most marginally acceptable of professional journals:

> The major part of psychology is nonempirical and thought is unthinkable for most psychologists. Three decades have seen only a slight increase in the inclination of psychologists to recognize that there is something amiss in having such a glaring discrepancy between myth and reality in their scientific efforts. So long as the foundational considerations for a psychological science are allowed to rest, almost entirely by default, on the currently existing set of historical "givens", psychology will continue to be a social arena where ignorant armies clash by night. (Ossorio, 1985, p. 21)

After listing so many things scientists do and avoid doing, perhaps this is the proper place to introduce into the picture a new role: that of philosophers of science. Questioning personal construct theory, Dennis Hinkle (1970) articulated three levels of psychological scrutiny envisioned by Kelly:

> Kelly liked to point out that most psychological theories fail to account for the behavior of those who devise and use such theories. He regarded construct theory as a theory about theorizing and recognized that a sufficient account of human behavior would necessarily include (1) the behavior of the observed person (subjects), (2) the behavior of observing (scientists), and (3) the behavior of observing observers (philosophers of science). This self-reflexive requirement of an adequate behavior theory means that whatever apparatus is proposed to account for a subject's behavior must itself be sufficient to account for the activities of persons in the number two and three positions (Note that a fourth position would simply be the conceptual duplicate of the third position—observing an observer; thus regress would be redundant). (Hinkle, 1970, p. 92)

The above quotation provides a useful context for the following remark: With all due respect, even Kelly himself, relying so much upon his model of person-as-scientist (implicitly bonding science with hypotheses testing, and role of scientist with every person who is immersed in the activity of testing hypotheses) did not commit himself fully to the aforementioned questions about quality of science. Besides emphasizing the difference between aiming at probability or necessity in the inquiry into "man-as-scientist," he himself did not elaborate upon the kind of science underlying his own model of person. The reasons for this are clear: scientists have no time to talk about the prerequisites of their work because they are busy working; they have little to say regarding the conditions of science because they are *using* it. What it is that they do, how good and how bad it is, is the province of another discipline: that of philosophy of science.

It would not be fair to Kelly to claim that he altogether ignored the nature of science in his writings. Actually, he talks about science in the context of the experimental testing of hypotheses. He summarized the psychotherapeutic approach of psychology of personal constructs as based on experimental science model where constructs are hypotheses and experimental method is the way to achieve it. But even more informative is the context in which Kelly puts his engagement with scientific experiments—that of psychotherapy:

> The psychotherapist helps the client design and implement experiments. He pays attention to controls. He helps the client define the hypotheses. He helps the client avoid abortive undertakings. He uses the psychotherapy room as a laboratory. He does not extort results from his client to confirm his own systematic prejudices nor does he urge his client, in turn, to seek appeasement rather than knowledge. Finally, he recognizes that in the inevitable scheme of things he is himself a part of the validating evidence which the client must take into account in reckoning the outcome of his psychotherapeutic experiments. (Kelly, 1955, p. 940-941/1991, vol. 2, p. 267-268)

The similarities between psychotherapy and science are even more elaborated in Kelly's writing:

> In psychotherapy, as in science, the object is to formulate questions in an answerable as well as in a relevant form. The task of the therapist is similar to that of the research adviser. He must help the client conceptualize variables which can be operationally distinguished. He must assist the client in making an experimental

design that lets the data—not personal wishes—choose between two or more alternatives. He advises the client how to keep commitments down to a size appropriate to the risks involved. He teaches him how to use laboratory facilities—in psychotherapy the principal laboratory is the interview room. (Kelly, 1955, p. 963/1991, vol. 2, p. 283)

But how can the client discover how scientists learn when scientists, as we saw previously, do not seem to be reflexive with this issue, appearing quite uninterested in the meta-issues of their work? Although Kelly highlighted the similarities between clients and scientists on the one hand, and the similarities between therapists and science supervisors on the other, it seems that a rather complicated set of relationships between science, empirical research, theory and philosophical meta-issues still does not provide a position reflexive enough for Kellyan standards—having a theory that is not only capable of accounting for the surrounding events of everyday life, but also capable of accounting for itself as well. It seems that we desperately need the third layer from Hinkle's cogent survey of psychological scrutiny in order to complete the picture: that of philosopher of science. The similar claim was already raised in Bannister's (1970) proposal to build a more reflexive science.

Right from the start Kelly (1955) was aware that some issues from the realm of philosophy of science are indispensable when talking about good theory—above all, an appropriate focus and range of convenience, which is expressed in terms of adequate abstractions tracing most of the phenomena with which psychology must deal, and being ultimately expandable—because even experimental results never conclusively prove a theory to be ultimately true. Unfortunately, it seems that these issues were not given detailed elaboration concerning their relevance in his theory (as well as in the rest of the psychology of his time), thus the reason that Hinkle accused Kelly of not being reflexive enough by his own standards (Hinkle, 1970). Therefore, it appears that a feasible way of elaborating the use of PCP is by proposing the counterpart to the *person-as-scientist*—and that is *psychotherapist-as-philosopher-of-science*. That is, in the spirit of PCP, a psychotherapist helps a client become an accomplished scientist instead of incipient one—enabling the practice of "good" instead of "bad" science. It is time now to elaborate the philosophy of science, exploring possible similarities between "pathology of science" and "pathology of conduct."

Approaching Science from a PCP Framework

Kelly's philosophy of science is grounded in his concept of validation:

> Validation represents the compatibility (*subjectively construed*) between one's prediction and the outcome he observes. Invalidation represents incompatibility (*subjectively construed*) between one's prediction and the outcome he observes. (Kelly 1955, p. 158/1991, vol. 1, p. 110; italics added)

First of all, this short quotation shows—perhaps better than anything else—that sensory stimuli and empirical facts do *not* constitute the subject matter of psychology as a science. Instead, it is the meaning that we attach to these stimuli in order to be able to process them as "empirical evidence"—an opinion strongly supported and sustained throughout constructivist and constructionist worldviews. Additionally, Kelly underscores the insight that validation entails "subjective" appraisal of compatibility between predictions and outcomes. This means that what different people may consider confirmation or disconfirmation of a prediction may be so diverse that it is practically impossible to predict it "objectively": the differences between subjectively construed compatibility or incompatibility of one's prediction can be limited only by the constraints of the human mind—thereby ensuring a generous degree of human diversity.

To illustrate this point, consider a brief quotation from a supervised case of psychotherapy. A young woman of 19 is seeing the therapist because she is insecure about her future career. She would like to study philosophy, but for reasons she refers to as "low self-esteem" she is not sure if she should make such a choice. The therapist suggests a little experiment—a philosophical literature review to meet requirements for graduation exam in high school. The client accepted the experiment, wrote the work and showed it to her teacher. She returned to her therapist thoroughly devastated, reporting that the whole experiment was a total disaster. The therapist was surprised but wanted to stay credulous. She asked her client for a verbatim report of what the teacher said. The client had written the following about her teacher's feedback:

> *Teacher:* Your thesis is good; I have not seen such a good piece of work for a long time. It does not need any change or editing and can be submitted straight away. Make one more version different from a graduate thesis in form, perhaps one which may be published. You are talented in this kind of work—it would be a shame if you did not pursue this career further.

The therapist was quite shocked because she had construed this feedback as a strong case of validation. Wishing to remain credulous again, she asked her client to clarify why she understood this as a case of invalidation. This is what the client wrote to account for her subjectively construed sense of being invalidated:

> *Client:* This is a fair interpretation for several reasons: First of all, it is strange to say that there is nothing that needs changing—perhaps my teacher thinks that there is not enough time for the revision, so she wants to prevent me from feeling guilty because I do not have enough time to correct the thesis. Second, there are correcting marks only on the first two pages of manuscript—so she probably did not bother to read it all. Furthermore, maybe the teacher has talked to my therapist (the client knows that her therapist and her teacher know each other) so she is not being

honest for some therapeutic reasons. Finally, my work does not contain anything new; I was just restating the comments of other writers. My teacher has surely recognized this, but she did not want to tell me this now—probably she is saving this for the oral examination!

Still trying to stay credulous, the therapist asked for further clarification:

Therapist: I must admit that it is very difficult for me not to see any hints of positive reactions in words of your teacher. Are you being too harsh on yourself?
Client: Oh no, my teacher is very capable of telling someone when they have written something that is not good. She rejected the thesis of a friend of mine from the class, and she told him to write it again—but this does not apply, because this was during the winter holidays and he had enough time to rewrite it.

The aforementioned case shows nicely what can happen when there is a strong vested interest in a certain core convictions—it represents a clear example of strong bias in result interpretation. The client's core construing firmly rested on the idea that she is not talented and that she is a failure—an idea that carried strong hidden advantages preventing her from further high aspirations leading to great disappointments—and therefore all of her work was interpreted commensurate with this line of reasoning. Her "strong bias" enabled her to construe (*subjectively*) the report of her teacher (seen as quite flattering by her therapist) as a proof of her hypothesis that she is a failure. This kind of reasoning, embedded in Kelly's theory, is also evident in depth oriented brief therapy, which is now called coherence therapy (Ecker & Hulley, 1996; 2008), emphasizing that people produce particular symptoms because these symptoms are germane to hidden, nonverbal and emotionally potent construction of reality held in implicit memory. The cure is simple: production of symptoms ceases if these constructions of reality in which the symptom is necessary to have ceases to exist. This illustration succinctly illustrates the importance of a priori factors in empirical "research," and justifies the importance of introducing the realm of philosophy of science to the psychotherapeutic enterprise.

It also shows that, generally speaking, scientific theories ought to be testable. Some people make great theorists, but poor empirical researchers. They preserve firm convictions about what is going to happen or what is not going to happen, but they are utterly unwilling to make the test themselves. Unfortunately, if there is no way to prove or disprove the validity of an hypothesis, this approach will not lead to genuinely scientific theories in the first place, as many different approaches to philosophy of science such as logical empiricism, falsificationism, even the paradigm approach contend (for a cogent survey on logical empiricists, Popper and Kuhn's approach to science see Couvalis, 1997). Theories have to be inspected in the light of their validational outcome—be it their closeness to truth (their *verisimilitude*) or their pragmatic status (their *viability*). Although the criteria of successful ways of testing hypotheses vary among different philosophers of science (just as they may vary among different persons-as-scientists who construe compatibility between their predictions and the outcome they observe *subjectively*—as in Kelly's opinion), constructs as guidelines for action have to be tested in action in order to evaluate their predictive potential.

Having that in mind, there are two common mistakes connected with the failure to test a hypothesis properly. The first mistake is based on the fact that some *hypotheses are not testable*. Consider the example of a man who is thoroughly convinced that his life would be a success if some event on which he ruminates had never happened. For example, a client reported that his mother had not picked him up from the nursery when he was small, and that he remembers this event clearly as the single cause of all the invalidation which has happened to him after that. Even if the therapist stays firmly in a credulous stance, it is obvious that there is no possible way to validate or invalidate such a statement. One of the reasons it is so firmly kept in the client's repertory of favorite rationalizations is that it cannot be tested and thus proved right or wrong—since our poor client could not be born again in order to test his hypothesis in an alternative scenario excluding his mother's negligence. Unfortunately, the fabric of time cannot be folded and unfolded on a whim, and there is no "reset" button to keep people safe from their biographical troubles. But on the other hand, it may feel good and comforting to stick with such a conviction, as it keeps him safely distant from facing his own responsibilities. One can not answer the simple question "Can we put four angels on the head of the pin," but we can endlessly debate the subject because it is difficult to find four angels willing to volunteer to test this hypothesis!

The second example deals with the case of *hypotheses that are not falsifiable* or construing based upon convictions so strong that it is virtually impossible to imagine the set of conditions enabling their falsification. If a person believes thoroughly in something it is difficult to find the situation or a context in which that hypothesis can be proved wrong. A client was absolutely convinced that he is gifted and talented translator, although he never had officially translated a text. His validation for that hypothesis rested on numerous mistakes in other translations he had inspected; but he has never ever had a translation published himself, thus making any potential invalidation (after inspection of correctness of his own translation) impossible. Therefore, as Kelly used to say, real scientists deal with probabilities, not with necessities. If there is only one outcome of hypothesis testing—that of validation—then the outcomes are not contingent but necessary, and do not represent the act of science.

It is also important to clarify another issue raised by philosophy of science—that of *incommensurability* of two different theories. At the level of metatheory (Madsen, 1985), many sciences can be described in terms of simultaneous theoretical pluralism (Royce; 1985), signifying the state where two or more rival theories try to explain the same realm with substantially different discursive repertories. The problem arises when one tries to compare two competing theories because they rest on different ontological and epistemological perspectives, and they structure the realm of their concern with different entities mediated by different discourses. Feyerabend (1978) states that such theories (also known as incommensurable theories) cannot be compared because there is no superordinate theory that we can use as the neutral realm enabling the scientist to compare them.

Although Kelly could not possibly have talked about Feyerabend's work in his writings, as the former predated the latter by decades, he nonetheless was well aware of this problem, since he was very clear in that new theories formed during the course of reconstruction in psychotherapy are not necessarily better than the old ones. In forming a new theory, a client has a chance to avoid the same mistakes he was facing from the perspective of his previous futile perspective—which led him to psychotherapy in the first place. The aim of constructivist therapy is not to discover the truth about the world, or to develop a single theory that corresponds to the world as it is, as realist philosophy of science suggests. Rather, it is to explore the functioning and implications of different theories in a world of many different perspectives. The goal of psychotherapy lies in creating and sustaining a *mobility of mind*, enabling clients to reconstrue and form new theories if the old ones are not functional in their effort at anticipation. This does not mean that new theories are only the product of accumulation of knowledge leading to stronger and stronger correspondence with the world as it is. It means that theories are the products of the ongoing effort of persons-as-scientists to fit their performances and resources with an ever changing world. The quest for truth is not aimed at producing a perfect, everlasting theory of the permanent world granting eternal bliss to the human race—an illusion that realist philosophers often share with clients who construe "therapy as a way to attain a fixed state of mind" (Kelly,

1955, p. 570/1991, vol. 2, p. 11). On the contrary, theories are much like dairy products in that they have an expiration date, although we hope they might last a little longer!

The philosophical thesis of realism states that objects in the physical, social and psychological world exist and have properties independently of our theoretical concepts and discourses about them. It has been said that "this general philosophical thesis is accepted by both scientific realists and traditional empiricists, and indeed, by most ordinary folk, including children above the age of two" (Greenwood, 1994, p. 16). We want to make a counterstatement here. The world is not always as it is. It changes. Thus our theories about it change. That way our knowledge also changes. This change affects the truth about the world upon which we act. That way we change. If this thesis of constructivism is still not accepted by scientists and children above the age of two, do not worry—it will be accepted soon.

Instructions for Ruining the Career of a Scientist: Logical Mistakes

If there are any instructions on how to approach science properly, then, at least in the realm of personal construct psychology, by the same token there must be an opposite pole. Let's imagine, then, that somewhere there are instructions in how to conduct science improperly and lose scientific credibility. And indeed there are—there are thousands of ways to do science improperly. The growing body of literature in philosophy of science offers evidence for this statement. However, the most prominent set of incorrect approaches to science is based on using inaccurate logical argument (inaccurate inference) which in philosophy of science and logic comes under the common name "logical mistakes."

In psychotherapy, work on logical mistakes was done as early as in the pioneering writing of cognitive therapists (Beck, 1963, 1964; Ellis 1962). According to the cognitive model, many forms of mental disorder are caused by difficulties in the effective processing of information, or, at another level, from errors or biases in thinking. An emotional condition such as anxiety or depression, for example, may reflect particular false beliefs held by the client, or errors in logical inference. The task of therapist, then, is to detect systematic errors—in terms of arbitrary inferences, selective abstraction, overgeneralization and distorted ideation—and help clients to formulate their experiences more realistically. The main differences between this model and Kelly's (1955/1991) constructivist approach is in the postulation of knowable reality in the first and the core conviction that reality in principle cannot be known in the latter. Without an observable reality there is no way to distort thinking process or abstract unselectively, so Kelly's person-as-scientist is very well aware that the mere notion of science can be construed in several, alternative ways—as is expected from the majority of philosophers of a science nowadays.

There are many types of logical mistakes, and it would be difficult to treat them all here. Therefore, what follows may be considered an abridged edition of some of the logical mistakes taken from a broader list of such errors (Couvalis, 1997; Ristic, 2006). Generally speaking, *logical mistakes imply an incorrect logical argument that some persons declare correct*. Usually, they are divided into two groups: formal and informal mistakes. Formal mistakes develop when a person does not follow logical rules. They depend on the form of logical reasoning and not on its content. In this case, the formula that represents the structure of logical argument is not analytically (logically) correct. On the other hand, informal mistakes do not depend on the form, but on the content of argumentation. Several examples of both groups of mistakes follow.

GROUP A: FORMAL MISTAKES

I: Affirmation of consequences
The first type of logical mistake on this list is connected to the formal mistakes in *modus tollens*.
  Premise 1: p → q (*If p happens, then it leads to q*)
  Premise 2: q (*q has happened*)
  ___
  Conclusion: p (*p has also happened*)

Consider a quite common example of a male adolescent with low self-esteem. He thinks of himself as a loser, being abandoned by girls because he is not worth anything. He meets a lovely girl, Mary, and starts to make passes at her and she utters a couple of unclear words and runs away. Many adolescents would take this as proof that they are losers by inferring that :
  Premise 1: *Girls run away from losers*
  Premise 2: *Mary ran away from me*
  ___
  Conclusion: *I am a loser*

The mistake arises because there are potentially innumerable reasons for running away from someone. Even if we agree that the first premise is "true" and that girls run away from guys who are not worth anything, in this particular example, Mary's retreat could have happened due to a myriad of other reasons: For example, she may be agoraphobic; she may have heard that there is a Tsunami wave coming soon and wanted to run for her life; or she has a terrible problem with diarrhea and wishes to reach the safety of the toilet. Construing is the guideline for action. The action can be seen, but not the construing underneath. The inference that the act that happened did actually happen says only that it has happened, but not *why* it has happened. They do not justify (*subjective*) constructions of intentions and reasons behind the act, and that does not follow from this kind of reasoning.

II: Negation of ascendants

This is quite a similar type of mistake, and it differs from the previous only because it has some sort of negation in it.

Premise 1: p → q (*If p happens, then it leads to q*)
Premise 2: -p (*p has not happened*)

Conclusion: -q (*q has not happened*)
For example, consider the following example:
Premise 1: *Girls run away from losers*
Premise 2: *Mary did not run away from me*

Conclusion: *I am not a loser*

Again, our poor adolescent might be in serious trouble, because his sudden optimism is unwarranted, because Mary may be the kind of girl who is for some reason unreachable by the male mind, attracted to losers. The fact of being not left by girls is not enough for making such an inference: it does not exclude the condition of "being a loser."

III: Mistake of disjunctive syllogism

If the first premise of the logical argument contains a disjunctive syllogism or non-excluding disjunction, then the following argument is incorrect:

Premise 1: p v q (*p or q will happen*)
Premise 2: p (*p has happened*)

Conclusion: -q (*q has not happened*)

Sometimes it is not possible to test hypotheses even with the wish to do so, because the hypotheses are not articulated clearly enough. They may be formed in a rather loose manner of construing, which allows the flexibility to conclude that an event has validated our construing whatever the outcome. For example, all constructions including a disjunction like "*I am quite a happy fellow or quite an unhappy fellow," for example, can be validated whatever the case of the experimental outcome—because the possibilities of the outcome were already contained within the question which does not allow the elimination of one of the conditions to be the evidence of invalidation of the other. Furthermore, disjunctive statements tend to be tautological and thus always true. Unfortunately, at the same time they are completely uninformative, since they do not tell us the proper condition we are in. Validation is always ensured but at a high price—that of anxiety. Simply stated, *vague questions lead to fuzzy answers.* In such a case persons-as-scientists do not know exactly what the hypothesis was that they have tried to test. They have done the experiment, but do not have a clear idea about what their design was. They cannot say exactly what the question they have been asking was and they cannot say clearly what the results are telling them. For example:

Premise 1: *I am a happy or an unhappy person*
Premise 2: *Peter says I am a happy person*

Conclusion: *This is what I am saying*
But at the same time:
Premise 1: *I am a happy or unhappy person*
Premise 2: *David says I am unhappy person*

Conclusion: *This is what I am saying*

GROUP B: INFORMAL MISTAKES

I: Error fundamentalis

First on the list of informal mistakes is *error fundamentalis*, belonging to material mistakes of making (necessary) wrong conclusions from wrong premises. Although a great deal of human conduct labeled as pathological is often construed as "irrational," this is not the case in PCP, due to Kelly's strong conviction that all behavior has some sort of idiosyncratic, ad interim logic for every specific person. What seems to belong to the realm of pathology is not due to a lack of rationality, but instead to invalid initial premises. Simply stated, if the premises are wrong, the conclusions reached through them must be wrong as well.

Consider the rather drastic example of a forensic case in which a man of 35 woke up one morning, took an axe, and cut off the heads, arms and legs of his wife and two children. After the act, accounting for his conduct he explained to the psychologist on duty in jail that "people are like plants and that he only wanted to trim his family in order to enable them to grow faster." Aside from being construed as monstrous, his behavior was also labeled irrational—which it certainly was not. It was a perfect example of immaculate rational inference drawn from a false premise.

Premise 1: *People are like plants*
Premise 2: *Plants need to be trimmed*

Conclusion: *People need to be trimmed*

It appears quite obvious that the conclusion is inaccurate because people do not need to be trimmed. This conclusion was drawn through rationally correct syllogistic inference, but it is incorrect in that the first premise was not correct, because people are not like plants in all respects; there are some rather important differences between them. Although the conclusion reached is reached through the correct process of rational reasoning, it cannot be true because the premises on which it stands are false.

II: Mistake of taking unproved for proved (Petitio principii)
This mistake appears when there is a premise in a logical argument that is taken for granted and true, although it has not passed any test of its veridical status. This argument is usually presented in the following way:

<u>Statements p, q, r are true</u>
Therefore, p is true.

A special case of *petitio principii* is "circular argument" (*circulus vitiosus*). It is a form of circular mistake which goes like this:

Statement p is true because statement q is true.
Statement q is true because statement r is true.
Statement r is true because statement p is true.

The conclusion is deduced from premises, and for the proof of one of the premises the same conclusion is used, which forms the circle in which neither a premise nor conclusion is proved. For example, consider the case of the client who was convinced that his mother hated him because she beat him badly when he was small. He was beaten badly because he was not receiving enough love and care from his mother. He did not have sufficient love and care from his mother because she hated him. It sounds logical, but the logic of this argument is actually unwarranted.

III: The mistake of argumentation pointed at a person (argumentum ad hominem)

One of the very common cases of logical mistake is a mistake known as *argumentatum ad hominem*. It is stated in a form of logical argument with the conclusion that a certain statement p is false, and evidence of that conclusion contains the critique of a person (or persons) which hold that statement, and not a critique of the statement itself. Although it represents a wrong logical way of deducing the arguments, it is very frequently used.

Statements in the book q are written by person p
As a person, p is immature and acts like an adolescent
―――――――――――――――――――
Therefore, statements in the book q are wrong

For example, during the thirties, Mendel's theory of genetics was discarded in the former Soviet Union as a creation of an Austrian priest, a holder of "bourgeois idealism." Furthermore, many adolescents will be utterly ready to discard viable advice just because it comes from their parents.

IV: The mistake of excessive proving (Qui nimium probat, nihil probat)

The one who proves excessively proves nothing! This mistake is based on the catch that from stated evidence for statement p follows not only statement p, which has to be proved, but also some other statements which may be false.

Perhaps a lot of behavior from the repertory of obsessive and compulsive clients—often referred to as 'tight construers' in PCP—may be considered from the standpoint of this logical mistake. Hours and hours spent in shopping trying to find the particular pair of shoes to fit a certain imagined criterion; or endless washing of hands may be seen as an illustration of this: Too much analysis leads to paralysis!

V: The mistake of imprudent generalization

This mistake consists of placing the general rules that are supposed to be valid for a certain class of cases on the basis of very small number of cases or on the basis of atypical cases belonging to that class.

<u>P has happened once or twice</u>
P will always happen

Consider the case of a client who thinks that all honest people are unhappy. This is the case with the client's mother, an obedient oppressed housewife, as well as with her father, a selfless and hardworking loser. This has happened with her grandmother and grandfather and she infers that it is happening to all other honest people. In this case, the client is prepared to see this statement as a general rule rather than a case of a family script that does not necessarily apply to all people. Or consider a woman who was refused by the boy she had asked for a date many years ago, who stayed unmarried because she has concluded that no one ever will take her out—an imprudent generalization made with an unrepresentative sample.

VI: Mistake ad verecundiam

The *ad verecundiam* mistake is represented by the logical argument in which the inference is claiming that a certain statement is true because a certain person (of importance, status or authority) says it is true. This argument looks like this:

<u>Person O states p.</u>
Therefore, p.

This is mistake probably belongs to the vast field of reasoning and behaving based on what is known in PCP as "imposed meaning," as well as the clear case of "introjects" in many other theories, such as psychoanalysis, client centered therapy, or gestalt therapy among others. Some clients do certain things without trying to access their validity for themselves. They do it because they are exposed to repeated messages from others which become important signposts in their life—sometimes even before they are capable of verifying them with their own criteria. A lot of human conduct is governed by early commands or prohibitions from parents, teachers or other persons of authority.

IF PEOPLE ARE SCIENTISTS, ARE THEY LOGICAL TOO?

This is the moment to try to draw some "transitive" inferences about the scientific basis of the human enterprise—its rationality and logic. Is the model of person-as-scientist broad enough to cover all the relevant nuances of human conduct? As a matter of fact, people often not only make logical mistakes in their reasoning, but sometimes they dismiss the entire project of logic from their anticipations. To get back to Kelly once more:

> Man does not always think logically. Some take this as a serious misfortune. But I doubt that it is. If there is a misfortune I think it more likely resides in the fact that, so far, the canons of logic have failed to capture all the ingenuities of man, and, perhaps, also in the fact that so many men have abandoned their ingenuities in order to think "logically" and irresponsibly. For each of us the exercise of ingenuity leads him directly to a confrontation with his personal responsibility for what happens. But, of course, he can avoid that distressing confrontation if, through his conformity to rules, he can make it appear that he has displaced the responsibility to the natural order of the universe. (Kelly, 1969, p. 114)

So it seems that Kelly was very well aware of the logocentric bias present in the evaluation of the human condition, an awareness surprisingly commensurate with recent postmodern voices questioning too flattering a role assigned to human rationality. On the other hand, dismissing the importance of human rationality in the fifties was perhaps too threatening a task, bearing in mind that the legacy of the enlightenment epoch was firmly rooted in the academic context of his time. But even as he opted for the person-as-scientist model, Kelly has never said that the person is *nothing but a scientist*—a point well made by Harter (2007).

So, why do our inferences go wrong? Is it purely a methodological failure or a fault based on other reasons? Is it because the events we are facing are not sufficiently known (anxiety), or not sufficiently articulated (loose construing)? Or perhaps our criteria for including events in our inferences are not demanding enough (overly permeable construing) or perhaps are too high (overly impermeable construing)? Could it be that our criteria are too biased towards some vested interest (hostility)? Is it simply because they are the only criteria matching our affordances at a time (disorder)? Perhaps all of these questions need further elaboration in order to highlight the paths leading to pathology without necessarily pathologizing individual clients.

The application of the relational ontology (Stojnov & Butt, 2002) to pathology may cast some new light on problematic inferences. Indeed, the whole process of inference presented above may appear too cognitive and solipsistic to the relationally oriented mind, as pathology can so easily be reduced to individual and internal deficit in syllogistic inference. Even if this chapter appears to some as a strong case of monadic psychology, it was not written with that intention in mind. The process of drawing the wrong inferences, connected herein to the problem of pathology, is, in the vast majority of cases, the result of the *relations* with other persons. It may be that the crucial importance of these relations is the fundamental reason for which people sacrifice their rationality, their *common sense*. In this case, the subject of sacrifice is the proper logical inference, even the rules of logic themselves. This represents the more acceptable choice to many humans, as opposed to the perceived alternative. Whatever this alternative may be, it is supposed that it is somehow connected to human relations—not only to the more pleasant relations of belonging, acceptance, mutuality and core validation, but also to the less pleasant opposites—relations of rejection, threat, hostility and invalidation. Untangling the threads of meaning of these relations and exploring their participation in what we used to call "pathology" will be an important future contribution to our inquiry into problematic inferences and the exercise of bad science.

THE MODEL OF PERSON-AS-SCIENTIST ITSELF: STILL COOL OR HISTORY?

Although some important understandings of the person-as-scientist have been elaborated in this paper, it seems that these lead to asking new questions rather than giving definite answers. Nevertheless, one question seems to be the most important at this point: Is Kelly's model of person as-scientist still useful and viable, or should it be replaced by a new one?

The question is big, but by no means premature. In spite of the central importance of the scientist model for his theory, even Kelly himself stated that "man might be better understood if he were viewed in the perspective of the centuries than in the flicker of passing moments" (1955, p. 39), as well as that the therapist should approach autobiographical data but considering the client as a historian who can "lift the vibrant themes out of the tumult of context" (1955, p. 989/1991, vol. 2, p. 301). Implicitly he is suggesting that the person-as-historian (versus person-as-chronicler) approach could upgrade the person-as-scientist's continuous meaning-making efforts. Furthermore, he was hinting at the consolidation of the "viewpoints of the clinician, the historian, the scientist and the philosopher" at the onset of his two volumes (Kelly, 1955, p. 5/1991, vol. 1, p. 5). And for more contemporary approaches to this question, there is a noticeable elaboration of the acquisition of personal knowing in the arts in considering "the implications of balancing Kelly's metaphor of person-as-scientist with the metaphor of person-as-artist" (Harter, 2007, p. 167). This particular paper notwithstanding, there is also an attempt to supplement the person-as-scientist with complementary metaphor of the person-as-philosopher-of science.

It would be rather premature to reconsider the status of Kelly's model of person-as-scientist without reconsidering the usual meaning of the concept of science. Trying to define "metascience"—a general term for all studies pertaining to science, Karl Madsen (1985) emphasized the essential need to articulate and define what science is in the first place. In his cogent description, he concludes that science contains three components. *Empirical research*, the first of them, is for most scientists and philosophers what the word "science" stands for. The results of empirical research are descriptions and observations, and some philosophers of science (like August Comte and the continental positivists, and John Stuart Mill and the English empiricists) believe that meaning of science should be identified exclusively in these terms. This restrictive conception of science was enlarged by the logical empiricists (neopositivists such as Bertrand Russell, Ludwig Wittgenstein, Rudolph Carnap, and other philosophers of the Vienna circle). To empirical research they added *theoretical thinking*, whose role was to produce theories conceived as a set of testable hypotheses together with explanatory models.

Scientific processes have grown into two groups—empirical research and theoretical thinking, which produce two kinds of scientific expositions: description and hypothetical theorizing. After the domination of neopositivists which lasted until the Second World War, again an enlarged conception of science was developed by Karl Popper, Thomas Kuhn, Michael Polanyi, Stephen Toulmin and many others. These philosophers of science added *philosophical thinking* to theoretical thinking and empirical research, by emphasizing, for example, the concept of *paradigm* by Kuhn and a *metaphysical research program* by Popper. Thus a new level, which Madsen calls the "metalevel," was introduced into the processes of science, which now includes sets of philosophical metatheses for any given scientific text. The metalevel includes two subparts, philosophy of the world and philosophy of science. First, *philosophy of the world* includes the ontological (metatheoretical) hypotheses that must be distinguished from scientific hypotheses, as the latter belong to the hypothetical, testable level of the scientific text, whereas the former do not. Nevertheless, in keeping with a metamodel, the world-hypotheses form an overall, generic background enabling empirical research and data-based descriptions, as well as theoretical explanations and hypothetical interpretations of the world. The second subpart of Madsen's metalevel, *philosophy of science,* includes metatheses about epistemological, metatheoretical and methodological problems. These metatheses are often called *rules, norms* or *ideals* in scientific research and the construction of scientific theories. Madsen concludes his brief exposition of the development of the conception of science by a summarizing definition that claims that "science can be defined as the social-cultural system of individuals who are engaged in empirical research, theoretical and philosophical thinking. It produces scientific texts which in their complete versions include three levels of abstraction: the philosophical metalevel, the theoretical hypothetical level and empirical data level" (Madsen, 1985, p. 3-4).

What Madsen's lapidary statement means is that scientists not *only* test their hypotheses, but also formulate them in accordance with the prevailing rules and norms of the philosophy of science, like testability or the possibility of falsification. With hypotheses that are validated in their research they formulate theories, meaning that they somehow have to interpret the events they are faced with. But this is not all. They also need to create the frame of reference in which their descriptions and hypothesis-testing and interpretation of the results will be possible. They have to construct a frame of reference in order to make sense of these—a *personal construct system*. But the sense is not only personal, it is above all common, and therefore it is called "common sense." They depend on other fellow humans in doing so—in an endless stream of human relations.

This further means that the realm of science is not "semantic-proof" as it used to be presumed in traditionalist discourse. It is not a realm exclusively filled with "hard facts" and "golden nuggets of truth." It also hosts the interpretative effort of trying to bind research findings with threads of meaning. This is not only an empirical enterprise, but an imaginative undertaking as well. Science cannot be viewed as a project of liberating empirical research from the chains of philosophical speculation, since every scientific project rests on the shoulders of certain metatheoretical issues. Even the assertion that empirical science is speculation-free is a metatheoretical statement. Furthermore, using imaginative effort to build the frame of reference which will enable the input of meaning in every research program is a slow process flowing through a diachronic plane, where common and dominant frames of reference, once they hit the walls of restraints, are replaced by alternative constructions providing the necessary meaning in order to carry on with the research. This means that these efforts are also historical in their nature. Therefore, science encompasses the research efforts of scientist, philosopher and historian at the same time. And this makes Kelly's effort in 1955 towards consolidation of the "viewpoints of the clinician, the historian, the scientist and the philosopher" quite prophetic, bearing in mind the dominance of positivist thinking in the academic world of his time.

So it seems that science is still a noble undertaking, but there is no science without scientists, and marked nobility is not their only feature. Scientists are not only noble persons, they are human too. This means that they do much more than test hypotheses. They are not only collectors of "hard facts"; they are also imaginative beings, and they cannot live without meaning-making skills. This, in turn, leads to a far-reaching statement: science is not semantic-proof anymore. In this, it is no less concerned with the meaning of life than is theology, philosophy or Monty Python.

In one of his last essays entitled "Ontological Acceleration," Kelly (1969) proposed that the scientific enterprise, broadly construed, has accelerated the course of evolution. He accounted for this rapidity as a result of the increased number of people experimenting daringly with new forms of behavior based on their personal constructions of events. But it should be emphasized that all these behavioral experiments are accompanied by hermeneutic efforts of equal importance—that of interpreting their implications and creating their meaning.

It is also important to add that Kelly formulated his model of person more than half a century ago. Perhaps his argumentation may sound too romantic in the light of more recent critique, which offers valid reasons to challenge too noble a picture of the scientist:

> To begin the tale, scientific psychologists have shared with the scientific community at large a particular view of the character of the scientist. This view, largely constructed with logical empiricist philosophy, paints a heroic picture of the scientist. In dramatic terms, the scientist is one whose skills in observation and reason enable him (as feminist critics point out, the role is traditionally gendered) to step outside the vagaries of common opinion and political prejudice, to press beyond the frontiers of the unknown and to carve truth from nature. (Gergen, 1998, p. 116)

Gergen assumes that the picture of the scientist is a product of "stereotyped thinkers." But assuming things is one thing, and assuming that things are not what we assume they are is another. Both processes foster potential deconstruction of traditional discourse about science and scientists. Is it possible that "there can be only one" way to define the role of scientists, or has it become an obsolete cliché, as Gergen (1998, p. 116) has so succinctly put in his caveat? Is the definition of science and the practice of scientists beyond the application of constructive alternativism? If not, what are the productive and stimulating alternatives to the traditional discourse? Could it be that there is some substantial difference between natural and social sciences—and their philosophies of science, respectively? Are "prediction and control" the only acceptable superordinate constructs for the person-as-scientist in PCP, or could we offer some other, equally viable superordinate positions?

Although this reasoning opens highly relevant discussion about the viability of privileged worldviews and the favored social status of the scientific enterprise, it does not diminish the importance and viability of the person-as-scientist model. But it also raises the need to reconsider its meaning and to construe it alternatively. The current chapter shows that the meaning of science was reconsidered and revised more than once. I do not see why it should not be reconsidered once more—and indeed—many more times. "People always reconstrue what they cannot deny"—be it the formulation of hypotheses, theories, metatheoretical issues, frames of reference, norms and standards in science, as in the case of "proper scientists," as well as core constructs, peripheral constructs or the whole system of constructs, as in the case of the person-as-scientist. Whatever the case, the intention is to show that this compatibility can be used as a viable metaphor for many years to come—if we accept the idea that scientists are more human than they often are willing to accept, and that humans in their daily functioning are far more scientific than we dare assume.

INSTEAD OF A CONCLUSION

As mentioned before, it does not seem feasible to reach any final conclusions concerning human projects that were developed for thousands of years with ever-changing insights in the meantime. It appears that Kelly's view of science and the scientist was commensurate with the *Zeitgeist* of his epoch, but at the same time surprisingly fresh and avant-garde. On the one hand, I do not see his construction of science as too outmoded or oppressive, since it can be applied to the other pole of science and used in the venture of psychotherapy as a way of elaborating another important question, that of pathology. It appears highly promising to continue this elaboration, because it seems much more human and emancipatory and more bearable to be diagnosed as a "bad scientist" than to be stigmatized as a "crazy," "neurotic," "psychopathic," "psychotic," or a "lunatic." Using the existing categorization of psychological disorders may be much more oppressive, even when disguised in scientific discourse, than analyzing someone's search towards knowledge in terms of the fruitfulness and viability of his or her scientific efforts.

Questioning Kelly's view of science and scientist does not necessarily make his model of person-as-scientist superfluous and redundant. Questioning the mere core of current discourse about science (as is done in philosophy of science) and elaborating it with different views on how science can be construed among different philosophers of science, as well as what a person-as-scientist actually does, confirms the core of Kelly's work—the philosophy of constructive alternativism. Therefore, there is no given, ready-made and clear cut edition of the person-as-scientist, except one using as many possible alternative constructions of science as come to mind. Even a thorough reconstruction of what Kelly saw as the proper science and the proper role of a scientist, done in the light of recent postmodern revision of science, would still make us proper constructivists busy in our reconstructive efforts—and I am glad of that!

REFERENCES

American Psychiatric Association (1994). *Diagnostic and statistical manual of mental disorders* (4th ed.). Washington DC: American Psychiatric Association.

Bannister, D. (1966a). A new theory in personality. In B. Foss (Ed.), *New horizons in psychology* (pp. 25-54). Harmondsworth: Penguin.

Bannister, D. (1966b). Psychology as an exercise in paradox. *Bulletin of the British Psychological Society, 19*, 21-26.

Bannister, D. (1970). Science through the looking glass. In D. Bannister (Ed.), *Perspectives in personal construct theory* (pp. 47-61). London: Academic Press.

Bannister, D. (2003). Kelly versus clockwork psychology. In F. Fransella (Ed.), *International handbook of personal construct psychology* (pp. 33-39). New York: Wiley.

Bannister, D. & Fransella, F (1986), *Inquiring man* (3rd edition). London: Routledge.

Bateson, G. (1972). *Steps to an ecology of mind.* New York: Ballantine Books.

Beck, A. T. (1963). Thinking and depression: Idiosyncratic content and cognitive distortions. *Archives of General Psychiatry, 9*, 324-333.

Beck, A. T. (1964). Thinking and depression: Theory and therapy. *Archives of General Psychiatry, 10*, 561-571.

Couvalis, G. (1997). *The philosophy of science.* London: Sage.

Ecker, B., & Hulley, L. (1996). *Depth oriented brief therapy: How to be brief when you were trained to be deep, and vice versa.* San Francisco: Jossey-Bass.

Ecker, B. & Hulley, L. (2008). Coherence therapy: Swift change at the roots of symptom productions. In J. D. Raskin & S. K. Bridges (Eds.)., *Studies in Meaning 3: Constructivist psychotherapy in the real world.* (pp.57-85). New York: Pace University Press.

Ellis, A. (1962). *Reason and emotion in psychotherapy.* Secaucus: NJ: Citadel.
Feyerabend, P. (1978). *Science in a free society.* London: New Left Books.
Fransella, F. (1983). What sort of scientist is the person-as-scientist? In J. Adams-Webber & J. Mancuso (Eds.), *Applications of personal construct theory* (pp. 127-137). Toronto: Academic Press.
Gergen, K. (1998). The ordinary, the original, and the believable in psychology's construction of the person. In B. Bayer & J. Shotter (Eds.), *Reconstructing the psychological subject* (pp. 111-126). London: Sage.
Greenwood, J. (1994). *Realism, identity and emotion.* London: Sage.
Harter, S. L. (2007). Visual art making for therapist growing and self-care. *Journal of Constructivist Psychology, 20,* 167-183.
Hinkle, D. (1970). The game of personal constructs. In D. Bannister (Ed.), *Perspectives in personal construct theory* (pp. 91-111). London: Academic Press.
Kelly, G. (1955). *The psychology of personal constructs.* New York: Norton/ London: Routledge & Kegan Paul.
Kelly, G. (1969). Ontological acceleration. In B. Maher (Ed.), *Clinical psychology and personality: The selected papers of George Kelly* (pp. 7-46). New York: Wiley.
Kelly, G. (1969) The strategy of psychological research. In B. Maher (Ed.), *Clinical psychology and personality: The selected papers of George Kelly* (pp. 114-132). New York: Wiley.
Kelly, G. (1970) A brief introduction to personal construct theory. In D. Bannister (Ed.), *Perspectives in personal construct theory* (pp. 1-31). London: Academic Press.
Leitner, L. & Phillips, S. (2003). The immovable objects versus the irresistible force. *Journal of Humanistic Psychology, 43,* 156-173.
Madsen, K. (1985). Psychological metatheory. In K. Madsen & L. Moss (Eds.), *Annals of theoretical psychology, 3,* 1-9. New York: Plenum Press.
Mancini, F. & Semerari, A. (1988). Kelly and Popper: a constructivist view of knowledge. In F. Fransella & L. Thomas (Eds.), *Experimenting with personal construct psychology* (pp. 69-80). London: Routledge and Kegan Paul.
Mischel, T. (1964). Personal constructs, rules and the logic of clinical activity. *Psychological Review, 71,* 180-192.
Neimeyer, R. A. (1987). An orientation to personal construct therapy. In R. A. Neimeyer & G. J. Neimeyer (Eds.), *Personal construct psychology casebook* (pp. 3-19). New York: Springer.
Ossorio, P. G. (1985). An overview of descriptive psychology. In K. Gergen & K. Davis (Eds.), *The social construction of person* (pp. 19-41). New York: Springer-Verlag.

Reid, F. (1979). Personal constructs and social competence In P. Stringer & D. Bannister (Eds.), *Constructs of sociality and individuality* (pp. 233-255). London: Academic Press.
Ristic, Z. (2006). *O istrazivanju, metodu i znanju* (On research, method and knowledge). Belgrade: IPI.
Royce, J. (1985). The problem of theoretical pluralism in psychology. In K. Madsen & L. Moss (Eds.), *Annals of Theoretical Psychology, 3*, 297-317. New York: Plenum Press.
Rychlak, J. (1985). *A philosophy of science for personality theory* (2nd ed., rev.). Boston: Houghton Mifflin. (Original work published 1968)
Rychlak, J. (1988).: *The psychology of rigorous humanism* (2nd ed.). New York: New York University Press. (Original work published 1977)
Stanislavski, K. (2004). *Sistem: Teorija glume* (System: Theory of acting, Serbian translation). Belgrade: Ethos.
Stojnov, D & Butt, T. (2002): The relational basis of personal construct psychology. In R. A. Neimeyer & G. J. Neimeyer (Eds.), *Advances of personal construct theory: New directions and perspectives* (pp. 81-113). Westport, Connecticut and London: Praeger.
Tschudi, F. (1983). Constructs are hypotheses. In J. Adams-Webber & J. Mancuso (Eds.), *Applications of personal construct theory* (pp. 115-127). Toronto: Academic Press.
Walker, B. (2002).: Nonvalidation vs. (In)validation: Implications for theory and practice. In J. D. Raskin & S. K. Bridges (Eds.), *Studies in meaning: Exploring constructivist psychology* (pp. 49-63). New York: Pace University Press.
Walker, B. & Winter, D. (2005): Psychological disorder and reconstruction. In: D. Winter & L. Viney (Eds.), *Personal construct psychotherapy* (pp. 21-34). London: Whurr Publishers.
Warren, B. (1990): Personal construct psychology and the Aristotelian and Galileian modes of thought. *International Journal of Personal Construct Psychology, 2*, 287-300.
Warren, B. (1998): *Philosophical dimensions of personal construct psychology*. London: Routledge.

❧ 14 ☙

The Status of the Individual in Pragmatism and Constructivism

Trevor Butt

In this chapter, I want to think about the nature of the individual in constructivism. For far too long, the individual was construed as a social atom in orthodox psychology. The advent of the constructivist family (I include social constructionism in this, as will be clear below) has led to a decentering of the self and the individual. Instead there is an emphasis on relationship: what goes on between people rather than "within" them. But sometimes this leads to the abolition of all choice and agency on the part of the individual. This dispute about the role of the person within the constructivist family is by no means new (see Mascolo & Dalto, 1995). Here I want to consider it in the light of the work of an earlier (and sadly mainly forgotten) psychology: pragmatism.

The Individual in Social Psychology: A Brief History

It took a long time for Anglophonic social psychology to recognize the social world. The behaviorist ascendancy a century ago ushered in a period in which the individual was seen as a social atom. Society was "out there." Individuals came together to make it up—they were real, observable, concrete. Society, by contrast, was merely a concept, abstract and invisible. Social psychology recognized that groups had a definite effect on individuals—usually a detrimental one. How was it that people fell under the spell of the crowd, lost their sense of conscience and generally misdirected when under the sway of the group? In the wake of the Second World War, social psychology pondered what had made the Germans so beastly. And of course it was their upbringing and social institutions that provided such firm grounding for the authoritarian personality. The implicit virtue of the individual contrasted with the crushing or even dangerous vision of society is visible in other fields of psychology as well. For Rogers (1967), individuals were like plants. Left to themselves, they are a credit to both themselves and others. They are creative, loving and essentially decent. Of course they needed facilitating conditions, just as a plant needs nourishing soil and light. But everywhere we see the damage done when the actualizing tendency is thwarted by the social world. In the enthusiastic reception of Rogers' work we can make out an ideological component: individual good, society bad.

So we owe a great debt to Kenneth Gergen. He was almost a lone voice in North American social psychology of the 1970s and early 1980s, insisting on a social and historical context for the individual. When he launched the social constructionist movement in 1985, it began a vital re-balancing of the discipline. The social world was not just there to get in our way, de-rail or transform us into neurotics and psychopaths. It was certainly as real as are individuals, and what went on between people was as (or more) important that what went in "within" them (See Gergen, 2010 [this volume]). It is not that individuals are social atoms that come together to form society. Instead, each is formed in relationship—the individual is a social construction. Rom Harré, a British philosopher of science had been criticizing the lack of the social in social psychology on something of a parallel course. He offers us an interesting and enlightening simile for the individual/society relationship (Harré, 1989). Individuals in the same society are like different farmers in the same neighborhood: they share climate and soil and are therefore restricted in producing some things while facilitated in producing others. So for example, in the Yorkshire Dales where the soil is shallow and the climate wet and cold, sheep are invariably produced, and never cereals. There will of course be differences between the farms. Indeed these differences will be very apparent to farmers themselves. Nevertheless, they are much more alike than different, as will be obvious to a farmer visiting from say the south of England.

Constructionism and Constructivism

These developments in the 1980s gave rise to a related set of movements that I will call the constructivist family. Gergen's work seems to have had more impact in the UK than in North America. British social psychology quite rapidly split into a cognitive social psychology orthodoxy, and a constructionist alternative. Discursive psychology and later "critical social psychology" dominated some university departments. Psychologists discovered that language was more than a matter of description and simple naming. Each individual is born into a world shaped by a language that both facilitates and restricts what can be talked about, and indeed, thought about. People *do* things with their talk; they cajole plead and bully with it. Philosophers such as Ryle, Austin and Wittgenstein began to be read by social psychologists, and cited as the basis of the new social psychology. In North America, constructivism began to take shape. Based on the work of von Glasersfeld, Maturana and Varela, it embraced the psychological thought of Kelly and Piaget.

How are we to understand the relationship between these different types of new social psychology? We can consider that at least they are a family of approaches. The notion of family resemblance comes from Wittgenstein. Family members share features in an overlapping way—they can be recognized as similar without there necessarily being a clear and identifiable core essence. In the case of the constructivist family, it is not difficult to spot important differences, as one might in any family. There are different emphases on the role of language, on the importance of social versus individual construction, and the centrality of personal interpretation. But there remain features that clearly separate them from an orthodox objectivist approach. They all contend that the world around us is never simply discovered through our contact with it. The process of construction silently interweaves with any investigation we carry out, so that reality is always made as well as found. Chiari and Nuzzo (1996) make a convincing case that this indeed points to a core essence of true constructivism albeit at a high level of abstraction: all share a rejection of the person versus world dualism. Let us look at what this means.

A naïve realist worldview sees a world populated by separate objects—computers, desks and books for examples. As I sit here trying to compose a text on the screen, I can see these things in front of me. It seems indisputable that this is the way things are. They impinge on my senses and are registered in my brain as separate objects. This is what Merleau-Ponty (1945/1962) referred to as the doctrine of objective thought: the idea that the world consists of separate objects with causal relationships between them. But as Merleau-Ponty argued, objective thought does not do justice to what he called "the lived-world"—the way things really appear to us. So suppose it were not me, but Julius Caesar, suddenly (and unfortunately!) resurrected, looking around him. Is this what he would see? I doubt it. Having had no experience of any of these objects, and having no idea at all of their function, how could he? The stimulus array might appear in any number of ways, perhaps connected in some strange fashion that we would marvel at. After all, he lived in a world populated by supernatural forces and omens. They appear *to me* as separate objects because of their uses to me, their roles in my life. In my perception, I anticipate my connection with them.

And anticipation involves more than expectation, its cognitive component. It incorporates action and interaction. This is what George Kelly (1969, p. 88) meant when he said of the person: "Always the future beckons him, and always he reaches out in tremulous anticipation to touch it. He lives in anticipation; we mean this literally: *He lives in anticipation!*"

Perception, then, is an act of construction, governed by our anticipation and interaction with the world. In contrast to the naïve realist, constructivists begin their analysis with the interaction between the person and the world. This is a dialectical relationship, that is to say one in which both poles emerge and develop as a result of the interaction between them. In this way, as Chiari and Nuzzo (1996) argue, constructivism rejects the person/world dualism.

THE DECENTERING OF THE SELF

It is important to remember that what is now seen as a constructivist world-view was not invented *de novo* by constructivists. In the early twentieth century, there were many strands in philosophy that proposed this: pragmatism in the USA, Macmurray in Scotland, phenomenology in France and Germany, and Ryle, Austin and Wittgenstein in England. All in their different traditions criticized the individualist approach in psychology. All recognized the importance of the linguistic community in which a person is embedded. And all stressed the interpersonal over the intrapersonal realms. In all these systems there is no "ghost in the machine," no self-entity at the center of each individual. Perhaps the most frequently cited quote of Merleau-Ponty's comes from his famous preface to *Phenomenology of Perception,* and expresses the phenomenological view:

> (The world) is the natural setting of, and field for, all my thoughts and all my explicit perceptions. Truth does not "inhabit" only the "inner man," or more accurately, there is no inner man, man is in the world, and only in the world does he know himself. (Merleau-Ponty, 1945/1962, p. xi)

All the same, the academic wheel is constantly reinvented. New generations develop their own theoretical frameworks, along with accompanying vocabulary and concepts in which to express things. But we must be aware that different theoretical frameworks, like languages, capture some meanings better than others. The problem with some members of the constructivist family (and I would include here social constructionism, discursive psychology and critical social psychology) is that the individual vanishes altogether as we move towards an appreciation of the interpersonal realm. It is not that the self is decentered; rather it is abolished. So for example, Gergen (2010 [this volume]) ends his chapter with a focus on what "understanding" means. I think he usefully points out that we appear to know when we have grasped another's meaning; understanding is an interpersonal phenomenon. But he also says that we never have access to other minds, what is in them is anybody's guess. Understanding, he concludes, is to do with knowing how to respond correctly to the other. We often know when we can and cannot do it, and this is when we say we either do or do not understand them:

> In effect, to understand each other is to coordinate our actions within the common scenarios of our culture. A failure to understand is not a failure to grasp the essence of the other's psyche, but an inability to participate in the kind of scenario the other is inviting. (Gergen, 2010 [this volume], p. 23)

As an example, he considers the case of responding to another person's grief and loss. I show a lack of understanding by trying to gloss over the other person's feelings, and by contrast, show understanding by softly murmuring words of condolence. I know and reproduce the formula in my culture and therefore I understand. But surely we know what it means to *pretend* to understand. Suppose I have no care or feeling for the person or her situation but go through the motions of the formula so as not to appear thoughtless. Is this what we mean by understanding? I think not. The social constructionist analysis begins to resemble that of the behaviorist, focusing only on what may be observed and quantified; what Skinner (1974) used to refer to as "verbal behavior."

Humanism is too easily scorned by some in the constructivist camp. It is not necessarily a move towards crude individualism. It is quite possible to recognize the importance of the social world and at the same time the importance of the individual within it. Of course the interpersonal realm is vital in understanding the individual self—this has been at the heart of the work of those streams in philosophy I listed above. No one sums this up more beautifully than does Merleau-Ponty:

> In the experience of dialogue, there is constituted between the other person and myself a common ground; my thought and his are inter-woven into a single fabric, my words and those of my interlocutor are called forth by the state of the discussion, and they are inserted into a shared operation of which neither of us is the creator. . . . In the present dialogue, I am freed from myself, for the other person's thoughts are certainly his; they are not of my making, though I do grasp them the moment they come into being, or even anticipate them. And indeed, the objections which my interlocutor raises to what I say draws from me thoughts which I had no idea I possessed, so that at the same time I lend him my thoughts, he reciprocates by making me think too. (Merleau-Ponty, 1945/1962, p. 354)

This quote nicely captures the experience of interaction; the way in which we are transformed in a particular dialogue through an inter-twining with another person. Gergen (2010 [this volume]) uses the example of a dance. One might add many others, and I think an ordinary conversation or dialogue is particularly potent. We do not just take turns in talking and listening, and neither do we decide in advance exactly what we are going to do or say. The conversation, as it were, outruns both of us, and we find as well as make ourselves in it. It is another example of a dialectical relation: both participants unfold in relation to each other as the interaction progresses.

This is what Mead (1910/1982) referred to as a social act, and following him, was elaborated by Blumer (1969) as joint action. But Merleau-Ponty makes the point that we remain separate individuals: "I am freed from myself, for the other person's thoughts are certainly his." I cannot *literally* feel your pain. But neither are the other's thoughts and feelings simply anybody's guess, as Gergen suggests—"I do grasp them the moment they come into being."

What is needed, surely, is an analysis that recognizes that the person is indeed embedded in the social world, and the individual is not a social atom. But at the same time we have to accord some power and agency of the individual; a notion of the individual self that is not an entity at the center of the person, but a social construction, albeit a center of choice and agency once constructed.

Pragmatism

For this I think we can turn to the tradition of pragmatism. This is now thought of as a philosophical movement, but it formed the basis of psychology in the USA before it was supplanted by Watson's behaviorism in the early twentieth century. Psychologists now think of William James and John Dewey as philosophers, while George Mead is sometimes seen as a sociologist. Of course, history is written by the victors, and the pragmatists' version of psychology was indeed defeated in psychology's rush to scientism. If we think in terms of George Kelly's proposition about constructs, we can see that pragmatism came to identify the contrast pole to the new scientific psychology, helping to define the emergent pole as such. Dewey had warned in the 1890s of the folly of taking the reflex arc as the paradigm for learning. Mead had helped supervise John Watson's Ph.D. and unsuccessfully tried to ward off the move to an entirely animal and experimentally based psychology.

It is difficult to define pragmatism. Its practitioners pursued independent paths and even called it by different names—pragmatism, pragmaticism and instrumentalism, for example. We can perhaps best see it as a movement whose members share a family resemblance (see Menand, 2002; Thayer, 1982). Perhaps the most prominent feature is an insistence on contextualizing the value and use of principles in human action. Instead of asserting universal principles concerning truth and the good life, there is a focus on what these mean in particular local conditions. So abortion, execution and euthanasia present very different problems about the value of human life. We can see this when members of "pro-life" political groups advocate execution. And of course many people who are pro-abortion and pro-euthanasia abhor execution. Pragmatism does not try to solve moral problems by recourse to overarching moral principles; there is no way of looking the answer up in the back of the book. We won't get the solutions from God. And neither will "rationality" replace divine authority, as some enlightenment thinkers had hoped. Life is messy, and the same action takes on different meanings in different contexts. This then, is iconoclastic philosophy, and it has been subject to a number of misunderstandings. I will very briefly look at two here: that pragmatism represents dangerous relativism, and that it provides a rationale for the worst aspects of monopoly capitalism.

Relativism

It is easy to see how this sort of thinking (in many ways similar to what is now termed postmodern thought) is easily accused of relativism. Anyone who is exclusively guided by a grand narrative, whether it is Christianity, Islam, Radical Feminism or Marxism, wants this sort of "bottom-up" thinking replaced by the imposition of their particular "top-down" principles. The lack of foundational thought in pragmatism allows for any abuse and oppression when we accept that one person's view is as valid as any other, they say. But as Richard Rorty (1999) points out, pragmatists are as opposed to abuse and oppression as are absolutists. It's just that they don't imagine that they will be abolished by the assertion of philosophical principles. Military juntas and dictators are unlikely to be swayed by a word or two about the thought of Jesus or Kant. It is the power of force or argument that is likely to count. If we want to argue against the abuses of a totalitarian regime, it does not detract from our argument that we are not asserting universal rights and instead arguing from the basis of beliefs in our society. Arguments are not won by pointing to an overarching principle, but by assembling a case that is convincing. If we propose (as does Rorty) that human suffering is an evil that we should avoid as far as it is possible, we state our premise and contextualize it. Absolutism presents more humanitarian dangers: when one is driven by abstract principles, context is ignored. It is worth remembering that it is not in the name of relativism that abortionists are murdered, adulterers and homosexuals executed, or heretics burnt at the stake.

Apologists for Monopoly Capitalism

This is a view that has been propagated by Marxists (see Joas, 1997). Because pragmatism rose to prominence along with the industrial might of the USA, it is seen as devoid of principle and ideologically driven. Its lack of foundational principles is seen as an excuse for exploitation. This was an objection that Dewey and Mead had to contend with a century ago.

> Pragmatism is regarded as a pseudo-philosophic formulation of that most obnoxious American trait: the worship of success; as the endowment of the four-flusher with a faked philosophical passport; the contemptuous swagger of the glib and restless upstart . . . the Ford efficiency engineer bent on the mass production of philosophical tin lizzies. (Mead, as quoted in Joas, 1982, p. 36)

Yet both Dewey and Mead were strongly committed social liberals, actively engaged in improving the lot of the poor and dispossessed. In 1931, Dewey (1931/1993b) called for the founding of a new political party in the USA, since he regarded the democratic process as being undermined by both parties being too influenced by big business. He recognized problems that had developed in the classical liberal stance on the position of the individual (Hildebrand, 2008). While the *laissez-faire* liberalism had the function of granting the individual economic freedom, this was at the cost of protecting resources for the few at the expense of the many. The result was what he called "the lost individual," one that is enslaved by economic forces and unable to develop his or her potential.

The Individual

Dewey's notion of individualism was decidedly not that of individual as social atom. The person is grounded in social practices in "law, industry, religion, medicine, politics, art, education and philosophy" (Dewey 1931/1993a, p. 86). It is not that individual atoms come together to form society. Instead, the individual is shaped by the social world:

> Individuality is at first spontaneous and unshaped; it is a potentiality, a capacity for development. Even so, it is a unique manner of acting in and with a world of objects and persons. It is not something complete in itself, like a closet in a house or a secret drawer in a desk, filled with treasures that are waiting to be bestowed on the world. Since individuality is a distinctive way of feeling the impacts of the world and of showing a preferential basis in response to these impacts, it develops into shape and form only through interaction with social conditions; it is no more complete in itself than is a painter's tube of paint without relation to a canvas. (Dewey, 1931/1993a, pp. 86-7)

So Dewey undercuts the person/world dualism; individuals are not separate from and in any way opposed to the social world, but of it. (Exactly the same point Merleau-Ponty made when quoted earlier: "man is in the world, and only in the world does he know himself"). The individual or self is not an essence at the center of the person, like a secret drawer in a desk, but a potentiality, to be shaped in interaction.

This socially based origin of the individual was a position that Dewey developed from his friend and colleague, George Mead. Mead's thought was influenced by Darwin's theory of evolution. He proposed that humankind participates in what he called three orders: the physical, the vital and the mental. All living forms are made up of atoms and molecules (the physical order), but the vital order of life imparts a new dimension on the physical. But unlike bacteria, fishes and most mammals, humans also participate in a mental order. They have consciousness. By this he means more than simply being awake of course. Consciousness here is an ability to reflect on things and to direct action in a deliberate way. So consciousness is an *emergent property*; participation in the mental order transforms action that might be blindly instinctive in the vital order. Actions take on meaning. So, for example, sexual activity might become lovemaking for human participants. We can see that emergence is the opposite of reductionism, where the mental order is bleached of meaning and is seen perhaps as the property of selfish genes, an explanation belonging to the vital order.

The evolution of consciousness lies for Mead in the importance of the social act. In the social act, the gestures of one participant lead to gestures in the other. In "lower animals" this can be a simple fixed-action pattern, where say, one fish's movements determine those of a mate or an antagonist. But in humans, the pattern is not fixed and determined, as there is a covert stage of the act in which the act is interpreted and responded to in terms of its construed meaning. A conversation of gestures then ensues. This is transformed by the immersion of participants in a linguistic community, where speaking adds nuances of meaning that extend gesture. We have noted how

Blumer (1969), following Mead, developed this idea into joint action, in which neither individual is in total control of the outcome of the act; the interaction has a life of its own that outruns the intentions of the individuals participating in it. For Mead, the evolutionary advantage of the social act is that it allows co-operation between members of the species. Through recognizing what the other is up to, and acting in the light of it, we are able to work together towards some end. Of course, it can also lead attempting to one individual outwitting another, or controlling them in some other way:

> We are conscious of our attitudes because they are responsible for the changes in the conduct of other individuals. A man's reaction towards weather conditions has no influence upon the weather itself. It is important for the success of his conduct that he should be conscious not of his own attitudes, of his own habits of response, but of the signs of rain or fair weather. Successful social conduct brings one into a field within which a consciousness of one's own attitudes helps toward the control of the conduct of others (Mead, 1910/1982, p. 348).

So the emergent property of consciousness is embedded in social interaction, and we can see that the individual is firmly rooted in the social world. However, this social origin of the minded individual must not blind us to the unique nature of each individual. The individual is indeed a social construction, but once constructed, each is a center for choice and agency. As Dewey points out, "individuality is a distinctive way of feeling the impacts of the world and of showing a preferential basis in response to these impacts" (Dewey, 1931/1993a, p. 87).

INDIVIDUAL AND SOCIAL CHANGE

I think the best analysis of how individual and social change occurs is still that of Berger and Luckmann (1967). Building on phenomenology, as well as on the social psychology of Mead, they proposed three moments in social change: internalization, externalization and objectivation (see Butt, 2004, for an extended discussion of this). All three occur simultaneously all the time, but for any individual, we can consider them in this sequence. Individuals are born into a social world that precedes them and they come to take it as natural as they internalize it. But society does change over time, and this is because each individual externalizes (talks and acts in various ways). This results in a variety of objectivations—writings, institutions, buildings and so forth that modify society. This leads to a new social world that future individuals internalize in their turn. Individuals, then, are socially constructed, and each society puts together different types of individuals. What we take as reasonable and acceptable is for example very different from that of citizens in our countries only a century ago.[1]

I think that personal construct theory (Kelly, 1955) is useful in understanding and elaborating the process of internalization; how different individuals make sense of what they find in the social world. As another approach grounded in pragmatism, it also has the advantage of being compatible and able to complement the work of Berger and Luckmann. Because of his clinical interest, Kelly's focus was on the individual. Nevertheless he understood the social groundedness of the individual (see Butt, 2001). He famously declared that the philosophy and psychology of Dewey was to be seen between the lines of personal construct theory (Kelly 1955, p. 154). We might see the quote from Dewey above ("individuality is a distinctive way of feeling the impacts of the world and of showing a preferential basis in response to these impacts") as right at the heart of Kelly's theory. The impact of the world is not passively internalized, but interpreted and felt differently

---

[1] Many commentaries on Gergen's social constructionism point out that he chose this nomenclature so as to preserve a link with the seminal work of Berger and Luckmann. It should be remembered, however, that this remains only a footnote in his 1985 article, and he chose not to elaborate this linkage.

by different individuals. What one sees as only a threat another sees also as grounds for hope and opportunity. And our "preferential basis in response" differs as well. The ways two people act in the face of what they both see as a threat can differ widely. Kelly's proposition was that each individual sees alternatives for action and then chooses that alternative that makes most sense to them in terms of their autobiography.[2] Of course this choice is not necessarily deliberated upon; in everyday life we simply don't have time for this—to choose our words carefully in conversation for example. Our experience is that we generally find ourselves acting and talking in a way that makes sense to us. But action represents intentional choice nonetheless.

The role of the social world is to supply us with dimensions along which to construe things. There are occasionally those creative acts when people think laterally, or "outside the box" as we now say. But most of the time, certain lines of thought and action are facilitated for us—ready to hand and easy to draw on. But still there remain always alternative constructions of any event, and the options within these construed dimensions that individuals take up differ in the light of the implications of individual choice.

Let us return to the example of the expression of grief that Gergen (2010 [this volume]) uses. The manner in which grief is expressed is certainly something that has changed quite suddenly (at least in the UK) in the last decade or so. Harré, and Gillett (1994) contrasted the display of emotion at British and Mediterranean funerals. Whereas stoicism was the order of the day in the UK, much more display of emotion was the rule in the Mediterranean region. As Gergen says, responding appropriately to another's grief depends on knowing the rules that apply in any given society. But the rules can and do change.

---

[2] See Kelly's Choice Corollary: "A person chooses for himself that alternative in a dichotomized construct through which he anticipates the greater possibility for extension and definition of his system" (Kelly, 1955, p. 62).

Just three years after Harré and Gillett were writing, Diana Princess of Wales died in a car crash in Paris. The resulting extraordinary outpouring of grief in the UK came as a shock to most commentators and also, it appears, to the royal family. People that had never known her wept and raged, while her family adopted what they saw as a dignified and measured response. Her loss was felt most truly by those who displayed least emotion, at least in public. Clearly we must not mistake emotional show for depth of feeling.

What brings about changes in the rules of emotional expression? It is hard to be certain, but what we can say is that this is part of a pattern that Giddens (1992) refers to as the rise of the "reflexive project of the self." In late modernity, there has been an increasing focus on people's reflecting on themselves: their feelings, ambitions and self-directed plans. The nineties saw a big increase in the demand for therapy and counseling; and psychological coaching appeared. "Getting in touch with one's feelings" became much more important. Old virtues like stoicism and dignity went out of fashion, and were even construed as emotional disabilities, while emoting was more accepted as authentic. However, it cannot be that there are some deterministic forces at play that produce this. It might well be true that economic prosperity provides the necessary ground in which this culture grows; we are unlikely to find the luxury of reflection in the third world, where keeping alive will provide focus enough. But prosperity has not in the past led to the same result. The ancient Greeks, supported by a state built on slavery, were prosperous enough. They produced philosophy that we still draw on today, but this did not result in the same type of reflexive project.

In Berger and Luckmann's (1967) model, the cultural values in which the individual is immersed are internalized. But individuals are not passive receptors of cultural values. If they were, how would the individuals of today have avoided simply internalizing the stoicism of the previous generations? It is because of the creative actions of individuals that culture changes. Old values are not merely taken in, but can be subject to critical scrutiny. The advent of the reflexive project of self, along with all its components, results in such a critical appraisal. This results in new externalization and objectivation. Confessionals in TV shows and magazines, people constantly being asked how they feel in news reports, "human interest" stories in newspapers—all are examples of the objectivation of the new rules of feeling expression. This is what new individuals find in their social world, and this is the framework within which they are invited to interpret their experience. But once again, it does not predict how any particular individual will act; there is no causal determination here. Individuals are not like blotting paper, passively soaking up the values around them. They choose a course of action that makes sense to them. The social world might suggest dimensions along which to construe and even strongly suggest which pole to adopt, but individuals choose that pole which best elaborates their self-theory. Individuals who prize stoicism and self-control are not easily persuaded to suddenly begin to act in a way they consider to be emotionally incontinent.

Gergen (2010 [this volume]) argues that the most we can mean by understanding another's grief is to see it as an appropriate social performance. I have argued that an appreciation of pragmatism's social psychology—in particular Kelly's personal construct theory—helps us do more than that. It is difficult to see the comment "Well, that's that. No sense in crying over spilled milk. Let's get a beer." (Gergen, 2010 [this volume], p. 22) as an appropriate response to grief, it is true. But I can imagine something similar, implying that we must not dwell on it, as a recommendation of a stoical world-view. And I can also imagine some attempts to empathize that would be just as clumsy and would seem phony and anything but understanding.

Kelly, following Mead's formulation of the social act, developed a concept of sociality. Here, understanding follows an attempt to construe the constructions of another person. This seems to me to present a much better grasp of what we mean by "understanding." We feel "understood" when we partake in a social act and recognize that other participants are acting in the light of our constructions. Gergen's example of responding to grief with quiet words of consolation is a good example of this and surely more than merely the performance of a social ritual. Yes, we need to see the individual as socially constructed and, yes, it is vital to appreciate the primacy of interactions in which individuals both make and find themselves. But we also need a psychology that recognizes the status of the individual. For this we don't have to delve into the demonology of the inner person. Dewey worked to undercut this sort of mind/body dualism and Kelly built on this to produce a psychology that attempts a true understanding of the person, without any recourse to an inner, essential self.

REFERENCES

Berger, P., & Luckmann, T. (1967). *The social construction of reality.* Harmondsworth: Penguin.

Blumer, H. (1969). *Symbolic interactionism.* Englewood Cliffs, NJ: Prentice-Hall.

Butt, T. W. (2001). Social action and personal constructs. *Theory and Psychology, 11,* 75-95.

Butt, T. W. (2004) *Understanding people.* Basingstoke: Palgrave Macmillan.

Chiari, G., & Laura Nuzzo, M. (1996). Psychological constructivisms: A meta-theoretical differentiation. *Journal of Constructivist Psychology, 9,* 163-184.

Dewey, J. (1993a). Individuality in our day. In D. Morris & I. Shapiro (Eds) *John Dewey: The political writings* (pp.81-88). Indianapolis: Hackett. (Original work published 1929)

Dewey, J. (1993b). The need for a new party. In D. Morris & I. Shapiro (Eds.), *John Dewey: The political writings* (pp.161-168). Indianapolis: Hackett. (Original work published 1931)

Gergen, K. J. (1985). The social constructionist movement in modern psychology. *American Psychologist, 40,* 266-75.

Gergen, K. J. (2010 [this volume]). Meaning in relationship. In J. D. Raskin, S. K. Bridges, & R. A. Neimeyer (Eds.), *Studies in meaning 4:* Constructivist perspectives on theory, practice, and social justice (pp. 9-24). New York: Pace University Press.

Giddens, A. (1991). *Modernity and self identity.* Cambridge: Polity.
Harré, R. (1989). Language games and the texts of identity. In J. Shotter & K. J. Gergen (Eds.), *Texts of identity* (pp. 20-35). London: Sage.
Harré, R., & Gillett, G. (1994). *The discursive mind.* London: Sage.
Hildebrand, D. (2008). *Dewey: A beginner's guide.* Oxford: Oneworld.
Joas, H. (1997). *George Mead: A contemporary re-examination of his thought.* Oxford: Blackwell.
Kelly, G. A. (1955). *The psychology of personal constructs* (2 vols.). New York: Norton.
Kelly, G. A. (1969). Man's construction of his alternatives. In B. Maher (Ed.), *Clinical psychology and personality: The selected papers of George Kelly* (pp. 66-94). London: Wiley.
Mascolo, M. F., & Dalto, C. A. (1995). Self and modernity on trial: A reply to K. Gergen's Saturated Self. *Journal of Constructivist Psychology, 8,* 175-192.
Mead, G. (1982). Social consciousness and the consciousness of meaning. In H. Thayer (Ed.), *Pragmatism: The classic writings* (pp. 341-350). Indianapolis: Hackett. (Original work published 1910)
Menand. L. (2002). *The metaphysical club.* London: Harper Collins.
Merleau-Ponty, M. (1962). *Phenomenology of perception.* London: Routledge. (Original work published 1945)
Rogers, C. (1967). *On becoming a person.* London: Constable.
Rorty, R. (1999). *Philosophy and social hope.* London: Penguin.
Skinner, B. F. (1974). *About behaviorism.* New York: Vintage Books.
Thayer, H. (1982). (Ed.). *Pragmatism: The classic writings.* Indianapolis: Hackett.

About the Editors

Jonathan D. Raskin is a professor of psychology and counseling at the State University of New York at New Paltz. His published work includes four co-edited books, including the first three *Studies in Meaning* volumes. In addition to serving as an associate editor for the *Journal of Constructivist Psychology*, he is licensed as a psychologist in New York and maintains a small private practice. A fellow of the American Psychological Association, Dr. Raskin is a past recipient of the State University of New York's Chancellor's Award for Excellence in Scholarship and Creative Activities.

Sara K. Bridges is an associate professor of counseling psychology at The University of Memphis. Her scholarship examines constructivism, sexuality, and depth focused approaches to psychotherapy. In addition to publishing extensively on constructivism, Dr. Bridges has co-edited all three previous *Studies in Meaning* volumes. She is the current president of both the Constructivist Psychology Network and the Society of Humanistic Psychology (Division 32 of the American Psychological Association). Dr. Bridges is a licensed psychologist and co-director of the Coherence Psychology Institute.

Robert A. Neimeyer is a professor of psychology at The University of Memphis, where he also maintains an active clinical practice. He has published 23 books, including *Meaning Reconstruction and the Experience of Loss* (with the American Psychological Association), *Constructivist Psychotherapy* (with Routledge), and *The Art of Longing,* a book of contemporary poetry (with BookSurge). The author of over 300 articles and book chapters, he is currently working to advance a more adequate theory of grieving as a meaning-making process, both in his published work and through his frequent professional workshops for national and international audiences. Dr. Neimeyer is the editor of *Death Studies* and the *Journal of Constructivist Psychology.*

Appendix:
About the Constructivist Psychology Network

Studies in Meaning is the official book series of The Constructivist Psychology Network (CPN). CPN is a network of persons interested in constructivist approaches to psychology, relationships, and human change processes. It is largely comprised of psychologists, but there are also members from related disciplines. Those interested in personal constructivism or related areas of constructivist, constructionist, narrative, or postmodern approaches to psychology are encouraged to join. CPN officially became a non-profit organization in July 2005. Up to date information about CPN is maintained on the organization's website: http://www.constructivistpsych.org

CPN membership is open to anyone. An annual membership includes a subscription to the *Journal of Constructivist Psychology* (4 issues per year) and receipt of the CPN newsletter the *Constructivist Chronicle*. Members often receive discounted rates for the biennial CPN conference held in even numbered years. CPN membership rates for 2010 are as follows:

Professional memberships: $70
Student memberships: $40

This is an excellent deal, especially when you consider that the current non-CPN member price for an individual subscription to the *Journal of Constructivist Psychology* alone is $242 US per year. Further, no matter where you live or what currency you use, you can pay your dues quickly and easily online using our secure online payments option.

How to Join CPN

The easiest way to join CPN is via our secure website using a credit card or PayPal account. Go to http://www.constructivistpsych.org and click the "Join or Renew" link. Then follow the easy instructions. Dues payments can also be made by check or money order (in US dollars made payable to CPN); instructions for paying by mail are available on the CPN website.

Index of Proper Names

[numbers in **bold** refer to listings in reference sections.]

Abousleman, T. M., 251, **275**
Abram, D., 230, 236, **243**
Adame, A. L., 227, 230, 236-237, **243**
Adams, W., 237, **243**
Aksoy-Toska, G., 308, **314**
Aldarondo, E., 247-249, **272**
Allen, K. R., 185, 187, 189-190, **203**
Allen, W., 125, **148**
Alon, N., 52, **63**
Alte, C., **246**
Alte, D., **246**
Alvarez, A., 189-190, **201**
Amodio, D. M., 258, **272**
Anderson, H., 134, **148**, 175, **181**
Anderson, T. M., 53, **64**
Angus, L. E., 43, 47, 54, **61-63**
Apted, M., 173
Arar, M., 159, **181**, 183
Arnold, M. B., 99, **121**
Atkinson, D., 185-186, **201-202**
Attig, T., 72, **89**
Austen, 10
Austin, J. L., 23-**24**, 363, 365
Averill, J. R., 94-95, 97, 117, **121-122**
Azuma, H., 305

Bahner, A., 188, **204**
Bakhtin, M., 126, 146, **148**
Baldwin, S. A., 72, **91**
Bannister, D., 233, **243-244**, 317-318, 321, 333, **357**
Barker, M., 309-310
Barkham, M., **62**, 136, **150**
Bar-On, D., 128, **148**
Barone, D. F., 300, **310**
Barrett, L. F., 94, 96, **121**, 302, 312
Barta, J., **246**

Bartky, S., 206-207, 212-213, 220-221, 224, **224**
Bateson, G., 30, **61**, 322, **357**
Batista, J, 35, **61**
Bauer, T., 198, **203**
Bavelas, J. B., 49, **64**, 139, **148**
Baxter Magolda, M. B., 285, **311**
Bearman, S. K., 205, **225**
Beck, A. T., 49, **61**, 340, **357**
Begley, E. A., 232, **245**
Belenky, M. F., 285, 288, 291, 294, 296, **311**
Bendixen, L. D., 282, **313**
Benjamin, L. T., 263, **272**
Berger, A. R., 67, **90**
Berger, J., 206-207, 212, 221, **225**
Berger, P., 125, **148**, 373-374, 376, **378**
Berman, J. S., 69, **89**
Berry, J. W., 287, 296-297, 305, 311-312, **314**
Biggs, J. B., 309, **311**
Billig, M., 24, **24**
Bird, J., 169, 170, **181-182**
Blaisure, K. R., 185, 187, 189-190, **203**
Blood, S. K., 206, 211, 221, 223-224, **225**
Blume, A., 189-190, **201**
Blumer, H., 368, 373, **378**
Boelen, P., 67, 69, **89**
Bohart, A. C., 241, **244**, 246
Bohm, D., 321
Bonanno, G. A., 68, 71, **89**
Bond, L. A., 285, 296, **311-312**
Bordo, S., 206, 212, 220, **225**
Boston, P., 130, **148**
Bouffard, B., 54, **61**
Bourdieu, P., 128, **148**
Bowlby, J., 66, 70, **89**
Bradford Ivey, M., 139, **150**
Brannon, L., 215, **225**

385

Brebner, J., 102, **121**
Bridges, S. K., 185, 193, **202**, **204**, **246**, 247, 381
Brinegar, M. G., 56, **61**
Brody, L. R., 102, **121**
Bronfenbrenner, U., 295, **311**
Brown, L. S., 258-259, **273**
Brown, M. C., 186, 188-190, 196, **202**
Bruner, J., 30, 36, 39, **61**, 70, **89**, 288, 301, **311**, **314-315**
Bryant, R. M., 248, **273**
Buber, M., 117, **121**, 231, 237, 239, 241, **244-245**
Burger, J. M., 263, **273**
Burr, V., 207, 209, 212, 215-216, 218-220, **225**, 251, **273**
Burstow, B., 172, **182**
Busch, R. S., 131, **151**
Bush, G. W., 159, **182**, 310
Butt, T. W., 257, **273**, 350, **359**, 361, 374, **378**
Bydawell, M., 302, **312**
Byrne, C., 296, **312**
Byrne, N., 169, **182**
Byron, G. G., **359**

Caesar, J., 364
Calhoun, L., 68, **89**
Callan, V. J., 309-**310**
Calogero, R., 216, **225**
Cameron, N., 232, **244**
Capretta, P., **246**
Carey, B., 262-263, **273**
Carnap, R., 352
Casas, A., 185-186, **201-202**
Castaneda, C. L., 251, **275**
Castonguay, L. G., 52, **61**
Cauce, A. M., 295, **313**
Ceccato, S., 6, **8**
Ceci, S. J., 288, **315**
Celentana, M. A., 228, **245**

Cervantes, J., 189-190, **201**
Chertoff, M., 310
Chiari, G., 364-365, **378**
Child, C., 309-**310**
Chomsky, N., 168
Clark, H. H., 145, **148**
Clinchy, B. M., 285, 291, **311**
Coates, L., 139, **148**, 159, 167, 180, **182**
Coleman, R. A., 68, **89**
Combs, G., 130, 134, 139, 142, 146, **149**
Comte, A., 351
Constantine, M. G., 248, **273**
Cook, T., 296, **311**
Coon, H. M., 290, **314**
Couture, S., 131, 147-**148**, **151**
Couvalis, G., 337, 341, **357**
Creswell, J. W., 306, **311**
Crethar, H. C., 251, **273**
Crites, F., 52, **61**
Crockett, K., 135, **150**
Croteau, J. M., 190, **203**
Cruz, G., 48, **62**
Cullen, D., 185-188, 191, **204**
Cummings, W., 186, 188, **202**
Cummins, P., **246**
Cunha, C., 29, 48, **63**
Currier, J. M., 68-69, 71, **90**
Cushman, P., 162, **182**

Daloz, L. A., 185, 187, 189, **202**
Dalto, C. A., 361, **379**
Danziger, K., 127, **148**
Darley, J. M., 263, **273-274**
Darwin, C., 372
Dasen, P. R., 297, **314**
Davidson, M. N., 190, 192, **202**
Davis, G. L., 186, 188-190, 196, **202**
Davis, K. E., 68, **89**
Day, R., 172, **182**
Deleuze, G., 128, **148**

INDEX OF PROPER NAMES

Denzin, N. K., 194, **202**
Derrida, J., 129, **148**
Detert, N. B., 53, **62**
Dewey, J., 300, **313**, 368, 370-374, 378, **378-379**
Diener, E., 97
Difranco, A., 168, **182**
Dimaggio, G., 31, **62**
Doan, R. E., 96, 117-119, **121**
Dohm, F., 186, 188, **202**
Dokecki, P., 251, **275**
Dornbusch, S. M., 297, **312**
Dubois, F., 167, **182**
Dunnett, N. G. M., 232, **244**, **246**

Eaton, J., 131, **148**
Ecker, B., 336, **357**
Edwards, D., 12, **24**, 131, 136, **148**
Efran, J. S., 247
Einstein, A., 321
Elkins, D., **246**
Elliott, H., 181
Elliott, R., 133, **149**
Ellis, A., 340, **358**
Ellis, B. J., 118, **121**
Ellsworth, C. P., 97, **123**
Emery, G., 49, **61**
Ephron, D., 262, **273**
Epston, D., 29, 31, 33, **64**, 125, 129, 135, 146, **149-150**, **152**, 177, 179, **182-183**
Epting, F. R., 232, **244**, **246**
Espinoza-Herold, M., 86, **202**

Faidley, A. J., 192, 195, **203**, 227-228, 230-232, 234, 238, 241, **245-246**
Fairclough, N., 128, **149**
Fassinger, R. E., 190, **203**
Fea, C., 215, **225**
Feixas, G., 193, 194, 197, **202**
Feldman, L. A., 96, **121**

Ferrara, K., 131, 143, 145, 147, **149**
Feyerabend, P., 339, **358**
Field, N. P., 67, 72, **89**
Fine, M., 194, **204**
Firth-Cozens, J. A., **64**
Fisch, R., 56, **64**, 126, **151**
Fischer, C. B., 189-190, **202**, **246**
Fish, S., 11-12, **24**
Fogel, A., 32-34, **62**
Forehand, R., 186-190, **202**
Forster, G., **246**
Forster, K., **246**
Foster-Johnson, L., 190, 192, **202**
Fouad, G., 247, 256, **276**
Foucault, M., 126-127, **149**, 176, **182**, 206, 212-213, 216, 220, **224-225**, 252, **273**, **275**
Fox, D., 251, 254, **275**
Frank, E., 91
Frank, J. D., 266-267, **273**
Fransella, F., 321, **357-358**
Fredrickson, B. L., 101, **121**, 206-210, 214, 217-218, 220-223, **225-226**
Freedman, J., 130, 134, 139, 142, 146, **149**
Freire, P., 181-182
Freud, S., 15, 72, **89**, 126, **149**
Frieden, G., 251, **275**
Friedman, L., 264, 266, **273**
Friedman, M., 240, **244**
Friedrichs, M., 72, **89**
Frijda, N. H., 100, **121**

Gadamer, H. G., 11, **24**
Gale, J. E., 146, **150**
Gallois, C., 309-310
Gao, B., 67, **89**
Gardner, C., 215, **225**
Garfinkel, H., 12, **24**, 131-132, **149-150**
Garvey, A., 32, **62**

Gasman, M., 190, **202**
Gelso, C., 197, **204**
Gendlin, E. T., 73, **89**
Georgas, J., 287, **312**
Gergen, K. J., 9-10, 12, **24**,125, 130, 149-**150**, 173, **183**, 193, **203**, 207, 218, **225**, 249, 250, 253, 257, 259, 272, **273**, 319, 355, **358**, 362-363, 366-368, 374-375, 377-378, **378**
Gerstein, L. H., 247, 268-269, **273, 276**
Giddens, A., 376, **379**
Gilbert, L. A., 186, 190, 192, **203**
Gillett, G., 375-376, **379**
Gillies, J., 72, **91**
Ginott, H., 185, **203**
Glasersfeld, E. von, 3, 6, **8**, 249, 253, **274**, 363
Goffman, E., 129, 131, **149**
Goldberger, N. R., 285-286, 298, 307, **311-312**
Gonçalves, J., 29
Gonçalves, M. M., 29, 31, 35-36, 40, 43, 46-48, 50-52, 57, **62-64**, 96, **123**
Gonzales, N., 295, **313**
Gonzalez, V., 186, **202**
Goodman, L., 189-190, 200, **203**, 247, 251, 254-255, **274, 276**
Goodman, S. J., 189, **202**
Goodwin, J., 299, **312**
Gottlieb, C. D., 130, **149**
Gottlieb, D. T. 130, **149**
Grabe, S., 205, **225**
Grant, K., 172, **182**
Green, A. G., 185, **203**
Green, S., 198, **203**
Greenberg, D. L., 70, **91**
Greenberg, L. S., 43, 47, 57, **61-63**, 97, 100, 117, **122**, 131-132, **149**
Greenfield, P., 298, **315**
Greenwood, J., 340, **358**

Griffith, J., 131, **149**
Griffith, M. E., 131, **149**
Grigorenko, E., 298, **314**
Grove, K., 295, **313**
Guattari, F., 128, **148**
Guilfoyle, M., 57, **62**
Gustafson, J. P., 57, **62**

Habermas, J., 127, **149**
Haerel, F. C., 282, **313**
Hage, S. M., 248, **273**
Hall, J. A., 102, **121**
Hamedani, M. G., 292-293, **313**
Hanley, J. H., 190, **204**
Harding, S., 282-283, 291, 305, **312**
Hardy, G. E., **62, 64**
Harkness, S., 297, **315**
Harré, R., 362, 375-376, **379**
Harter, S. L., 349, 351, **358**
Have, P. ten, 131, 133, 139, 144, **149**
Hawley, G. C., 185, **203**
Hawxhurst, D. M., 251, **275**
Hayek, F. A., 271, **274**
Hebl, M. R., 222, **225**
Heilman, N., **246**
Heilman, T., **246**
Helms, J. E., **203, 274, 276**
Herbozo, S., 216, **225**
Heritage, J., 131, **149**
Hermans, H. J. M., 31, **62**, 70, **89**, 93-94, 98, 102-104, 117-118, 120, **122**
Hermans-Jansen, E., 104, 118, **122**
Hermans-Konopka, A., 93
Hersh, R. H., 263, **274**
Hildebrand, D., 371, **379**
Hill, C. E., 52, **61**
Hill, M. S., 205, 215, **225**, 247
Hinkle, D., 331, 333, **358**
Hinkle, S., **246**
Hiraga, Y., 295, **313**
Hirschfeld, A., 190, **202**

Hitler, A., 242
Hofer, B. K., 283, 285-287, **312**
Hoffman, L., 135, **149**, 171, **182**
Hofstede, G., 290, 292, **312**
Hofstede, G. J., 290, 292, **312**
Holland, J., 68-69, 71, **89**
Hollingsworth, M. A. 190, **203**
Holmes, T. R., 281, 296, **312**
Homer, 187
Honos-Webb, L., 53, **62**
Horne, S. G., 185, 189-191, 196, **204**
Houch, P. R., **91**
Hsu, H. C., 32, **62**
Huang, Y., 217-218, **226**
Huebner, D. M., 222, **225**
Hulley, L., 336, **357**
Humble, A. M., 185, 187-191, 197, 199, **203**
Hutchby, I., 147, **149**
Huwe, J. M., 190, **203**
Hyde, J., 205, **225**

Israel, T., 247, **276**
Ivey, A. E., 139, **150**
Izard, C. E., 99-100, 118, **122**

Jackson, D., 49, **64**
James, W., 121, **315**, 368
Janoff-Bulman, R., 67
Jefferson, G., 136, **151**
Jenkins, D., 246
Joas, H., 370, **379**
Johnson, A. G., 260-261, **274**
Johnson, F., 205, **226**
Johnson, M. P., 185, 187, 189-190, **203**
Johnson, S. M., 100, **122**
Johnson, S., 247, 270, **274**
Johnson, T., 139, **148**
Johnson, W. B., 186-188, 190, **203**
Jones, E., 309-**310**
Jones, L., 188, **204**

Jost, J. T., 258, **272**
Kagitcibasi, C., 287, **312**

Kant, I., 6, **8**, 321, 370
Kaschak, E., 206-207, **226**
Katz, A., 161, 172, **182**
Keesee, N. J., 68, 71, **90**
Kelly, G. A., 30, 56, **62**, 67, 126, **150**, 194, **203**, 227-230, 236-239, 241-, 242, **244**, 249, 253, 265-267, **274-275**, 317-322, 324-329, 331-334, 336-339, 341, 344, 348-351, 354, 356-357, **357-358**, 363, 365, 368, 374-375, 377-378, **379**
Kelly, S., 189, **203**
Kemmelmeier, M., 290, **314**
Khadr, O., 159, **183**
Khine, M. S., 287, **313**
Kidder, L., 195, **204**
Kierkegaard, S., 239
Kille, M. F., 93, **122**
Kindaichi, M. M., 248, **273**
King, E. B., 222, **225**
King, P. M., 286, 291, **313**
Kinman, C., 129
Kirkman, M., 211, **226**
Kirkpatrick, D., 268-269, **273**
Kiselica, M., 189-190, 200, **203**
Kissling, E., 215, **226**
Kitayama, S., 289, 294, **313**
Kitchen, M., 161, **183**
Kitchener, K. S., 286, 291, **313**
Klass, D., 72, **90**
Knudson, R., 246
Kogan, S., 128, 146, **150**, 153
Kohlberg, L., 263, **274**
Kohn, M. L., 294, 297, **313**
Konopka, A., 102, **122**
Koocher, G., 191, 196-197, **203**
Kopko, K. A., 288, **315**
Koshik, I., 141, 145, **150**

389

Knaevelsrud, C., **91**
Kramarae, C., 215, **226**
Krieger, S., **246**
Kuhn, T., 10, 12, **24**, 337, 352

Lamb, M. E., 298, **314**
Lamborn, S. D., 297, **312**
Lampert, M., 303, **312**
Landfield, A. W., **246**
Langlois, A., 167, **182**
Lark, J. S., 190, **203**
Larochelle, M., 6, **8**
Larsen, R. J., 97, **122**
Latane, B., 263, **273-274**
Latour, B., 12, **25**
Latta, R. E., **203**, 274, **276**
Lax, W. D., 272, **274**
Lazarus, R. S., 99, 100, **122**
Lee, C. C., 247, **274**
Lee, J., 308, **314**
Lehman, D. R., 292, 303, **315**
Lehner, G. F. J., 266, **274**
Leitner, L. M., 192, 195, **203**, 227-232, 234, 236-238, 241-243, **243-245**, 320, **358**
Leitner, M., **246**
Lepper, G., 53, **62**
Levitt, H. M., 88, **90**
Lewin, J., 54, **61**
Liang, B., **203**, 274, **276**
Liddell, C., 302, **312**
Lin, J., 222, **225**
Lincoln, Y. S., 194, **202**
Lindberg, S., 205, **225**
Lindblom-Ylanne, S., 301, **313**
Linell, P., 140, **150**
Llewellyn, S. P., **62**, 64
Lonka, K., 301, **313**
Love, K., 188, **204**
Lovell, C., 307, **313**
Luckmann, T., 125, **148**, 373-374, 376, **378**

Luna, G., 185-188, 191, **204**
Lyddon, W. J., 308, **313**
Lyman, S. M., 194, **204**
Lyons, A., **246**

Machado, C., 29, **63**
Maciejewski, P. K., 67, 71, **91**
Macmurray, J., **365**
Maddux, J. E, 300, **310**
Madigan, S., 163, 169, 177, 181, **183**
Madill, A., 136, **150**
Madsen, K., 338, 351-353, **358**
Maercker, A., **91**
Magai, C., 93, 95, **122**
Mahoney, M. J., 49, **62**, 70, **91**, 253, **274**
Malamuth, N. M., 118, **121**
Malkinson, R., 72, **91**
Mancini, F., 321, **358**
Mancuso, J., **246**
Maracek, J., 194, **204**
Markus, H. R., 289, 292-294, **313**
Martin, J., 73, **90**
Martín-Baró, I., 177, 181, **183**
Martinez, E., 205, **225**
Martins, C., 35, **63**
Mascolo, M. F., 361, **379**
Mason, C., 295, **313**
Master, S. L., 258, **272**
Matos, M., 29, 35, 43, 46, 48, **62-64**
Maturana, H. R., 249, 253, 263, 267, **275**, 363
May, R., 227, 231, 239, **245**
Mazzetti, M., 264, **275**
McAdams, D. P., 30, **63**, 70, **90**
McAuliffe, G., 307, **313**
McCarthy, I., 169, **182**
McClendon, S. A., 186, 188-190, 196, **202**
McFadden, S. H., 93, 95, **122**
McIlvried, J., **246**
McIlvried, S., **246**

McNamee, S., 130, **150**, 173, **183**, 193, **204**
McWilliams, S., **246**
Mead, G., 368, 370-373, 377, **379**
Meira, L., 48, **63**
Mellinger, W. M., 141, 145, **150**
Menand, L., 369, **379**
Mendel, G., 346
Mendes, I., 29, 35, 43, 47, **62-63**
Mergenthaler, E., 53-54, **62**
Merleau-Ponty, M., 364-365, 367-368, 372, **379**
Meshot, C. M., 53, **64**
Miettinen, R., 300-301, **313**
Milgram, S., 263, **272-273**, 275
Mill, J. S., 351
Miller, G, 130, **150**
Minuchin, S., 49, **63**
Mischel, T., 324, **358**
Monk, G., 135, 145, **150**
Montes de Vegas, A. Y., 251, **275**
Moodie, T., 282, **313**
Moore, W. S., 284-285, **313**
Moradi, B., 217-218, **226**
Morgan, C., 97, 117, **122**
Morrow, S. L., 251, 252, **275**
Mounts, N. S., 297, **312**
Muis, K. R., 282, 288, **313**
Myerhoff, B., 163, **183**

Nash, S., 251, **273**
Neighbors, L. A., 205, **226**
Neimeyer, G. J., **246**, 308, **314**
Neimeyer, R. A., 33, **63**, 65-73, 87-88, **89-91**, 126, **150**, 193, **202**, **204**, **246**, 247, 320, **358**, 381-382
Nesse, R. M., 71, **89**
Neville, H., 185-186, **201-202**
Nickman, S., 72, **90**
Nilsson, J., 188, **204**
Nisbett, R. E., 290, **314**
Noblet, B., **246**

Noblet, C., **246**
Noll, S. M., 221, **225-226**
Norris, C., 126, 129, 134, 147, **150**
Norton, D. L., 93, **122**
Nsamenang, B. A., 298, **314**
Nuzzo, M. L., 364-365, 378

Oades, L., **359**
Obama, B., 269
Obuchowski, K., 90, **122**
Ochs, E., 128, **150**
Ogbu, J.U., 298, **314**
Ogden, C. K., 9, **25**
O'Hara, M., **246**
Olson, D. R., 288, **314**
Omer, H., 52, 57, **63**
Omoregie, H., 289, 294, **313**
Orbach, S., 206, 212, 215, **226**
Osatuke, K., 53, **63**
Osgood, C. E., 96, **122**
Ossorio, P. G., 331, **358**
Ota Wang, G., 251, **275**
Oyserman, D., 290, **314**

Paderna, L., 67, **89**
Panepinto, A. R., 238, **245**
Parker, I., 131, **150**, 254, **275**
Paulsen, M. B., 304, **314**
Peltier, L., 173-174, **183**
Pennebaker, J. W., 71, **91**
Perry, W., 283-285, 291, **314**
Person, E. S., 93, 95-96, 117, **122**
Pfenninger, D. T., 230, 237-238, **245**
Phillip, D., 308, **314**
Phillips, S., 320, **358**
Piaget, J., 363
Pinsof, W. M., 131-132, **149**
Pintrich, P. R., 285, **312**
Plutchic, R., 99, **122-123**
Poerksen, B., 249, 253, 264, 267, **275**
Polanyi, M., 352
Polkinghorne, D. E., 30, **64**

Pomerantz, A. M., 134, 136, **150**
Poortinga, Y. H., 287, 297, **312**, **314**
Popper, K., 321, 337, 352, **358**
Potter, J., 12, **24**, 131, 136, **148**
Presnell, K., 205, **225**
Prigerson, H. G., 67, 71, **91**
Prilleltensky, I., 251, 254, **275**
Pritchard, S., 232, **244**
Prowell, J., 177, **183**

Quinn, D. M., **225**

Rabinow, P., **225**, 252, **275**
Radke, C., 161, **183**
Raskin, J. D., 70, **91**, 190, 193, **202**, **204**, **246**, 247, 257, **275**, 381
Redford, R., 173
Reid, F., 324, **359**
Rennie, D., 131, **151**
Reutter, L., 128, **152**
Reynolds, C. F., **91**
Reynolds, V., 157, 161, 177, **183**
Ribeiro, A. P., 29, 35, 43, 47, **62-64**
Ribeiro, E., 47, **64**
Richards, I. A., 9, **25**
Richardson, C., 177, 181, **183**
Ristic, Z., 341, **359**
Robbins, S., **246**
Roberts, T., 206-210, 214, 217, 220-223, **225**
Robinson, M., 189-190, 200, **203**
Rodin, J., 205, **226**
Rodrigues, G., 29
Rogers, C., 362, **379**
Rogoff, B., 293, 294-296, 299, 301-302, **314**
Rohrbaugh, M. J., 56, **64**
Romanyshyn, R. D., 230, **245**
Rorty, R., 10, **25**, 125, 129, **151**, 272, **275**, 370, **379**
Rosenthal, D., 211, **226**
Rossman, K. M., 186, 190, 192, **203**

Roth, S., 166, **184**
Rotondi-Trevisan, D., 54, **61**
Roy, B., 252, 254, **275**
Royce, J., 338, **359**
Roy-Chowdhury, S., 136, **151**
Roysircar, G., 247, **276**
Rubin, D. C., 70, **91**
Rubin, S. S., 72, **91**
Rush, A. J., 49, **61**
Russell, B., 352
Russell, G. M., 185, 189-191, 196, **204**
Russell, J. A., 94, 96-97, **121**, **123**
Ruzgis, P., 298, **314**
Rychlak, J., 321, **359**
Ryle, G., 10, 363, 365
Rynearson, E. K., 69, **91**

Sacks, H., 136, **151**
Salgado, J., 29, 31, 48, **63-64**, 96, **123**
Salvatore, S., 46, **64**
Salvi, L. M., 56, **61**
Sanders, S., 181
Santos, A., 29, 35, 46, 51-52, **62-64**
Sarbin, T. R., 30, 52, **61**, **64**
Sartre, J. P., 213
Schack, M., 178, **184**
Schegloff, E., 136, **151**
Schiffrin, D., 138, **151**
Schlosberg, H., 97, **123**
Schlosser, L., 197, **204**
Schlutsmeyer, M. W., 230-231, **245**
Schoenfeld, A. H., 304, **314**
Schultz, L., 125
Schut, H., 69, **91**
Schweitzer, J., 189, **203**
Segall, M. H., 297, **314**
Semerari, A., 321, **358**
Shane, S., 264, **275**
Shannon, C., 7, **8**
Shapiro, D. A., **64**

Shaw, B. F., 49, **61**
Shear, K., 69, **91**
Shermis, S. S., 254, **276**
Shoham, V., 56, **64**
Shotter, J., 12, **25**, 129, 161, 172, 175, **182**, **184**, 219, **226**
Silberstein, L., 205, **226**
Silverman, D., 138, 141, **151**
Silverman, P. R., 72, **90**
Simpson, J. A., 263, **272**
Sinclair, R., 178, **184**
Sinha, D., 305, **314**
Skinner, B. F., 367, **379**
Sloan, W., 53, **64**
Slusky, C. E., 52, **64**
Smith, A., 211, **226**
Smith, C. A., 97, **123**
Smith, L. T., 282, 305, 307, **314**
Smith Kemp, N., 6, **8**
Snyder, C. R., 300, **310**
Sobal, K., 205, **226**
Solomon, C. R., 185, 187, 189-190, **203**
Solomon, R. C., 98, 120, **123**
Sparks, E., **203**, 274, **276**
Speedy, J., 130, **151**
Speight, S. L., 254, 258, **275**
Spence, D., 125, **151**
Spencer, D., 376
Stanislavski, K., 322, **359**
Steele, J., 190, **204**
Steinberg, L., 297, **312**
Steup, M., 282, **315**
Stevens, C., **359**
Stice, E., **225**
Stiles, W. B., 53, 56-57, **61-64**
Stojnov, D., 257, **275**, 317, 350, **359**
Stone, R., 300, **315**
Striegel-Moore, R., 205, **226**
Stroebe, M., 69, **91**
Strong, T., 125, 127, 130-132, 139, 142, **151**

Strongman, K. T., 94, 118, **123**
Super, C. M., 297, **315**
Surber, D., **246**
Sutherland, O., 308, **315**
Suzuki, D. T., 126, **151**

Tallman, K., 241, **244**
Tamasese, K., 172, **184**
Tarule, J. M., 285, **311**
Taylor, C., 128, **150**
Tedeschi, R. G., 68, **89**
Tegarden, B., **246**
Tegarden, S., **246**
Tellegen, A., 97, **123**
ten Have, P.
    See Have, P. ten.
Thayer, H., 369, **379**
Thomas, J. C., 227, 230-231, **245**
Thomas, L., 189-190, **201**
Thompson, C. E., 254, **276**
Thompson, K., 216, 225
Thomson, A., **246**
Tilsen, J., 175, **184**
Todd, M., 180, **182**
Tolman, D., 211, **226**
Tomm, K., 136, 142, **151**
Toporek, R. L., 247-249, 251, 254, **276**
Torres Rivera, E., 251, **273**
Toulmin, S., 125, **151**, 352
Townsend, S. S. M., 289, 294, **313**
Triandis, H. C., 290, **315**
Tschudi, F., 324, 329, **359**
Tulviste, P., 298, **315**
Turner, V., 162, **184**
Tweed, R. G., 292, 303, **315**
Twenge, J. M., **225**

Uchida, Y., 289, 294, **313**

Vaihinger, H., 250, **276**
Valsiner, J., 31, 55, **64**

van den Bout, J., 67, **89**
van den Hout, M., 67, **89**
van Dyke, J. G., 71, **91**
Varela, F. J., 249, 253, 267, **275**, 363
Vera, E. M., 254, 258, **275**
Verberg, N., 68, **89**
Vidich, A. J., 195, **204**
Vijver, F. J. R. van de, 287, **312**
Viney, L. L., **246**
von Glasersfeld, E.
    See Glasersfeld, E. von.
Vultaggio, J., 190, **202**
Vygotsky, L. S., 130, **151**

Wade, A., 159, 162, 167, 172, 176-178, 180-**182**, **184**
Wadlington, W., **246**
Wagner, B., 69, **91**
Waldegrave, C., 172, **184**, 252, 259, **276**
Walker, B., **246**, 321-323, **359**
Walker, K. L., 190, **204**
Walker, L., 178
Walter, J. W., 239, **245**
Walz, G. R., 247, **274**
Wang, Q., 288, **315**
Wardle, J., 205, **226**
Warren, B., 321, **359**
Watson, J. B., 368
Watson, D., 97, **123**
Watson, J., 43, **62**
Watzlawick, P., 49, 56, **64**, 126, **151**
Weakland, J., 56, **64**, 126, **151**
Weingarten, K., 148, **151**
Weinstock, J. S., 285, 296, **311**
Weintraub, S. R., **274**, **276**
Wells, C. T., 304, **314**
Wertz, F. J., 189, **202**
West-Stroming, D., 32, **62**
White, C., **184**

White, M., 29, 31, 33, 49, **64**, 125, 127, 128-130, 142, 146, **152**, 162, 172, **184**
White, R., 246
Widdicombe, S., 136, **150**
Williams, D. C., 88, **90**
Williams, R. A., 251, **276**
Williams, W. M., 288, **315**
Williamson, D. L., 128, **152**
Winslade, J., 129, 131, 135, **150**, **152**
Winter, D., 321, **359**
Wittgenstein, L., 4, 5, **8**, 10, 126, 132, 136, **152**, 162, 167, **184**, 352, 363, 365
Witztum, E., 72, **91**
Wohl, M. J. A., 68, **89**
Wolf, N., 205, 212, **226**
Woods, D. K., 134
Wooffitt, R., 131, 147, **152**
Woolgar, S., 12, **25**
Wortham, S., 31, **64**
Wortman, C. E., 71, **89**
Wright, G., 190, **204**

Yee, C. M., 258, **272**

Zambrano, I., 298, **315**

Subject Index

Abortion, 369, 370
Absolute Knowing, 285-286
Absolutism, 370
Accountability, 173
    cultural and collective, 171-174
    individual vs. collective, 173
Acquired Immune Deficiency
    Syndrome. See AIDS.
Action, 229
Action i-moments, 36, 39, 41, 46, 47, 49-50, 51, 56
Action tendencies, 99-100
    general, 103, 111-112
    negative, 103, 115-116
    positive, 103, 113-114
Activism. See Social activism.
Ad verecundiam, 348
Adaptive grievers, 68
Affirmation of consequences, 342
AIDS, 235, 302
Al-Qaeda, 159n
Alternative media, 167n
Ambiguity, 169, 169n
American Psychological Association (APA), 186, 258
    Ethics Code of, 258
    position on torture, 262
Anger, 118
Anti-essentialism, 218
Anticipation, 365
Anxiety, 329, 341, 344, 349
Appearance-related compliments, 215, 216-217
APA. See American Psychological Association.
Argumentum ad hominem, 346
Arts, 351
Assimilation of Problematic Experiences Scale (APES), 53, 54
Association of Marriage and Family Therapy, 247
Assumptive world, 67
Attachment, 70, 88
Australia, 181n
Autobiographical meaning, 67
Autonomous media, 167

Behavioral terms, 128
Behaviorism, 361, 368
"Being held up," 161
Belonging, 177-178
Biases in thinking, 341
Bodies as objects, 222
Body dissatisfaction, 205
    cognitive distortions in, 206
    sociocultural influences, 206
Botswana (Africa), 181n
Buddhist view of meaning, 126, 129

Canada, 157, 160, 173, 173n
    government of, 159n
Capitalism, 260, 369, 370
Case of Bill, 235
Case of George, 231-232, 233
Case of Shannon, 199-200
Center for Strategic and International Studies (CSIS), 159
Central Intelligence Agency (CIA) See CIA
Child abuse, 234
Chile, 181n
China, 292, 304
Choice corollary, 227, 375n
Christianity, 369
Chronic grievers, 68
CIA, 159
Circulus vitiosus (circular argument), 346
Client-centered therapy, 35, 348
Cognitive distortion, 49

Cognitive schemas, 9
Cognitive therapy, 49, 249
Cognitive-behavioral therapy, 35, 50
Coherence therapy, 336
Collectivism, 290
Colonization, 171-172
Commitment, 285
Common sense, 350, 353
Communication, xi, 3-8, 14
    Shannon's formal theory of, 7
Communication theory, 12
Communicative interchange, 10
Community psychology, 248
Complicated grief, 67, 69, 71, 73
Confucian model of knowledge, 292, 304, 309
Consciousness, 372-373
Consciousness-raising, 250-251
Conservatives, 258-259
Contextual knowing, 285-286, 287-288
Contextual relativism, 284-285
Constructed knowing, 285
Construction of "others," 5-6
Constructionist, 334. *See also* Social constructionism.
Constructive alternativism, 228, 357
Constructivism, 88, 253, 361, 363-364
    and humanism, 367
    model of supervision, 193, 194-195, 197
    as a postmodern position, 193
    problems in, 366
Constructivist, 334
Constructivist mentoring, 192-201. *See also* Mentoring.
    case of Shannon," 199-200
    egalitarian aspects of, 192
    and role relationships, 192-193
Constructivist theory of bereavement, 67

Constructivist therapy, 65, 193-194, 339
Continuing bond, 65, 72, 78
Core beliefs, 318
Core constructs, 356
Core-ordering processes, 49
Corporate media, 167, 168
    as preferred term to mainstream media, 167n
Corporate power, 162, 167
Corporations, 164
Correspondence, 339
Counseling, 125
    and deconstruction, 127-130, 125-148
    as distinct from social justice, 249, 265-269
    cognitive, 250
    humanistic, 250
    psychoanalytic, 250
    range of convenience of, 265-267
    as social constructionist, 130-131
Counseling profession
    lacking singular political viewpoint, 261-262, 264-265
Counseling psychologists
    as social justice agents, 247, 248
    as more just than others, 263-264
    politics of, 264-265
Counseling psychology, 189, 190
Critical pedagogy, 181n
Critical psychology, 248, 254
Critical social psychology, 363, 366
Cultural reverence, 232-234
Cultural values, 289-292
Culture, 292
    as "recipe" for thought and action, 289-290
Death penalty. *See* Execution.
Deconstruction, 125, 126, 146

Subject Index

Deconstructive conversations, 127, 128-129
Deconstructive questioning, 129, 132, 135-136, 139
　case examples, 137-140, 140-142, 142-145
Deconstructive practice, 126, 127, 129
Democrats, 258
Department of Homeland Security, 310
Depression, 205, 341
Depth oriented brief therapy, 336
Developmental niche model, 297-298
Dharamsala, 181n
Dialogical self theory, xii, 94, 98, 120
Differential Emotion Theory, 100
Disciplinary power, 219, 220-221
Discourse analysis, 131-132, 136, 147
Discourse markers, 138
Discourse(s)
　defined, 211
　dominant, 212, 222-223
　"romance narrative," 211, 212
　of male sex drive, 216
　and self-objectification, 211-212
　and social structures, 212-213, 223
　and subjective experience, 215
　"women as sexual objects," 212, 215
Discursive psychology, 12, 131-132, 136, 363, 366
　research methods of, 131
Disjunctive syllogism, 343
Disorder, 328, 349
Distorted ideation, 341
Doctrine of objective thought, 364
Doing justice, 160

Dominant discourses. *See* Discourses, dominant.
Dualism, xiv, 284, 378. *See also* Mind-body problem.
　individual/society, 224
　individualism/collectivism, 290
　person/world, 364, 365, 371
Dualists, 307

Eastern philosophies, 239
Eating disorders, 205, 206
Ecological model, 295
Embodied knowing, 169
Emergence, 372
Emotion
　and change in self, 97-99, 101, 104-110
　and change in motivation, 99-101
　dynamic nature of, 96-97, 101
　evolutionary perspective on, 99
　rules for expression of, 375-377
　Frijda's model, 100
　Greenberg and Johnson's model, 100-101
　verbs as best way to convey, 102-103
Empirical research, 351
Empirically supported treatments, 241, 262
Empty chair, 69
England, 363, 365. *See also* United Kingdom.
Epistemological beliefs, xiv, 281, 291-292, 310
　impact of parent's beliefs on children, 296-298
　and psychotherapy, 307-308
Epistemological development, 281, 299-300
　and ability to craft arguments, 291

biases in studying, 286-289
and pragmatism, 300-302
Epistemological elitism, 282-283
benefits of, 302-304
consequences of, 304-309
Epistemological perspectives, 285, 287
on a developmental continuum, 289
Epistemological Reflection Model, 285-286
Epistemological staircase, 283-286
Epistemology, 10, 329, 339, 352. *See also* Personal epistemology.
defined, 282
rationalist vs. constructivist, 308
"West" as epistemological bully, 282-283
Equality, 165
Error fundamentalis, 344
Errors in logical inference, 341
Essentialism
defined, 217
and objectification theory, 217-219
Ethic of resistance, 160, 165
Ethical responsibilities, 161-162
Ethical sanctions, 258
Ethics, 160-161, 168-169
Ethiopians, 234
Ethnographic listening, 135
Ethnomethodology, 12
Euthanasia, 369
Evolution, 354
Evolutionary theory, 372
and emotion, 99
Execution, 369
Existential guilt, 240
Existential writers, 238
Exosystem, 295
Experience cycle, 322

Experiential personal construct psychology, xiii, 227-228, 237. *See also* Personal construct psychology.
Experiential psychotherapy, 35
Externalization, 374
Externalizing questions, 139-140, 146

Fairness, 165
Faith, 241-242
False consciousness, 251
Falsificationism, 337-338
Fatal accident, 69, 71
FBI, 173n
Fear, 118, 326
Federal Bureau of Investigations. *See* FBI.
Feeling
in social constructionism, 19-20
Felt sense, 73
Feminism, 369
Focus of convenience
defined, 265
Foreclosed survivors, 68-69
Formal mistakes, 341-342
Four operations of language, 167
France, 365
Freedom
constrained rather than determined, 16-17, 18
Freudian terms, 128. *See also* Psychoanalysis.

Galilean modes of thought, 321
Gaze, 220, 222. *See also* Male gaze.
Geneva Conventions, 262, 263
Germany, 365
Gestalt therapy, 348
"Ghost in the machine," 10, 365
Global warming, 236
Graduate students

mentoring of, 186-189, 196-201
    subordinate status of, 191
Graduate study in psychology. *See*
    Psychology, graduate
    study in.
Grand narratives, 369
Grief, xii
    Butt's response to Gergen,
        375-378
    as example of syncrhonization,
        23
Grief therapy, 65-91
Guantanamo Bay, 159n
Guided object frames, 32
Guilt. *See* Existential guilt.

Habitat for Humanity, 269
Health care, 233-234
Heterosexism, 233, 258
Heuristic model of therapeutic
    change, 48-52
Heuristic model of therapeutic
    stability, 55-61
History of science, 12
Homelessness, 233
Homicide, 69, 71
Homosexuality, 258
Homosexuals, 370
"Horizon of understanding," 11
Hostility, 324, 327-328, 349-350
Human understanding, 11
Humanism
    and constructivism, 367
Humanistic counseling, 250
Humanistic scholars, 20, 239
Humility, 242-243
Hypothesis testing, 319
"I-it" relationships, 237
i-moments. *See* Innovative moments.
i-positions, 98, 117, 120
Identity, 70
Imagery, 73

Imaginal dialogue, 81
Impermeable construing, 349
Imprudent generalization, 347
Incident at Oglala (film), 173n
Incipient scientist, 324, 326, 329
Incommensurability, 338
India, 181n
Individual
    in constructivism, 361
    in humanism, 367
    in orthodox psychology, 361
    in pragmatism, 371-373
    Rogerian view, 362
    and social change, 373-378
Individualism, 260, 290, 365
Individualist ideology, 12
Indonesia, 235
Inferiority, 118-119
Infinite repsonsibility, 172
Informal mistakes, 341, 344
Information theory, 7
Information transfer, 7-8
Innovative moments (i-moments),
    xii, 31, 35-36, 45-46, 47, 48,
    56, 58-60, 61
    coding of, 40-43
    as exceptions to the rule, 35
    emergence of, 42
    and frames, 32
    model of change in
        psychotherapy, 52
    temporal salience of, 41-42, 45
    types of, 36-40
    and unique outcomes, 31-32
Ingenuity, 349
Innovative Moments Coding System
    (IMCS), 40-43, 48, 53, 54, 55,
    56
Integral universe, 228-230, 237, 238,
    241
    as co-constructed, 229
Intentionality, 9, 319

Interconnected reality, 229
Internalization, 373
International Tibet Independence
    Movement (ITIM), 268
Interpersonal reverence, 231-232
Interpretive communities, 11
Introjects, 348
Invalidation, 321, 334-335, 350
Iran, 157
Iraq War, 168n, 235
Irrationality, 344
Islam, 369

Joint action, 368
Just. *See* Social justice.
Just practice, 161

Kantian theory, 321
Knowers
    connected vs. separate, 291
Knowing
    and cultural values, 289-292
    in ecocultural context,
        296-299
    in ecological context, 295-296
    in psychology research
        methods texts, 299
    in sociohistorical context,
        293-295
Knowledge, 281
    "body knowledge," 298, 305
    Confucian vs. Socratic
        conceptions, 292
    cross-cultural aspects, 287-288
    experiential, 298

Laissez-faire liberalism, 371
Language, 3-8, 127, 363, 364
    ability to communicate
        meaning, 126
    and construction of "others," 5-6
    cybernetic constraints on, 5
    four operations of, 167
    and social adaptation, 5
    and meaning of individual
        utterances, 13
    meaning as never fixed in,
        209-210
    and power, 127-128
Language games, 5, 126
Legacy, 78, 81
Leonard Peltier Defense
    Committee, 173n
Letters to the deceased, 69
Levels of change, 32-35
Liberation psychology, 177, 181n,
    248
Life narrative, 87
Linguistic communication. *See*
    Communication.
List of Emotional Verbs, 102
Literary theory, 12
Lived world, 364
Logical empiricism, 337, 352, 355
Logical mistakes, 340
Loose construing, 343, 349
Loss narrative, 67
Love, xii, 93-121
    complexity of, 93, 94-95
    in contrast to anger, inferiority,
        and fear, 118-119
    and general action tendencies,
        111-112
    and general change in self, 103,
        104-106, 120
    and negative action tendencies,
        115-116
    and negative change in self, 103,
        109-110
    and positive action tendencies,
        113-114
    and positive change in self, 103,
        107-108
    and self-organization, 93

as a syndrome, 94
transforming features, 93, 95-96
"Luxury of obliviousness," 261

Macro-narrative, 67
Making sense, 71
Male gaze, 211. *See also* Gaze.
   as maintaining power of men, 213
   ways women make meaning of, 214-217
Marginalized groups, 189, 190
Marxism, 157, 369, 370
Mathematics, 303-304
Meaning, 3, 9
   continuous reconstitution of, 21-22
   as coordinated action, 12-22
   as local, 17
   origin of, 126
   shift from within to between, 11-12
   as within individuals, 9, 10, 12, 19
   as within relationship, 11-12, 13-14
   and traditions of coordination, 18-20
   search for, 68
Meaning-makers, 67, 71
Meaning-making, 72, 351
Mechanistic beliefs, 283
Media. *See* Alternative media, Autonomous media, Corporate media.
Medical model, 249
Mentor
   defined, 187
Mentoring, xii, 185-201
   academic vs. emtional needs of students, 186-187
   case of "Shannon," 199-200
   constructivist approach to as form of social justice, 192-198
   feminist perspective on, 191-192
   of graduate students, 186-189, 196-201
   impact of deficiencies in, 190
   as moral obligation, 185-186
   multicultural perspective on, 191-192
   relationship to social justice, 189-192
   traditional perspectives on, 190
Metaphor, 73
Metaphysical research program, 352
Metascience, 351
Metatheory, 338, 352, 356
Method acting, 322
Micro-narrative, 67
Microsystem, 295
Middle-class families, 294, 301
Mind-body problem, xiv, 10, 222, 224, 378
   dichotomozing mind and body, 222-223
Mobility of mind, 339
Modernism
   and universal truth, 125
Modus tollens, 342
Monty Python (comedy troupe), 354
Moral righteousness, xii
More-than-human world, 229, 236-237
Motivation
   and emotion, 99-101, 117, 120
   and inferiority, 119
Multiculturalism, 251
Multinational corporations. *See* Corporations.
Multiplicity, 284
Mutual in-feeding, 55-60
   case examples, 58

Naïve realism xii, 364, 365
  and social justice counseling, 248, 250-251
Narrative
  as performative act, 31
Narrative intervention, 75
Narrative therapy, 29-61, 125, 146
  and deconstructive practice, 129-130
  externalizing questions, 139-140
  good and poor outcome cases, 43-48
  theoretical assumptions, 30-39
  unique outcomes, 29-30, 31
Naure vs. nurture, 262
Negation of ascendants, 343
Neopositivism, 352
New York Yankees, 268-269
New Zealand, 181n
No One Is Illegal (activist group), 172
Non-guided object frames, 32
Nonvalidation, 321
Normative discontent, 205

Objectification, xiii
  contribution of research to, 221-223
Objectification theory, 205, 206. *See also* Sexual objectification.
  core tenet of, 207
  essentialism of, 217-219
  and objectifying gaze, 207-208
  and sexual objectification, 208-209
  and social constructionism, 208, 223-224
Objectivation, 374
Objective thought. *See* Doctrine of objective thought.
Obsessive compulsive disorder, 347

O'Connor report, 159n
Odyssey, 187
Ontological hypotheses, 352
Ontology, 339
Optimal functioning, 237
Overgeneralization, 341

Paradigm, 352
Parenting, 295-298, 301-302
Patriarchal desires, 220
Performing change i-moments, 38-39, 41, 45, 46, 47
Permeable contruing, 349
Person-as-artist, 351
Person-as-historian, 351
Person-as-philosopher-of-science, 323
Person-as-scientist, xiv, 317, 321-324, 331, 337, 339, 341, 348, 350-351, 355-357
Personal construct psychology, xiv, 317, 329, 331, 340, 374-375. *See also* Experiential personal construct psychology.
Personal construct system, 353
Personal growth, 68
Personal epistemology, 281, 283
Petito principii (taking unproved for proved), 345
Phenomenology, 365, 373
Philosophical thinking, 352
Philosophy of science, 352, 356
Philosophy of "as if," 250
Philosophy of science, xiv, 321, 332-334, 337-338, 340, 344
Political violence, 157-181
"Politics of meaning making," 128
Positivist beliefs, 283
Postmodernism 193, 357
  and research, 194
Post-structuralism, 126

Subject Index

Posttraumatic stress disorder (PTSD), 235
Poverty, 128
Power, 127, 176n, 190, 213, 216, 224, 290, 291-292
Power Distance Index, 292
Pragmatism, xiv, 361-378
 and activity theory, 301
 defined, 300, 368-369
 as devoid of principle, 370-371
 and epistemological development, 300-302
 in evaluating epistemologies, 303
 and the individual, 371-373
 lack of foundational thought in, 369-370
Pre-reflective reasoning, 286
Prescription privileges, 258, 262
Private meaning, 19
Privilege, 260-261
Procedural knowing, 285, 304
Protest i-moments, 37, 41, 46, 47, 50-51, 53, 56
Psychoanalysis, 125, 129, 249, 250, 257, 348
Psychoanalytic theory, 15
Psychological disorders, 320, 324, 327, 356
Psychological states
 problem of "inner access," 11, 22
Psychology
 graduate study in, 188-189
 lacking singular political viewpoint, 261-262, 264-265
 openness to women and minorities, 190
 research methods textbooks, 299
 Western bias of, 305
Psychopathology, 320, 350, 356
Psychotherapist
 as philosopher-of-science, 317-359

Psychotherapy, 332, 356
 defined, 266-267
 and epistemologies, 307-309
 as experimentation, 324
 range of convenience of, 265-267
 and relational ethics, 160-161
 supposed neutrality of, 162
Psychotherapy manuals, 262
Public meaning-making, 19-20

Qualitative research, 306
Quantitative research, 306
Quasi-reflective reasoning, 286
Qui nimium probat, nihil probat (excessive proving), 347

Racism, 173, 174, 233, 258
Radical constructivism, xi
 and communication, 3-8
Radical feminism, 369
Radical psychiatry, 254
Range of convenience
 of counseling and psychotherapy, 265-267
 defined, 265
 and social justice counseling, 248, 265-269
Rape, 238-239
Rationality, 349
Reader response theory, 11
Realism
 naïve, xii, 248, 250-251
Realist philosophy of science, 339
Received knowing, 285
Reconceptualization i-moments, 37-38, 41, 45, 46, 47, 48, 51, 52, 53, 60
Reductionism, 372
Reflection i-moments, 36, 39, 41, 46, 47, 49-50, 51, 53, 56
Reflective Judgment Model, 286

403

Reflective reasoning, 286
Reflexivity, 169, 169n
Reification, 249
Relational ontology, 350
Relativism, 369-370
Relativists, 307
Repressed memory debate, 257
Republicans, 260
Research methods
    discursive, 131-132
    quantitative vs. qualitative, 306
Resilience, 68, 71, 88
Resilient survivors, 67
Resistance, 176, 176n
Restoration-oriented coping, 69
Retelling, 69
Reverence for humanity, 234-236
Reverence for the planet
    lack of as psychopathology, 236
Role relationships, 192-193, 195, 196
Romance narrative, 211, 212
Royal Canadian Mounted Police (RCMP), 159n

Santiago (Chile), 181n
Scotland, 365
Search for meaning, 68
Second World War, 352, 362
Selective abstraction, 341
Self
    as community of voices, 53
    decentering of, 365-368
    and emotion, 97-99, 101
    general change in, 103, 104-106
    and i-positions, 98
    negative change in, 103, 109-110
    positive change in, 103, 107-108
    "reflexive project of," 376
Self-acceptance, 119
Self-Confrontation Method, 103-104
Self-healing, 241

Self-Objectification Questionnaire (SOQ), 221
Self-discipline, 220
Self-esteem, 119
Self-narrative, 67-68, 70
Self-objectification, 208
    as a discourse, 211-212
Self-organization, 100, 101, 118
Self-surveillance, 220-221
Sense making, 68
Separation distress, 71
Sexism, 233, 258
Sexual assault, 217
Sexual harassment, 217
Sexual objectification, 208-209, 217. *See also* Objectification theory.
    defined, 210
    as a discourse, 224
    individual meanings of, 224
    potential benefits of, 214-217
    as a social construction, 209-212, 218-219, 223-224
    treated as objective reality, 210, 218
Sharing power, 254-255
Silenced knowing, 285
Social act, 368, 372-373, 377
Social activism, 267
    conflation with counseling, 268-269
    with torture survivors, 157-181
Social change, 373-378
    three moments in, 373-374
Social constructionism, xi, xiii, 9-24, 125, 126, 271, 272, 361, 366, 374n
    anti-essentialism of, 218
    assumptions of, 207
    and communcative interchange, 10
    and counseling, 130-131
    critique of isolated

Subject Index

individualism, 12
  and epistemological beliefs, 293
  freedom in, 16-17, 18
  and individual vs. society dichotomy, 219, 224
  and "keeping the conversation going," 272
  language in, 209-210
  and meaning in relationship, 9-24
  and objectification theory, 208, 223-224
  and sexual objectification, 209-212, 218-219
Social justice, xiii
  and advocacy for marginalized groups, 189-190
  as an appealing and agreeable idea, 248, 256
  defined, 247
  and mentoring, 189-192
  psychotherapist determinations of, 165
  reification of, 249
  risk in criticizing, 248
  and unethical practice, 259
  witnessing stance toward, 157-181
Social justice advocacy, 189, 190
Social justice counseling, 248-272
  defined, 249-250, 255-256
  definitional problems of, 255-256
  hubris of, 248, 260-265
  as going beyond psychology's range of convenience, 248, 265-269
  as imposing values, 248, 257-259
  as naïve realism, 248, 250-253
  six principles of, 254
  as a theoretical orientation, 249-250, 270-271
  as theoretically unelaborated, 248, 253-256

Social practices, 293
Social psychology, 361-363, 373
Social structures, 212-213
Sociality corollary (sociality), 227, 377-378
Sociology of knowledge, 12
Solidarity, 162, 163, 177-178
  contested definition of, 162n
  groundless approach to, 172
  supervision of, 168
Somalia, 166
South Dakota, 173n
Spirituality, 65, 68, 71, 87
Subjective knowing, 285
  and socioeconomic status, 294
Subjectivity, 9
Subjectivity assumption, 19
Suicide, 69, 71
Supervision
  constructivist model, 193, 194-195, 197
Supervision of solidarity, 168
Supplementary action, 13-14
  as a candidate for meaning, 14-15
  as constraining rather than deterministic, 16-17
  and continuous reconstitution of meaning, 21-22
  as creating and constraining meaning, 15-16
  prefigurative potential of, 15-16
  therapeutic example of, 14-15
Survivors of torture and political violence
  accommodating suffering of, 162
  placing on pedestals, 166
Syllogistic inference, 350
Synchronized action, 23

Target (store), 268
Theoretical pluralism, 338
Therapeutic cycles mode, 53-54

Therapeutic homework, 75
Thought
    as silent argument, 24
    in social constructionism, 19-20
Threat, 326, 350
Tibet, 228, 268, 269
Torture, xiii, 157-181, 185, 262, 263, 264
    defined, 158
    resisting, 176, 176n
    vs. tortuous, 158
Tradition of act and supplement, 15
Traditions of coordination, 18-20
Transana software program, 134
Transpersonal responsibility
    as an act of faith, 241-242
    as an act of humility, 242-243
    care and commitment in, 238-240
    and existential guilt, 240
    overview of, 237-238
Transpersonal reverence, xiii, 230-237
    and case of George, 231-232, 233
    and lack of culutral reverence, 232-234
    and lack of interpersonal reverence, 231-232
    and lack of reverence for humanity, 234-236
    and lack of reverence for more-than-human world, 236-237
    overview of, 230-231
Treatment manuals, 258
Trojan War, 187
Truth, 329
"Truths within traditions," 250

Understanding, 22-24
    critique of Gergen's view, 366-367
    and dance metaphor, 22-23, 367-368
Unique outcomes, 29-30, 31
    and i-moments, 31-32
United Kingdom, 363, 375. *See also* England.
United Nations, 158
United States of America (USA), 159n, 173n, 287, 294, 303, 304, 365, 368, 370, 371
United States Congress, 159, 258
United States government, 173n
United States Marines, 235-236
University of Calgary, 132-133
University of Wisconsin-Madison, 134
Upper-class families, 294
Utterances, 13-14
    source of meaning of in social construction, 13-14

Validation, 334-335, 338
Validation-invalidation circle, 322
Valuation Theory, 118
Vancouver, 181n
Verbs
    as best way to convey emotion, 102-103
Verisimilitude, 337
Viability, 337
Violent death, 69

War on terror, 178
Witness. *See* Witnessing stance.
Witnessing, 161
Witnessing position, 158. *See also* Witnessing stance.
Witnessing principles, 158, 170-181
    belonging, community, and solidarity, 177-181
    collaboration, 175-176

cultural and collective
   accountability, 171-174
  honoring resistance, 176-177
  immeasurable outcomes, 180-181
  structuring safety, 170-171
  witness rather than gossip,
   178-179
Witnessing stance, 157-181
  as addressing power, 164-165
  non-heroic nature of, 174, 174n
  and ongoing supervision,
   168-169
  and understanding language,
   165-168
  and understanding political
   world, 165-168
Women
  bodily dissatisfaction of, 205
"Women as sexual objects"
   discourse, 212, 215
Women's ways of knowing, 291
Women's Ways of Knowing Model
   (WWK), 286-287
Word salad, 18
Words, 11
  in Derrida's philosophy, 129
  as indicative of psychological
   states, 11
  as polysemic, 17
Working-class families, 294, 295-298
Working with survivors of torture
   and political violence
   useful assumptions about,
   163-164
World assumptions, 69
World-hypotheses, 352
World War II. *See* Second World
   War.

Yugoslavians, 234

Zeitgeist, 356

Lightning Source UK Ltd.
Milton Keynes UK
UKOW042112170113

205052UK00008B/303/P